ANNUAL REVIEW of NURSING EDUCATION

Volume 2, 2004

ANNUAL REVIEW of NURSING EDUCATION

Volume 2, 2004

Marilyn H. Oermann, PhD, RN, FAAN, Editor
Kathleen T. Heinrich, PhD, RN, Associate Editor

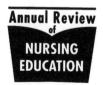

 Springer Publishing Company

Order ANNUAL REVIEW OF NURSING EDUCATION, Volume 3, 2005, prior to publication and receive a 10% discount. An order coupon can be found at the back of this volume.

Springer Publishing Company, Inc.
536 Broadway
New York, NY 10012-3955

03 04 05 06 07 / 5 4 3 2 1

ISBN-0-8261-2445-3
ISSN-1542-412X

ANNUAL REVIEW OF NURSING EDUCATION is indexed in *Cumulative Index to Nursing* and *Allied Health Literature and Index Medicus*.

Printed in the United States of America by Maple-Vail Book Manufacturing Group.

This volume is dedicated to the University of Arizona nursing professors, Robin E. Rogers, MSN, RN, CPNP; Cheryl McGaffic, PhD, RN, CCRN; and Barbara S. Monroe, MS, RN, CCRN, who died on October 28, 2002. The authors whose stories of innovative teaching, research, and assessment projects fill these pages honor their slain colleagues in the best way possible—by facing the challenges of educating nurses for the new millennium with caring, commitment, and creativity.

Contents

Part III: Simulation Labs in Nursing Education

Part IV: Innovative Strategies for Teaching in Nursing

Part V: Development of Students, Nurses, and Teachers

Contributors

Mary Ann Anderson, PhD, RN, APRN, BC
Instructor
Nursing Department, College of Health Professions
Weber State University
Ogden, Utah

Diane M. Billings, EdD, RN, FAAN
Chancellor's Professor
Professor of Nursing and Associate Dean, Teaching, Learning, and Information Resources
Indiana University School of Nursing, Center for Teaching and Lifelong Learning
Indianapolis, Indiana

Donna L. Boland, PhD, RN
Associate Professor and Associate Dean for Undergraduate Programs
Indiana University School of Nursing
Indianapolis, Indiana

Peggy L. Chinn, PhD, RN, FAAN
Professor Emeritus of Nursing
University of Connecticut
Storrs, Connecticut

Margaret O. Doheny, PhD, RN, ONC
Professor
College of Nursing
Kent State University
Kent, Ohio

Judy Boychuk Duchscher, MN, RN
Faculty, Nursing Education Program of Saskatchewan
SIAST Nursing Division
Saskatoon, Saskatchewan

Bonnie W. Duldt-Battey, PhD, RN
(retired)
Antioch, California

Adeline R. Falk-Rafael, PhD, RN
Associate Professor
York University School of Nursing
Toronto, Ontario

Nedra Farcus, MSN, RN
Instructor of Nursing
Pennsylvania State University Altoona Campus
Altoona, Pennsylvania

Carol Gilbert, PhD, RN
Associate Director
National League for Nursing
   Accrediting Commission
New York, New York

Barbara R. Grumet, JD
Executive Director
National League for Nursing
   Accrediting Commission
New York, New York

Kathleen T. Heinrich, PhD, RN
Professor
Division of Nursing
University of Hartford
West Hartford, Connecticut

Donna D. Ignatavicius, MS, RN,
   Cm
President, DI Associates, Inc.
Placitas, New Mexico

Marianne R. Jeffreys, EdD, RN
Professor, Nursing
The City University of New York
   College of Staten Island
Staten Island, New York

Marilyn Blau Klainberg, EdD,
   RN
Associate Professor
Interim Dean
Adelphi University School of
   Nursing
Garden City, New York

Felissa R. Lashley, PhD, RN,
   ACRN, FAAN, FACMG
Dean and Professor
College of Nursing
Rutgers, The State University of
   New Jersey
Newark, New Jersey

Kathleen Mastrian, PhD, RN
Associate Professor and Program
   Coordinator for Nursing
Pennsylvania State University
   Shenango Campus
Sharon, Pennsylvania

Magdalena A Mateo, PhD, RN,
   FAAN
Associate Professor
School of Nursing
Northeastern University
Boston, Massachusetts

Cheryl P. McCahon, PhD, RN
Associate Professor
Director, Undergraduate Nursing
   Program
Cleveland State University
Cleveland, Ohio

Dee McGonigle, PhD, RNC,
   FACCE
Associate Professor of Nursing
   and Information Sciences and
   Technology
Pennsylvania State University
New Kensington and University
   Park Campuses
Editor-in-Chief, *Online Journal of
   Nursing Informatics*
New Kensington, Pennsylvania

Eileen McMyler, MS, RN, BC
Nursing Education Specialist
Mayo Clinic and Mayo
   Foundation
Rochester, Minnesota

Helen I. Melland, PhD, RN
Professor
College of Nursing
University of North Dakota
Grand Forks, North Dakota

Patricia Gonce Morton, PhD,
  RN, ACNP, FAAN
Professor and Assistant Dean for
  Master's Studies
University of Maryland School of
  Nursing
Baltimore, Maryland

M. Ruth Neese, MSN
Staff Nurse
Emergency Department
Jupiter Medical Center
Jupiter, Florida

Wendy M. Nehring, PhD, RN,
  FAAN
Associate Dean for Academic
  Affairs and Associate Professor
College of Nursing
Rutgers, the State University of
  New Jersey
Newark, New Jersey

Sheila A. Niles, MSN, RN, CS
Director, Community Projects
  and Elder Health
Director, Healthy Town
Visiting Nurse Association
  Healthcare Partners of Ohio
Cleveland, Ohio

Carol A. Rauen, MS, RN, CCRN
Assistant Professor
Georgetown University School of
  Nursing and Health Studies
Washington, D.C.

Janet Hoey Robinson, PhD, RN
Professor and Associate Dean,
  Graduate Program
School of Nursing
Medical College of Ohio
Toledo, Ohio

Alicebelle Rubotzky, PhD, RN
Associate Professor
Department of Nursing
Rhode Island College
Providence, Rhode Island

Carol A. Sedlak, PhD, RN, ONC
Associate Professor
College of Nursing
Kent State University
Kent, Ohio

Lori Stier, EdD, RN
Administrative Director, Quality
  Management
North Shore-Long Island Jewish
  Health System
Great Neck, New York

Preface

A fter years of invisibility, these are exciting times for nurse educators! With news of the national shortage of nurse educators competing with headlines about the nursing shortage in the popular press, forward-looking administrators of colleges and universities across the country are beefing up or opening graduate and doctoral programs in nursing education. Moneys are being allocated for preparing nurse educators for teaching in schools of nursing, and in staff development and continuing education programs, and for funding educational research.

Amidst this ferment, nurse educators are being asked tough questions. How are nursing programs responding to local, regional, and national shortages of nurses? How are they addressing the current faculty shortage? In what ways are faculty adapting their curricula to prepare students to meet patient needs in a rapidly changing health care system? How are educators in clinical settings helping the nursing staff develop and maintain competencies? What innovative teaching strategies are educators using in the classroom and in clinical practice to best meet learner needs? The *Annual Review of Nursing Education* will help you respond to questions like these with the most up-to-date information available. Unique in focusing on the practice of teaching across settings, this review is written for nurse educators in associate, baccalaureate, and graduate nursing programs, as well as in staff development and continuing education programs.

The first part of this volume explores current trends in nursing education. In chapter 1 Barbara R. Grumet and Carol Gilbert report on findings from recent accreditation reviews and from information provided by the National League for Nursing Accrediting Commission. Faculty can learn about a program initiative or an innovation in a particular school of nursing by searching the literature or attending a nursing education conference. Rarely, however, are there reports available on the current status of nursing education in the United States. Prepared especially for the *Annual Review of Nursing Education*, this chapter tells how programs and faculties are responding to the nursing shortage, to the faculty shortage, and to other challenges they face in nursing education. For example, you will learn about student enrollment in schools of nursing, diversity of students, NCLEX pass rates and how faculty are preparing students for the NCLEX, curriculum trends, how faculty are using distance education in their programs, program resources, and how schools are responding to budget cuts. Throughout the chapter the authors cite examples of new initiatives, innovations in nursing education, and program responses to the challenges facing schools of nursing.

Nursing workforce needs are rapidly changing, and new career paths are emerging. The knowledge and skills gained in traditional nursing programs are no longer sufficient for employment in many settings. Certificate programs in nursing are one solution for preparing nurses for the current work environment. In chapter 2, Diane M. Billings describes different types of certificate programs, discusses their advantages and disadvantages, and examines how they contribute to fostering service-education collaboration in the age of the knowledge worker. As learner and employer demand for specialized education increases, nurse educators and their potential partners in clinical agencies are faced with considering the merits of developing certificate programs. Billings identifies factors to consider in deciding whether to offer a certificate program, and how to define and measure the quality of certificate programs in nursing. If you are thinking about developing an academic or a professional (noncredit) certificate program, this chapter will be of value to you and your colleagues.

Through service learning students provide meaningful service to a community and at the same time meet student and course outcomes. In chapter 3, Helen I. Melland describes the experience of planning and implementing a service learning project in Bolivia. She reviews the literature on service learning and its current status in nursing education, the cultural implications of such an experience for both the learners and the recipients of the service, and the implications of service learning projects for nursing education, practice, and research. Melland discusses the practicalities of planning and implementing service learning and uses the students' experience in Bolivia to illustrate these. The chapter presents valuable strategies for preparing students to provide culturally sensitive care. If you are considering integrating service learning into your curriculum, this chapter will assist you in meeting that goal.

The focus of Part II of the *Annual Review* is evaluation and assessment of programs and students. Chapters in this part examine program evaluation in nursing and public accountability, present innovative assessment strategies that faculty can adopt for their programs, and offer a new perspective on grading.

Program evaluation models and plans need to respond to the calls for program accountability, including a renewed emphasis on professional standards as a best practice guide to building curricula and defining learning outcomes, a philosophical shift from the evaluation of teaching to the assessment of learning, and the expectation that outcome data will be benchmarked against expected results to support quality improvement activities. In chapter 4, Donna L. Boland analyzes these and other changes and how they are affecting program evaluation in nursing education. She discusses the evolution of program evaluation, which provides a background for readers to better understand current trends; the goals of program evaluation in nursing education; a number of program evaluation models and the need for faculty to make an informed choice of a model in their own program; assessment of learning and different methods of assessment faculty can use; and evaluating distance learning. Program evaluation is an area in which many faculty are inadequately prepared. This chapter provides the background to understand and implement program evaluation and assessment across all levels of nursing education.

In chapter 5, Kathleen T. Heinrich and Ruth Neese offer a unique perspective on why nurse educators often shy away from program assessment. They suggest that educational phenomena like learning, critical thinking, and perspective transformation are often in the realm of the ineffable. By definition, ineffable educational phenomena are real, but not tangible. This means that traditional, quantitative assessment strategies alone are inadequate for assessing such phenomena. Based on a review of the educational literature, the authors conclude that ineffables are best assessed when they can be given a concrete form using a combination of assessment strategies drawn from quantitative, qualitative, and aesthetic-expressive approaches. The exemplar of an assessment of an evidence-based course presented in this chapter will help you to collaborate with students to identify, give form to, and assess ineffable phenomena.

Peggy L. Chinn sets the framework for chapter 6 with comments such as "If it weren't for having to grade students, I would love teaching" and "All students think about are their grades, not what and how they are learning." These concerns around grading are familiar to nurse educators. In this chapter Chinn presents some underlying thoughts and responses that have helped her deal with the difficult issue of grades and grading. She discusses issues related to traditional practices of grading and suggests practices that are consistent with values about human interactions that are generally claimed in nursing. She identifies reasons to examine traditional grading approaches and consider alternatives, and explores issues of grade inflation, pass/fail grading, and the power imbalances inherent in traditional grading. The chapter guides faculty in building a philosophic foundation for their grading practices and offers specific conceptual definitions for grades that can be used in undergraduate and graduate nursing courses.

Testing is a predominant means of measuring the outcomes of learning and providing data for arriving at grades in nursing courses. The focus of chapter 7, by Marilyn Blau Klainberg, is computer testing in nursing education. While many faculty in other programs use some form of technology to score tests and provide an item analysis, few schools of nursing are using computer technology for classroom testing of students. In this chapter, Klainberg provides an overview of available computer testing software and discusses its potential use in nursing education. She presents computer adaptive testing (CAT) and CAT software available for classroom testing, computer technology for creating tests that can be given on the computer itself or in the traditional paper-and-pencil format, benefits and drawbacks for faculty and students of computer testing, issues and solutions to maintain test security, and research in nursing education that compares computer and paper-and-pencil testing.

Online learning is an educational delivery tool being adopted by many nurse educators. In volume 1 of the *Annual Review*, we included a number of chapters on how faculty were using online learning and distance education in their nursing programs. In chapter 8, Dee McGonigle, Kathleen Mastrian, and Nedra Farcus emphasize the need for usability testing to help ensure the quality of online learning materials. They illustrate the adaptation of usability testing techniques, explain the reasons behind the need for this important validity check, and suggest a simple way to conduct two usability tests: simplified thinking aloud and heuristic evaluation. The authors also provide guidelines for faculty who want to conduct these tests on their online materials.

Part III includes two chapters on simulations in nursing education. To prepare students with competencies to meet the challenges of the work environment, and for nurses to maintain their clinical skills, educators have turned to simulation as a teaching method. With simulated experiences learners can focus on developing critical thinking, problem solving, and psychomotor skills in a risk-free environment.

In chapter 9, Patricia Gonce Morton and Carol A. Rauen describe how their schools of nursing developed patient simulation laboratories and implemented simulation in basic and graduate nursing programs. One facility houses 24 state-of-the-art patient simulation laboratories, including health assessment laboratories, a basic hospital unit, a 10-bed adult critical care unit, a pediatric unit, a neonatal intensive care, a labor and delivery unit, and an operating room. Each lab contains a variety of mannequins including fully automated, high-fidelity human simulators. A computer is at each bedside for students to review computer-assisted instruction as part of the learning experience. The authors also describe how the other facility acquired funding for its new simulation center, complete with patient simulators; how it integrated simulation in courses in the undergraduate and graduate nursing programs; and how it developed the role of simulation coordinator. If you are planning on developing and implementing simulation in your program, this chapter has the information you need to get started and carry the project to completion.

Wendy M. Nehring and Felissa R. Lashley had an opportunity to remodel their psychomotor laboratory with state-of-the-art equipment, including an adult and a pediatric Human Patient Simulator™ (HPS). The HPS is composed of a life-size mannequin and computer system, with preset scenarios that can be used for different disease conditions or new ones that can be added to fit the learning objectives of the course. With the HPS, students can develop knowledge, critical thinking, and psychomotor skills, and learn to work with the "patient" and health care team. In chapter 10, these authors describe the use of the HPS in nursing education and how they developed and now implement the HPS in the undergraduate program and throughout the nurse anesthetist specialization in the graduate program. The HPS is used to teach students about the nursing management of critical incidents using scenarios. Even if you are not planning on purchasing a HPS, the authors present their model for teaching nursing practice using critical incidents and provide a sample scenario that illustrates the model.

In Part IV the authors present innovative teaching strategies for use in the classroom and in clinical practice. Several chapters describe and illustrate teaching methods for critical thinking, provide a framework for using the principles of *Peace and Power* in the classroom with examples of how those principles are translated into actual teaching practices, and present innovative technology applications in a community health course.

Over the last decade there has been a wealth of literature on critical thinking. The authors of chapter 11, Carol A. Sedlak and Margaret O. Doheny, believe that the development of critical thinking should start with beginning nursing students. In this chapter the authors discuss and present examples of five active teaching/learning strategies that help students develop critical thinking in both the classroom and clinical setting. These include (1) Socratic questioning, (2) journal writing, (3) developing service learning activities, (4) conducting peer-review experiences, and (5) dressing up to portray nursing diagnoses to learn the nursing process. The chapter is valuable for teachers at all levels of nursing education and in staff development because it explains how to develop and implement each strategy and provides actual examples.

Many educators focus on giving information to students rather than on facilitating their learning. Learning is promoted through innovative teaching strategies such as concept mapping. A concept map is a visual learning tool or schematic device that organizes information or concepts and shows their relationships. Donna D. Ignatavicius, in chapter 12, describes how students learn, the relationship of critical thinking to learning, and how concept mapping enhances both learning and critical thinking. Ignatavicius explains and illustrates how concept maps can be used for teaching in the classroom, the skills laboratory, and clinical courses.

Chapter 13 moves beyond the discussion of innovative instructional methods to provide a framework for teaching in nursing. In this chapter Adeline R. Falk-Rafael, Mary Ann Anderson, Peggy L. Chinn, and Alicebelle Rubotzky describe their collective experiences in using the principles of *Peace and Power* in the classroom. They also give examples of how those principles can be translated into actual teaching practices and report some of the students' reactions to this framework, which is a new experience for most students. The authors present strategies for encouraging active participation in the classroom and how they can be adapted even for large classes. They also describe how to use SOPHIA, an acronym that stands for Speak Out, Play Havoc, and Imagine Alternatives, to introduce a topic for discussion in a class. This chapter provides a valuable framework for educators in all types of programs.

Over the past 10 years, the Cleveland State University Department of Nursing (CSU) and Visiting Nurse Association Healthcare Partners of Ohio (VNAHPO) developed its education/practice partnership, *Vision on 22nd Street*. The purpose of chapter 14, by Cheryl P. McCahon and Sheila A. Niles, is to describe selected VNAHPO technology initiatives and how they were subsequently integrated into the CSU community-based nursing curriculum. The authors present three phases of technology development: telehealth initiatives, point of care technology integration, and future initiatives. For each phase, they discuss curricular applications and issues for implementation including recommendations to guide faculty considering these initiatives.

Part V begins with a chapter on promoting academic integrity and using well-planned and proactive communication with students about academic dishonesty. Other chapters examine the transition experience of new graduates, what we can do to improve that process, and the development of nursing staff through orientation, ongoing competency development, and staff development programs. Two final chapters provide frameworks for preparing new teachers, and for educating nursing students.

There is growing concern that nursing student academic dishonesty is widespread. Chapter 15, by Marianne R. Jeffreys and Lori Stier, addresses this problem and provides academic administrators and faculty with strategies for effectively dealing with it. Nurse educators are in a key position to promote academic integrity and discourage dishonesty. A PROACTIVE communication strategy to prevent academic dishonesty is presented. It emphasizes the importance of: Policy, Responsibility, Ongoing action, Accountability, Commitment, Trust, Initiative, Values, and Expectations. The authors also suggest actions to take when faced with dishonest academic behavior such as cheating on exams and tests, plagiarism, fabricating data, and falsifying records. Through the use of case exemplars from a variety of academic and clinical settings, the authors illustrate how nurse educators can promote student academic integrity through the use of effective communication.

Considering the nursing shortage throughout North America, and the need to retain new graduates in the workforce, chapter 16, by Judy Boychuk Duchscher, will be of great interest to readers. This chapter guides readers in understanding the impact of an increasingly demanding work environment on the transition experience of new graduate nurses and the implications of shifting workloads and more intense practice environments on their professional self-concept, stress levels, and work satisfaction. The chapter also provides insight into the impact of these workplace characteristics on the quality of patient care. Duchscher emphasizes the importance of the relationship between senior nursing staff and novice nurses during the process of transition, and she proposes initiatives for both educational and service institutions to optimize their responses to issues in workforce recruitment and retention.

Nurse educators in clinical settings assume vital roles in the transition of new graduates and continued development of experienced nursing staff through orientation, ongoing competency development, and staff education programs. In chapter 17, Magdalena A. Mateo and Eileen McMyler present strategies for evaluating staff competency and development in orientation and throughout employment. In preparation for writing the chapter, they surveyed hospitals to inquire about their practices in relation to these programs, and they include these findings throughout the chapter. The authors present examples of program components and forms that can be adapted by other educators.

As America faces a nursing shortage, new faculty are needed in schools of nursing. The ability of nursing programs to increase the numbers of graduates is compounded by a critical nurse faculty shortage. Schools of nursing need aggressive faculty recruitment plans, multifaceted orientation programs, and caring leaders to direct, mentor, and develop nurse educators of the future. Janet Hoey Robinson, in chapter 18, describes the role of the academic leader in preparing new faculty for teaching. She examines the needs of new faculty and how academic leaders and faculty can meet them. Robinson has developed and uses a "caring coach with a vision" philosophy and leadership style to foster the development of new faculty for their teaching role.

In chapter 19, Bonnie W. Duldt-Battey shares her holistic framework for teaching in nursing. She describes holism, as it applies to students, as humanizing communication in the teacher-student relationship, forming a "spiritual connection" with students, and encouraging students to think critically and communicate persuasively. Students' evaluative comments are included to document the effectiveness of applying the holistic paradigm to teaching.

We hope you agree that Volume 2 of the *Annual Review of Nursing Education* has met the goal of keeping you updated on the latest innovations in nursing education across all settings. A special thanks is extended to Dr. Ursula Springer for recognizing the need for an annual review of nursing education and making it happen, to Ruth Chasek for her support and editorial assistance, and to Pamela Lankas for her assistance during production. We appreciate the hard work of the authors who were generous enough to share their innovations for the benefit of educators everywhere. And a heartfelt thanks to you for reading and recommending the *Annual Review of Nursing Education* to other nurse educators!

Marilyn H. Oermann, Editor
Kathleen T. Heinrich, Associate Editor

Part I

Current Trends

Chapter 1

An Overview of Trends
in Nursing Education

Barbara R. Grumet and Carol Gilbert

A nalyses of the latest nursing shortage are once again focusing on nursing education programs. What are nursing education programs of all types doing to respond to local, regional, and national shortages of registered nurses and licensed practical nurses? How do nursing educators adapt to changes in patients, health providers, and managed care? How do students learn in the "sicker and quicker" patient care environments of today's acute care system? How do faculty and students address the challenges of older patients, chronic illness, and the increasing diversity of patients? These and many other questions are being addressed by nursing leaders, educators, and policy makers.

As the accrediting body responsible for all types of nursing education, including master's, baccalaureate, associate, diploma, and practical nursing programs, the National League for Nursing Accrediting Commission (NLNAC) is in a good position to assess the state of nursing education around the country and across all program types. This chapter reports on findings from recent accreditation reviews, as well as information provided by all NLNAC accredited programs as part of ongoing monitoring activities.

ABOUT NLNAC

Accreditation is a voluntary and self-regulatory process by which non-governmental associations review educational institutions or programs and recognize those that meet or exceed standards and criteria for educational quality (NLNAC, 2002a). The NLNAC began in 1997, as a division of the National League for Nursing (NLN), which had been recognized as a specialized accrediting agency for nursing education by the United States Department of Education since 1952. In 2001, NLNAC became an independent subsidiary corporation of NLN, incorporated under the laws of the State of New York. The NLNAC accredits all types of nursing education programs—master's, baccalaureate, associate, diploma, and practical nursing. There are 1,494 nursing programs accredited by the NLNAC.

The Commission is governed by 15 elected commissioners, representing nursing education, nursing practice, and the public. The NLNAC is fully recognized as an accrediting agency by the United States Department of Education and recognized by the Council for Higher Education Accreditation. Each year NLNAC reviews approximately 200 programs; in the 2001–2002 academic year, it reviewed programs from 43 states, the District of Columbia, the Commonwealth of Puerto Rico, Guam, and the Virgin Islands.

The accreditation process reviews nursing education programs against national standards and criteria covering:

- Mission and Governance
- Faculty
- Students
- Curriculum and Instruction
- Resources
- Program Integrity
- Program Evaluation.

Steps in Accreditation Review Process

The accreditation review process for each program consists of the following steps:

1. Submission of a self-study document by the program.
2. A site visit by a team of peers, lasting 2 to 3 days, applying the accreditation standards and criteria within the context of the specific program type. The site visitors prepare a report and recommendation for accreditation status.

3. Peer review by an Evaluation Review Panel (ERP) for each program type. The ERP reviews the self-study document and site visit report, applying the standards and criteria for that program type. Following the peer review, the ERP makes a recommendation to the Commission for accreditation. Each ERP is chaired by a commissioner.
4. Discussion and decision on accreditation status made by the Commission. The commissioners review each program and make accreditation decisions across all program types.

The accreditation cycle is eight years for continuing accreditation and five years for initial accreditation. The NLNAC also conducts annual monitoring of all accredited programs through an annual report. Significant program changes are reported separately to the Commission.

CURRENT STATUS OF NURSING EDUCATION PROGRAMS

This chapter highlights some of the findings from NLNAC accredited programs that were reviewed during the Spring 2002 accreditation review and ongoing monitoring of all accredited programs (NLNAC, 2002c). Examples of specific programs are illustrative and not necessarily exclusive to these programs. Since more than 100 programs were reviewed during the Spring 2002 cycle, space does not permit citing specifics from each program reviewed.

Fewer Students

The United States Department of Health and Human Services (USDHHS) indicated in its July 2002 report on the nursing workforce that "after growing steadily during the first half of the 1990s, the number of new RN [registered nurse] graduates fell annually in the last half of the decade, resulting in 26 percent fewer RN graduates in 2000 than in 1995" (USDHHS, 2002, p. 3). Data from NLNAC accredited programs confirm this phenomenon. Table 1.1 shows graduates from all NLNAC accredited program types.

However, this trend may be reversing. Tables 1.2 and 1.3 report data on student enrollments in NLNAC accredited programs. More

TABLE 1.1   Mean Number of Graduates Reported by Accredited Programs by Program Type

Program type	2000–2001	1999–2000	1998–1999	1997–1998
Master's	37.0	36.2	40.0	38.4
Baccalaureate	58.3	59.7	66.0	70.0
Associate	55.0	55.1	63.0	65.0
Diploma	35.1	32.3	35.0	39.0
Practical Nursing	40.4	41.4	46.0	41.0

Multiple modes exist. The smallest value is shown.
Note: Trended across 1998–2002 NLNAC Annual Reports.

TABLE 1.2   Student Enrollment Reported by Accredited Programs by Program Type

Program Type	2001		2000		1999		1998	
	Mean	Mode	Mean	Mode	Mean	Mode	Mean	Mode
Master's	102.0	24.0	112.6	31.0*	123.0	40.0	116.9	26.0
Bacca-laureate	192.0	139.0	190.4	95.0*	203.0	74.0*	236.8	49.0
Associate	152.1	108.0	129.1	104.0	144.0	90.0	172.0	114.0
Diploma	113.7	79.0*	93.0	28.0*	94.0	44.0*	121.0	74.0
Practical Nursing	74.0	36.0	62.6	34.0*	80.0	30.0*	78.0	30.0

*Multiple modes exist. The smallest value is shown.
Note: Trended across 1998–2002 NLNAC Annual Reports.

programs reported significant increases than decreases in enrollment during 2000–2001, for the first time in three years. A 20% or more change in enrollments is considered to be "significant change." This phenomenon cuts across all program types. For example, 19% of baccalaureate programs report an increase in enrollments, while 14% report a decrease. The number of programs (67%) with "no change" in enrollment since the previous year also is the lowest in three years. The NLNAC accredited associate degree programs also report increased or

TABLE 1.3 Percentage of Significant* Change in Enrollment Reported by Accredited Programs by Program Type

Program type	2000–2001 (in %)			1999–2000 (in %)			1998–1999 (in %)			1997–1998 (in %)		
	Increase	Decrease	No change	Increase	Decrease	No change	Increase	Decrease	No change	Increase	Decrease	No change
Master's	13	16	70	7	12	80	7	13	80	13	8	79
Baccalaureate	19	14	67	7	13	80	5	15	80	5	14	81
Associate	19	6.4	75	7.5	9	84	3	14	83	1.3	16	83
Diploma	36	4	58	12	10	78	8	26	66	8	30	62
Practical Nursing	19	11	74	5	14	81	4	16	80	6	19	76

Significant = > 20% change.
Note: Trended across 1998–2002 NLNAC Annual Reports.

stable enrollments; 19% had increased enrollments, and only 6% had a decrease. The remaining 75% report no change in enrollment.

The nursing shortage is cited as one reason for significant increases in enrollment. It also is suggested as a reason for significant decreases or stability in enrollment—students are too busy working to attend school!

More Diverse Students

The student bodies are becoming more diverse—older, more males, and more racial and ethnic minorities. Many programs experienced an increase in part-time students who are combining school with work and family responsibilities. The NLNAC requested data on part- and full-time status for the first time in 2002. Results from the 2000–2001 academic year indicated that 28% of master's students, 18% of baccalaureate, 22% of associate, 21% of diploma, and 22% of practical nursing students are part-time students. While at least some of the baccalaureate students and all of the master's students are already RNs, part-time learning presents different challenges for nursing educators preparing basic RN students.

Some nursing programs, particularly those located in community colleges, are required to accept their students in an institution that mandates open admission. Many of these individuals are students from educationally disadvantaged backgrounds—poor high-school preparation, English as a second language, and many years out of school. These students, though, are not necessarily incapable of mastering a rigorous nursing curriculum. Programs in open-admission environments frequently report "selective admissions" to the nursing program, typically by mandating certain liberal arts "pre-nursing" courses in science, math, and English, and requiring a minimum grade of C or higher in each course. Many also require prospective students to take the NLN Pre-Admission-RN exam and achieve a minimum score set by the faculty.

Northern Virginia Community College in Annandale, Virginia, has a comprehensive array of student support services to maximize retention. Students must score at least in the 50th percentile on the NLN Pre-Admission-RN exam. The college requires all students to take the ACT COMPASS Test. Orientation programs are mandated for both the College and the Nursing program. In 2000, the nursing faculty decided to use the College Survey Inventory (CSI): Retention Management System with its first-year students. Students identified as high risk for dropping out of the program are referred to the College's Counseling Department and Nursing Department faculty for academic advisement. The faculty formed a Retention Committee whose members meet with students on a regular basis.

Students are encouraged to form study groups and to seek assistance from faculty and peer tutors if they need help with coursework. In addition, Inova, the area's largest health care system, has a formal mentoring system in place for nursing students. Students are encouraged to take advantage of this mentoring opportunity. These interventions have improved the retention rate considerably.

An example of outstanding mentoring and support for disadvantaged baccalaureate nursing students, both basic and RN, is found at Texas A&M, located on the Mexican border in Laredo, Texas. Eighty percent of their students come from disadvantaged, non-English-speaking families. The faculty and community have developed an extensive network of student advisement, mentoring, tutoring, and support, so that 90% of their students graduate, and 86% pass the NCLEX the first time. Courses include Web-assisted instruction, interactive video, computer-based tutorials, frequent testing, and quick feedback on test results. NLN Mobility Profile and NCLEX-RN review materials also are provided. Test review and feedback are part of almost every course. Students are notified mid-semester if they are at risk of failing, and are informed of the remediation needed to achieve a passing grade. These examples are illustrative of the many ways that our accredited programs are working to help students succeed in their program and achieve their goal of becoming a registered nurse.

Faculty Shortages

The nursing shortage and the "aging of the workforce" reported by the U.S. Department of Health and Human Services (2002) are affecting nursing education as well. Programs all across the country report faculty leaving academia because of retirement or for higher paying jobs in nursing service. They also report difficulty in hiring new faculty because salaries offered by the colleges and universities cannot compete with higher salaries available in many practice environments. Faculty shortages are cited as one of the barriers to increasing enrollments in nursing programs despite increased interest in nursing as a career and local nursing shortages.

Over the past five years, 21 percent of the 1,116 programs reviewed by NLNAC had an identified "pattern of concern" regarding faculty qualifications, utilization, or workload. A "pattern of concern" does not indicate a violation of accreditation standards, but rather suggests that a nursing program is at risk of being in violation if the situation does not change. The "good news" is that this percentage actually declined slightly in spring 2002, to 19%, in spite of the aging of faculty and the "wave" of faculty retirements being reported anecdotally.

An additional symptom of the faculty shortage is that the nursing program administrator (dean or chairperson) often does not have sufficient time to perform her/his duties. While most nursing education leaders find themselves in this situation, 7% of the NLNAC accredited programs reviewed during spring 2002 had the excessive workload of the program administrator listed as a concern.

Some schools are finding help with the faculty shortage from logical partners—local health care providers. A few schools reported that local health care systems have contributed funds for increased faculty salaries so that nursing faculty salaries are competitive with service. A few hospitals are sharing experienced, master's prepared nurses with local nursing education programs while paying their full salary.

Most nursing programs continue to rely on part-time, adjunct, and clinical faculty to deliver parts of the nursing curriculum. Some schools are making a significant effort to assimilate the part-time faculty into the nursing program. Some schools report inviting part-time faculty to attend faculty meetings as well as important events such as pinning ceremonies. Others report more extensive activities. For example, Niagara County Community College, located in upstate New York, has a comprehensive orientation and mentoring program for its part-time faculty. The nursing program prepares an orientation packet for part-time faculty, which includes complete information about the program, curriculum, faculty, and policies and procedures, which supplements the college's part-time faculty handbook. In addition, each part-time faculty member is assigned a mentor from the full-time faculty.

NCLEX

The NLNAC accredited programs report average NCLEX pass rates that are higher than the national average, and have done so consistently over the past five years (NLNAC, 2002b). Data provided to NLNAC confirm the findings of the National Council of State Boards of Nursing that the decline in NCLEX scores that began several years ago seems to be leveling off and is perhaps reversing a bit (Marks, 2002). Tables 1.4 and 1.5 present NCLEX and certification pass rates for NLNAC accredited programs. These data also confirm national findings that the pass rates are no different for graduates of baccalaureate and associate degree programs.

The pressure to produce graduates capable of passing the licensing examination is felt across the country, in all program types. More schools are putting in place minimum grade requirements such as a minimum C grade in each nursing course, or higher scores needed to pass a particular course. In addition, schools are requiring success on "pre-NCLEX" tests, typically given during the last weeks of the nursing program, for graduation. Some schools are increasing tutoring, test preparation, and NCLEX review support services. Others provide limited support, expecting the students to prepare themselves for both the "pre-NCLEX" and actual licensing examinations.

In some programs faculty are implementing curriculum changes and student support programs to enhance NCLEX success. Courses are reviewed to assure that the content tested by the NCLEX is addressed in the nursing curriculum. More critical thinking exercises are being incorporated into classroom activities and course examinations.

Curriculum

Nursing programs are responding in a variety of ways to the challenges of the nursing shortage and changes in health care. Although acute care is still a major focus of clinical and classroom instruction, nursing programs are revising curricula to incorporate changes in nursing practice and the health care system, including more gerontology, cultural diversity, ethics, death and dying, chronic care, community care, and managed care in courses. Nursing programs are incorporating more culturally relevant information into their curriculum particularly about health beliefs, attitudes toward sickness and death, and cultural practices and remedies. This is seen most frequently in programs located in regions where there is a strong presence of a particular racial or ethnic group. All programs are trying to make students more aware of the roles that culture and beliefs play in the response of patients and families to illness.

TABLE 1.4 NCLEX and Certification Pass Rate Percentages (2000–2001 Academic Year)

Program type	First-time exam takers (Percentage)					Repeat exam takers (Percentage)				
	National mean 2000*	Mean	Median	Mode	Range	National mean 2000	Mean	Median	Mode	Range
Master's certification**	—	96.0	100	100	75–100	—	—	—	—	—
Aggregate (NCLEX-RN)	83.8	87.0	88.2	100	42.9–100	48.5	69.0	74.0	100	0–100
Baccalaureate†	83.9	86.3	88.0	100	48–100		73.3	79	100	5–100††
Associate†	83.8	87.0	89.0	100	42.9–100		67.0	70.0	100	0–100
Diploma	83.4	89.0	90.0	100	50–100		68.1	67.0	100	0–100
Practical Nursing (NCLEX-PN)	85.0	89.0	92.0	100	51–100	41.6	73.0	75.0	100	7.14–100

*National data from the National Council of State Boards of Nursing. *1999 Licensure Statistics On-Line* (http://www.ncsbn.org/).

**25% of cases missing

†Data exclude NCLEX results from programs located in Puerto Rico as the exam is not required for practice.

††In several cases the percentage reported appears to be the percentage of students who were not successful in their first attempt rather than the success rate of the repeaters.

TABLE 1.5 NCLEX and Certification Mean Pass Rate Percentages for First-Time Examination Takers Reported by Accredited Programs by Program Type

	Year				
Program Type	2000–2001	1999–2000	1998–1999	1997–1998	1996–1997
Master's certification	96.0	96.3	94.0	93.5	—
(Response rate of graduate programs)	(75%)*	(80%)*	(77%)*	(60%)*	—
Baccalaureate	86.3	84.8	86.3	85.4	89.0
Associate	87.0	86.4	86.6	87.0	91.0
Diploma	89.0	86.6	87.7	89.0	94.0
Practical Nursing	89.0	89.2	89.0	88.4	93.0

Note: In percentages. Trended across 1997–2002 NLNAC Annual Reports.

Baccalaureate and master's programs have traditionally included courses and experiences in leadership, management, and supervision. As a sign of the times, increasing numbers of associate degree programs report adding course content in these areas in response to feedback from recent graduates and local employers. In some parts of the country, particularly rural areas, and in practice environments such as long-term care, associate degree nurses are assuming more supervisory and leadership responsibilities.

Technology is incorporated throughout the curriculum in all program types, requiring basic computer literacy. Faculty in baccalaureate and master's programs, and increasingly in associate degree and diploma programs, use the Internet for course assignments and classroom activities. Many programs require students to prepare Power Point presentations as part of their course assignments. Nursing labs are becoming more and more high tech, frequently using donati from local health care agencies to give students access to the latest patient care equipment. As another example of "learning partnerships," hospitals allow nursing programs to use their staff orientation equipment and rooms for student labs.

Bachelor's programs for RNs (RN to BSN) base their curricula on the recognition that their students are already licensed nurses, frequently with a number of years of clinical experience. Curricula are being re-designed to eliminate redundancy with associate degree programs. Classes are scheduled in a year round, "fast track" format, with classes frequently meeting evenings and weekends to accommodate work schedules. Course content focuses on liberal arts and integrating the liberal arts into clinical practice, community health, family, group, and change theories and application, patient education, and management.

As an example, the University of New England has a Two plus Two BSN program originally developed for students from their own associate degree nursing (ADN) program. Formal articulation agreements are in place from a number of regional ADN and diploma programs. The curriculum builds on the focus of individual and family as client to family as a structural/functional unit of service, the community as a client, and the health care organization as a system. Health promotion, disease prevention, adaptation to chronic illness, and population-based care are stressed. The role of the nurse expands to advocate, referral agent, counselor, change agent, leader, and researcher.

Many states require, or encourage, articulation between nursing program types. The National Council of State Boards of Nursing reports that seven states mandate and 43 states encourage articulation (Marks, 2002). The idea, of course, is to make it easier for associate degree graduates to complete baccalaureate and eventually master's degree programs, and for licensed practical/vocational nurses to become RNs.

Programs are providing more "real world" nursing experiences. Faculty practices are becoming a more common way for students to learn, and for faculty to keep, their clinical skills current while providing needed health care services to typically underserved populations. The University of Maryland School of Nursing developed a "clinical enterprise" to provide clinical experiences in patient settings other than acute care as well as expand opportunities for faculty practice and research, and development of new models of nursing care. The practice settings provide teaching opportunities, research environments, models of interdisciplinary care, and community health care. Both baccalaureate and master's students participate. Some of the practice environments include a nurse-managed primary care center in a medically underserved neighborhood in Baltimore, school-based wellness centers, mobile health care, a senior care center, and family and pediatric ambulatory centers. The focus of these environments is to develop and implement new models of nursing care emphasizing family, community, and interdisciplinary practice.

As another example, faculty at Texas A&M at Laredo School of Nursing have students in the community health nursing course work with residents of colonias, small, unincorporated communities on the Texas-Mexico border with high numbers of poverty-stricken residents. These are but two of the many examples of innovative programs combining nursing practice to underserved populations, clinical experience for students, and exposure to cultural diversity.

Both associate and baccalaureate programs are requiring a clinical preceptorship as part of their curricula to provide a transition into professional practice. The preceptorships are typically 1–2 months in length but may be longer. This type of experience is similar to the internship recommended in the Joint Commission on Accreditation of Healthcare Organizations (JCAHO) White Paper on the Nursing Shortage (JCAHO, 2002).

Distance Education

The NLNAC uses the definition of distance learning found in the Higher Education Amendments of 1998: "An educational process that is characterized by the separation, in time or place, between instructor and student" (NLNAC, 2002a, p. 70). Distance learning can include television, audio or computer transmission, audio or computer conferencing, video, or correspondence.

One form of distance learning in NLNAC accredited programs is a branch campus, where the entire curriculum is delivered, or an extension site, where a portion of the curriculum is delivered. Thirty programs reported that they added a branch campus/extension site in 2000–2001.

While some programs offer an entire degree online, most commonly the master's degree, many more offer courses, or units in courses, online. Ten percent of the master's, eight percent of the baccalaureate, and four percent of the associate degree programs added distance learning to their nursing programs during the 2000–2001 academic year. It should be noted that "distance learning" does not necessarily mean that an entire degree is available online.

As an example, the Minnesota State University at Mankato has developed an innovative, distance-based, master's program with clinical nurse specialist and Family Nurse Practitioner tracks to serve primarily the rural areas of Minnesota and neighboring Iowa. Interactive television is used to deliver the curriculum to up to 5 locations at a time, 60 to 120 miles from campus. Many courses are online, and the entire program is offered on a full- or part-time basis.

More RN to BSN programs are being developed using distance education. In these distance education programs, clinical courses are minimal; faculty recognize that students enter with baseline knowledge and clinical expertise.

Resources

Money is tight in higher education, and nursing programs are not exempt from institutional pressures to decrease expenses. Many public institutions report cuts in budgets, sometimes mid-year. Private institutions experience challenges to keep tuition affordable and deal with declining revenues from tuition, donations, and endowments. The financial pressures on higher education make it difficult for programs to hire faculty, upgrade technology, and add classroom and office space to increase enrollments or maintain program quality. During the spring 2002 accreditation cycle, 22% of the programs reviewed had a concern about resources, which includes learning resources (library, laboratory, and technology); fiscal resources (adequate budget to support the nursing program); physical resources (primarily classroom, office, and lab space); and support staff. This was an increase from the 5-year average of 15%.

Some nursing programs, however, are exempt from an institutional faculty hiring freeze. Another phenomenon beginning to take hold is a recognition that nursing faculty are "highly desired" and therefore may need to have salaries higher than the overall salary scale in the institution. Borrowing from the experience of other disciplines such as business, computer science, and physical therapy, a few baccalaureate and master's programs report paying faculty salaries higher than the institutional scale or offering a "bonus" to faculty at the end of the academic year.

The health care community is responding to the nursing shortage by providing increased support to nursing programs. Some programs in Texas, for example, report that hospitals are donating funds to nursing programs to supplement faculty salaries, provide professional development support, and purchase equipment, software, and library holdings. Many health care facilities have traditionally provided some tuition reimbursement to staff; this support is continuing. Other facilities are working directly with nursing education programs to provide "fast track" programs for practical nurses, nurse's aides, and other hospital staff to become RNs. These partnerships include full tuition payment for the staff, classroom space, mentors, tutoring, and other support. Still others have formal mentoring programs for nursing students, providing mentoring and often recruiting.

CONCLUSIONS

Based on the data provided to NLNAC by its accredited programs, it is safe to conclude that nursing education is alive and well, and adapting to the ever-changing environments in higher education and health care. Faculty and administrators are adjusting to the challenges of changing students, aging faculty, decreased resources, and increased interest in nursing as a career. Programs around the country are responding with imagination, flexibility, and creativity to adapt to changes in students, patients, and providers. Nurse educators are committed to the highest quality in nursing education.

The time and energy devoted to accreditation and peer review are a testimony to the desire of nursing educators to promote the highest quality in nursing education. Everyone involved in accreditation, from nursing faculty and institutional leadership to peer reviewers and commissioners, are concerned with one goal: to assure that every nursing program in the country that is accredited by NLNAC achieves the highest possible quality for the benefit of patients and their families.

ACKNOWLEDGMENT

Thanks to Dr. Susan Abbe, Director of Accreditation Services, NLNAC, and Mr. Anthony Bugay, Special Assistant, NLNAC.

REFERENCES

Joint Commission on Accreditation of Healthcare Organizations (JCAHO). (2002). *Healthcare at the Crossroads: Strategies for Addressing the Evolving Nursing Crisis.* Retrieved November 25, 2002, http://www.jcaho.org

Marks, C. (2002, August). National Council of State Boards of Nursing, Profiles of Member Boards: 2000, 2001. Report presented at the National Council of State Boards of Nursing Annual Meeting, Long Beach, CA.

National League for Nursing Accrediting Commission (NLNAC). (2002a). *Accreditation manual and interpretive guidelines by program type 2002.* New York: NLNAC.

National League for Nursing Accrediting Commission (NLNAC). (2002b). *NLNAC ongoing systematic program of review status report Spring 2002 accreditation cycle.* Unpublished document. New York: NLNAC.

National League for Nursing Accrediting Commission (NLNAC). (2002c). Self-study documents submitted to the NLNAC for the Spring 2002 accreditation cycle. New York: NLNAC.

U.S. Department of Health and Human Services (USDHHS). (2002, August). *Projected Supply, Demand,and Shortages of Registered Nurses: 2000–2020.* Retrieved November 25, 2002, http://phpr.hrsa.gov/healthworkforce/rnproject/report.htm

Chapter 2

Certificate Programs in Nursing: Service-Education Collaboration in the Age of the Knowledge Worker

Diane M. Billings

N ursing workforce needs are rapidly changing: jobs are in flux, new career paths in nursing are emerging rapidly, and the knowledge and skills needed for practice are becoming even more specialized. Employers are seeking employees with proven competencies and who are prepared for rapid transition to the work environment (Kohl, 2000). Traditional degrees in nursing (associate, baccalaureate, and master's) may no longer be sufficient for some positions, and nurse educators are being urged to consider new and flexible models of education to prepare nurses for the current workforce needs (Advisory Board Company, 2001).

Certificate programs are one solution for preparing nurses for the current work environment. Formerly marginalized and viewed with skepticism, certificate programs are becoming closer aligned with the missions and economic futures of academic institutions and health care agencies (Irby, 1999). Post-baccalaureate certificate programs are one of the growth areas in higher education, and certificate programs in health-related fields represent major increases in enrollment and interest in returning to schools for advanced degrees (Arora et al., 1996; LaPidus, 2000; Marchese, 1999; Patterson, 1999). The purpose of this chapter is to discuss the advantages and disadvantages of certificate programs and their contributions to fostering service-education collaboration in the age of the knowledge worker.

CERTIFICATE PROGRAMS

Certificate programs, like academic programs with defined outcomes and assessment criteria, are occupation-oriented courses or sequences of courses that constitute a coherent body of study in a discipline (Craven & DuHamel, 2002; Holt, 1991; Irby, 1999; Marchese, 1999) but unlike traditional academic programs, tend to be shorter in length, modular, convenient, and customized. They are often interdisciplinary, but they do not confer a degree (LaPidus, 2000; Kohl, 2000). The primary purposes of certificate programs are to prepare employees for emerging areas of workforce need, to advance careers or assist career transitions, and to prepare employees for specialization within a field. Certificate programs also may serve as recruitment strategies for enticing participants to seek advanced degrees.

Certificate programs appeal to adult learners, most of whom are employed and are seeking career advancement (Kerka, 2000). These learners are self-directed, have specific career goals, and are seeking education that is flexible and will prepare them for career advancement. Because of learners' needs for access and convenience, certificate programs increasingly use educational technology and distance learning strategies to offer the program.

Certificate programs appeal to employers because the employee who has met outcomes of the certificate program brings to the workplace an assurance of a minimum set of competencies, which may result in a shorter orientation time, be a better match between the employee's interests and skills and the institution's needs, and improve job satisfaction and retention. Additionally, as the nursing profession grapples with the issue of multisite licensing, certificates can serve as evidence of attainment of standardized competencies across state or institutional lines. With declining numbers of educators and increases in demand for education and training, the value of external validation of knowledge and skills becomes increasingly appealing, and many employers are reimbursing employees for successful completion of certificate programs.

Certificate programs have the potential for fostering collaboration among health care agencies and schools of nursing. Employers with large numbers of nurses and expanding areas of specialized health services often seek education partners to whom they can outsource the costs of expensive, short-term education. Many schools of nursing are positioned to meet these needs and can develop certificate programs that can award academic credit or contact hours. Benefits of educational collaboration include reduced educational costs, effective use of nurse educators, and improved educational and career transitions for the participants in the program (Billings, Jeffries, Stone, Rowles, & Urden, 2002; Dreher, Everett, Hartwig, et al., 2001).

Types of Certificate Programs

There are various types and models of certificate programs. Certificate programs can be described by their purpose, the authority by which they are offered, and the type of credit awarded.

Purpose

The primary purpose of a certificate program is to lead to or supplement a degree, for example, a teacher education certificate program in the master's nursing program or a postmaster's certificate option in nursing informatics. Another purpose of certificate programs is to recognize mastery in a specific content area, for example, a sequence of courses leading to a gerontology certificate in an undergraduate nursing program. Certificate programs also can be designed to focus on specific job-related skills such as a certificate in critical care nursing or financial management.

Degree and nondegree programs have coexisted in many institutions of higher education, but until recently they have served different audiences and existed as separate entities within the organization. The current direction is toward learner-centered planning to meet learners' needs in an integrated design, with courses that can be offered for both academic and nondegree credit (Arora et al., 1996; LaPidus, 2000).

Offering Authority

Certificate programs can be described as being university or nonuniversity based. Programs offered *within the university structure* tend to focus on a body of knowledge defined primarily by the faculty. The program may be "free standing," existing within a university that does not have a degree program in the content area of the certificate program, or an "add on," in which it is combined with an existing degree program

(Patterson, 1999). The certificate may be a postbaccalaureate or postmaster's degree, and may confer academic credit. Certificate programs may be offered by providers of noncredit education such as professional schools, schools of continuing studies, or offices of lifelong learning within a school of nursing or a college or university.

Certificate programs also are offered *in nonuniversity* settings such as programs by employers, the so-called "career universities" or "corporate universities." Certificates can be provided by licensing bodies or professional organizations (Irby, 2000). These programs tend to focus on job relevance, competency for workforce needs, and emphasis on competency assessment.

Credit

Certificate programs confer several types of credit. Certificate programs offered through or in collaboration with academic institutions confer *academic credit* such as in baccalaureate, postbaccalaureate, master's degree, and postmaster's degree programs. Faculty curriculum committees generally specify the number of courses or credits required to be designated as a certificate program and may offer opportunities for students to enroll in a sequence of courses both in the major and outside of the major to acquire competencies in a specialized area. Postmaster's certificate programs in nursing are relatively common. These programs prepare participants for specialized roles such as educator or nurse practitioner. Here learners must be enrolled in the institution of higher education in order to participate in the certificate program.

Certificate programs also can be offered as *noncredit programs*, usually for professional continuing education. Although often perceived as being less rigorous than academic credit, these certificate programs, in fact, can be quite similar to certificate programs offered for academic credit, as shown in Table 2.1.

ADVANTAGES AND DISADVANTAGES OF CERTIFICATE PROGRAMS IN NURSING

Certificate programs present a variety of advantages and disadvantages for nursing education and nursing service. To the extent that the advantages outweigh the disadvantages, certificate programs can offer substantial benefits for all stakeholders.

TABLE 2.1   Attributes of Academic vs. Professional (Noncredit) Certificate Programs in Nursing

Attributes	Academic certificate (offered for academic credit)	Professional certificate (offered as noncredit)
Certificate program has: • Purpose • Objectives/outcomes • Learning activities	Yes	Yes
Sequence of content in certificate program is clearly defined	Yes	Yes
Evaluation plan includes evaluation of: • Course(s) • Faculty • Clinical faculty/ preceptors • Teaching methods • Learning outcomes	Yes	Yes
Participant must be admitted to academic program to enroll	Yes	No
Participant must meet admissions requirements/ prerequisites	Yes	Yes
Participant must meet specified entry requirements (e.g., language, computer skills, licensure, experience)	Yes	Yes
Cost to participate	Tuition + fees	Fee
Clinical practicum (if appropriate)	Yes	Yes
Involves clinical preceptors	If appropriate	If appropriate

Advantages

Certificate programs are *learner-centered* because they are designed with a specific focus, are outcomes based, and prepare participants for real-world work. Within existing curricula, certificate programs provide learning options or serve as electives. If offered using distance education technologies, certificate programs also are convenient. Certificate programs provide an opportunity for learners to test their success in college-level programs or establish new career paths without a large investment of time or resources.

For schools of nursing and their offices of lifelong learning, certificate programs provide *opportunities for faculty to teach in their area of expertise*. Courses may be offered as electives or as part of an interdisciplinary sequence of courses in educational programs that do not offer courses in the faculty's area of interest or specialization.

Offering a certificate program provides *curriculum flexibility* and serves as one way to *establish the need/demand for the courses* prior to establishing them within the curriculum itself. In this regard, the certificate program serves as a testing ground for the curriculum. Certificate programs that involve interdisciplinary planning and extensive course management can be tested prior to integration into the curriculum. From the learner's perspective, certificate programs offer curricular flexibility when there are portfolio options or opportunities to use the certificate toward academic credit. Finally, the curriculum itself can benefit when standards and learning outcomes can be evaluated prior to integrating courses into the curriculum according to curriculum approval processes.

There are *economic advantages* of certificate programs. Because the programs are shorter than a degree program or a major within the program, they are easier to develop and offer. In addition, they are one way to be responsive to learner needs and create interest in or loyalty to the school (Patterson, 1999).

Certificate programs offer opportunities for *workforce partnerships* among clinical agencies, schools of nursing, and professional organizations (Advisory Board Company, 2001; Billings, Jeffries, Stone, Rowles, & Urden, 2002). Here, educator and agency resources are leveraged to develop certificate programs to prepare nurses for particular workforce needs and serve as mechanisms for recruitment of nurses in areas of short supply.

Finally, offering certificate programs is one way to be responsive to the nursing community, employers, and graduates of academic programs. In this regard, certificates represent *value added* to the school or clinical agency.

Disadvantages

There are disadvantages of certificate programs. Educators should consider costs, need, and curriculum planning as they consider benefits and opportunities for developing certificate programs.

Educational Need

The need for the certificate program must be documented, and workforce needs can fluctuate rapidly. The use of technology can expand geographic access and thus serve widely dispersed students with similar educational needs.

Cost

Certificate programs can be costly to develop and offer. Faculty need lead time to develop courses and reimbursement for course development time. If the program is technology mediated, additional software, hardware, instructional design, and maintenance costs must be accounted for in strategic plans.

Curriculum Planning Concerns

Certificate programs are not degree programs, and they are not a substitute for degree programs that develop a broad base for professional nursing. Integrating certificate programs within existing curricular structures may not be simple or even appropriate, and faculty must make program decisions in view of their educational institution's philosophy, mission, and purpose.

CONSIDERING CERTIFICATE PROGRAMS IN NURSING

As learner and employer demand for specialized education increases, nurse educators and their potential partners in clinical agencies are faced with considering the merits of developing certificate programs for workforce development and expanding opportunities for career and academic advancement. Additionally, nurse educators must consider how to match academic and/or continuing professional education with learner and workforce needs.

Educators should consider the following issues when determining the merits of certificate programs:

- Admission standards: What are the admission requirements? What are the minimum and maximum requirements for enrollment? What prerequisites must be completed?
- Curriculum: What are the intended program outcomes of the certificate program? How many credit hours are involved? What is the relationship of the certificate program to other degree programs within the institution?
- Relevancy of content: Will the content meet the needs of learners and employers?
- Competition: Do other certificate programs exist? Will this one be sustainable?
- Quality: How will the quality of the program be assessed?
- Faculty: What are the requirements for the faculty? Is there sufficient faculty in the area of need?
- Fiscal: Will development expenses be offset by enrollment?
- Partnerships: Is a partnership feasible? Would a partnership extend the fiscal and/or applicant base?
- Value to employer: Will there be a workplace need for the content and competencies of the program?
- Convenience: Can the program be offered in a way that is convenient to learners and employers?
- Type of credit to award: Academic credit? Contact hours? Both?

QUALITY ASSURANCE FOR CERTIFICATE PROGRAMS

As certificate programs proliferate, nurse educators and employers as well as the nurses and students who are potential participants in them must define and discern quality. What constitutes quality in certificate programs and who is assuring it? On what basis can the consumer choose the appropriate certificate program? On what basis can the employer be assured of the meaning of the certificate?

Currently there is no comprehensive system for quality assurance for "stand alone" certificate programs. Many programs rely on review by external accrediting agencies or are tied to industry standards (Irby, 1999). In other instances, it is the "global student," who by enrolling in certificate programs that may or may not be offered by accredited schools, are setting standards by creating demand (Adelman, 2000). Schools of nursing and their offices of lifelong learning benefit from having access to external reviews of their certificate programs through their national accreditation bodies for academic or continuing education programs.

Although there are a variety of quality indicators described by different agencies, the following are common elements of a quality assurance review of certificate programs:

- A defined mission guides the program
- Curriculum integrity
- Evidence of learning outcomes
- Methods of appropriate instruction, pedagogy, and course delivery
- Faculty and faculty support
- Qualified learners and student support services
- Program flexibility
- Plans for evaluation, assessment, or accreditation (Billings, 1999; Crowe, 2000; Higher Learning Commission, 2002; Walshok, 1991).

These criteria also guide the development, evaluation, and continuous quality improvement of the certificate program.

SUMMARY

Certificate programs bridge the gap between the employer's needs and formal degree programs by providing nursing professionals with current, content-specific knowledge in a particular area. When provided by an accredited source, the benefits include a learner-centered, outcomes-based educational experience. These programs could eventually assist nursing professionals in their transition to graduate level education.

Although certificate programs are costly to develop, collaboration among educational institutions, health care providers, and professional nursing organizations could be fostered. This partnership has the potential for enhancing the learning experience by providing each entity's diverse viewpoints and resources. This curricular integration, in turn, would provide the learner with the knowledge to meet the needs of their clients.

REFERENCES

Adelman, C. (2000, May/June). A parallel universe: Certification in the technology guild. *Change,* 20–29.

Advisory Board Company. (2001). *Building bridges: Towards more productive hospital-school partnerships.* Washington, DC: Advisory Board Company.

Arora, S., Blackburn, J., Goldstein, L., Goodman, M., Gratz, R., Kaleta, R., et al. (1996). *Adult Access Working Group Report and Recommendations.* University of Wisconsin-Milwaukee Current Initiatives. Retrieved February 13, 2003, from http://www.uwm.edu/Dept/Acad_Aff/archive/adultaccess.html

Billings, D. (1999). Program assessment and distance education in nursing. *Journal of Nursing Education, 38,* 292–293.

Billings, D., Jeffries, P., Stone, C., Rowles, C., & Urden, L. (2002). A partnership model of nursing education to prepare critical-care nurses. *Excellence in Nursing Administration, 3*(4). Retrieved February 13, 2003, from http://www.nursingsociety.org/publications/EXCEL_NA4Q02.pdf

Craven, R. F., & DuHamel, M. B. (2002). Certificate programs in continuing professional education. *Journal of Continuing Education in Nursing, 34*(1), 14–18.

Crowe, S. D. (2000). Assessing the quality of post-baccalaureate learning in the new higher education marketplace. In K. J. Kohl & J. B. LaPidus (Eds.), *Post baccalaureate futures, new markets, resources, credentials* (pp. 136–150). Phoenix, AZ: Oryx Press.

Dreher, M., Everett, L., Hartwig, S. M., & Members of the University of Iowa Nursing Collaboratory (2001). The University of Iowa Nursing Collaboratory: A partnership for creative education and practice. *Journal of Professional Nursing, 17,* 114–120.

Higher Learning Commission. (2002). *Best Practices for Electronically Offered Degree and Certificate Programs.* North Central Association Commission on Institutions of Higher Education. Retrieved February 13, 2003, from http://www.ncahigherlearningcommission.org/resources/electronic_degrees/Best_Pract_DEd.pdf

Holt, M. E. (1991). A rationale for certificate programs. *New Directions for Adult and Continuing Education, 52,* 3–10.

Irby, A. J. (1999). Post baccalaureate certificates. *Change, 31*(2), 36–41.

Irby, A. J. (2000). Certification for employability: What's new? In K. J. Kohl & J. B. LaPidus (Eds.), *Post baccalaureate futures, new markets, resources, credentials* (pp. 151–180). Phoenix, AZ: Oryx Press.

Kerka, S. (2000). Career certificates: High quality and cutting edge. *Trends and Issues Alert*, no. 16. (ERIC Document Reproduction Service).

Kohl, K. J. (2000). The post baccalaureate learning imperative. In K. J. Kohl & J. B. LaPidus (Eds.), *Post baccalaureate futures, new markets, resources, credentials* (pp. 10–30). Phoenix, AZ: Oryx Press.

LaPidus, J. B. (2000). Post baccalaureate and graduate education: A dynamic balance. In K. J. Kohl & J. B. LaPidus (Eds.), *Post baccalaureate futures, new markets, resources, credentials* (pp. 3–9). Phoenix, AZ: Oryx Press.

Marchese, T. (1999). The certificates phenomenon. *Change, 31*(2), 4.

Patterson, W. (1999). *Analyzing Policies and Procedures for Graduate Certificate Programs*. Washington, DC: Council of Graduate Schools. Retrieved February 13, 2003, from http://classic.cgsnet.org/pdf/analyzingpolicies.pdf

Walshok, M. L. (1991). Evaluation and quality control in certificate programs. *New Directions for Adult and Continuing Education, 52*, 23–31.

Chapter 3

A Service Learning Experience at One School

Helen I. Melland

"Let's take some students to Bolivia"—thus the words were spoken that began an 18-month project and resulted in a 3-week service learning project to the country of Bolivia, a small country land-locked in central South America. I was a grieving mom trying to be brave as I hosted a farewell reception for my daughter as she prepared to leave for a 2-year service stint in the Peace Corps. Kathy, a friend and colleague who was attending the reception to bid my daughter best wishes, had the brilliant idea to take students to Bolivia while my daughter was there, hopefully using her as a contact person for planning and implementing the experience. As a nursing professor at the University of North Dakota (UND), a school that prides itself in valuing experiences that expose students to different cultures, I knew in my head that this was a good thing for my daughter to do. But my motherly instincts told me differently. I was seeking solace and support from Kathy as she spoke those fortuitous words—and now as I look back—I'm so thankful she did.

This chapter describes the experience of planning and implementing an international service learning experience. Literature is reviewed describing what service learning is and its current status in nursing education, the cultural implications of such an experience for both the learners/servers and the recipients of the service, and the implications of service learning projects for nursing research, practice, and education. The concluding section of the chapter focuses on the practicalities of planning and implementing such a project.

SERVICE LEARNING

The term "service learning" is relatively new to the discipline of nursing. However, historically the practice of educating nurses reflects some processes consistent with the current concept of service learning. In the apprenticeship or diploma model of education, the primary emphasis was on service; hospitals often relied on students to meet their staffing needs. As nursing education moved into the higher education setting, pedagogy more strongly emphasized student learning. Clinical learning was designed to meet the needs of students; it was almost heretical to admit that students were providing a service during their assigned clinical learning experiences (Peterson & Schaffer, 2001).

Service learning represents a middle ground in which the concepts of student learning and service are both valued and an integral part of the learning. Service learning differs from clinical learning, field studies, and internships that focus on learning rather than service and from volunteerism that emphasizes the service and service recipient but not the student and learning (Tomey, 2001).

Definitions

The literature is replete with definitions of service learning. This variety of definitions allows for flexibility in applying the concept in a variety of settings and under the umbrella of different disciplines. A common thread in all definitions is that community service is integrated into academic study. Bittle, Dugglby, and Ellison (2002) defined service learning as "a teaching strategy that balances meaningful service to the community and the learning goals of nursing students" (p. 129). According to the American Association of Higher Education (AAHE), service learning is a "method under which students learn and develop through thoughtfully organized service which is conducted in and meets the needs of a community, is coordinated with an institution of higher education and with the community, helps foster civic responsibility, is integrated into and enhances the academic curriculum of the student enrolled, and includes structured time for students to reflect on the service experience" (Meek, 2000, p. 2).

Collaborating with Community Partner

The community service inherent in service learning requires the planner of the learning experience (the faculty) to communicate and collaborate with the community partner when designing the experience. Being acquainted with the community partner prior to the service learning project is ideal. Joint participation in planning the experience is essential. The community partner must understand the difference between voluntary service, in which the focus is on the service and the service recipient but not on the student or learning, and service learning. The faculty member must understand the difference between service learning and clinical learning, in which the focus is on learning rather than service. Both parties need to be good listeners so they can clearly understand each other's needs and priorities.

Methods of communication that keep faculty, students, and community personnel in contact throughout the experience must be identified. Student and volunteer lists should be developed and available to all who need them. Evaluation procedures for the conclusion of the experience need to be stated at the beginning with evaluative criteria made available to students and the community partner from the outset.

Outcomes of Service Learning

The faculty member must consider if the course content lends itself to the service learning paradigm—not all courses do. Student learning objectives that are consistent with the objectives of the community partner should be developed. The objectives should be measurable, clearly outlining the knowledge, skills, and abilities that students are to develop. Additionally, they should be attainable, realistic, and time specific. Frequently objectives related to increasing a sense of civic responsibility, self-awareness, and diversity are relevant. It also is appropriate for the service partner to identify two or three service objectives that complement the learning objectives.

When considering service learning, it is important to consider whether the experience will be mandatory in a curriculum or if students will have the option of participating in it without registering for academic credit. The AAHE definition states that the service learning project or assignment is to enhance the student's curriculum. That implies that service learning is part of a course and mandatory. To maintain rigor and academic integrity, Barber and Battistoni (1993) supported the idea that service learning should be an integral part of an academic course and be offered for full academic credit.

Another perspective is that service learning is not a mandatory component of the curriculum but is designed to provide the student with elective credit. A third approach is that the service learning experience not result in academic credit but that students enroll voluntarily out of a desire for the experience. This third approach is different from volunteerism in that the student's activities would be guided by a faculty member and the student would provide service while meeting clearly outlined learning goals.

Reflection

A concept that several authors (Bittle, Dugglby, & Ellison, 2002; Cauley et al., 2001; Eyler, 2000; Meek, 2000) include in their definition of service learning is *reflection*. Reflection refers to the intentional processing of the service learning experience by the student. This usually occurs because of some required assignment such as a written daily or weekly journal, minipapers, or discussion in which the student reflects on the service learning experience. Students should be encouraged to write freely in their journals and not become overly focused on grammar and spelling as they write. Honesty is important, and faculty need to help students trust that there will be no repercussions for thoughts or experiences shared in their reflections.

Specifically, students should reflect on the attainment of course objectives, actual experiences, and their feelings. Examples of questions and activities that can stimulate students to gain insight into the service learning experience include:

- What most surprised you about this experience?
- What was the most valuable aspect of your learning?
- How do you think this experience will influence your future involvement in your community?
- Briefly discuss the meaning of this experience in the context of each learning objective.

If a student was participating in the service learning project but not receiving academic credit, it still would be important for that student to participate in reflective exercises.

Reciprocity

Reciprocity, the idea that the experience should be of value both to the provider and the service recipient, is an important concept when considering service learning. The benefits to students are often reflected in improved academic performance, refinement of values, increased clarity in career choice, and a commitment to service throughout life. Benefits to community partners may not always be as obvious. Some documented benefits from service recipients include the provision of high-quality care to clients and also the access to academic resources such as library holdings, technological equipment, and faculty resources (Peterson & Schaffer, 2001).

CURRENT STATUS OF SERVICE LEARNING

It is impossible to state how many institutions or nursing programs currently integrate service learning into their curricula. Within the past decade this form of pedagogy has become more prevalent and current estimates are that hundreds of colleges and universities are implementing service learning (Cohen & Milone-Nuzzo, 2001). Many national groups have established service learning initiatives. The AAHE has undertaken a multiyear initiative to enrich service learning practice in eighteen disciplines, one of which is nursing. The primary activity of the initiative is the writing of a series of monographs by scholars in each of the 18 disciplines discussing the design, implementation, and outcome of specific service learning programs (Zlotkowski, n.d.).

A second national group is Campus Compact, which is a coalition of approximately 850 college and university presidents. The mission of Campus Compact is to promote community service that encourages partnerships between campuses and communities, and to assist faculty to integrate community engagement into their teaching and research. Members of Campus Compact, for example, promote legislation that creates opportunities for student service; create partnerships with business, community, and government leaders; provide information to schools on model service programs; research findings and trends related to service learning; award grants to faculty to assist in developing curricula; provide funds and awards for outstanding service work; and organize conferences and forums that provide a mechanism for the exchange of ideas and information on service learning (About Campus Compact, 2002).

TRANSCULTURAL CONSIDERATIONS

It is common for service learning experiences to occur in settings where individuals and groups reflect culturally diverse backgrounds. This includes experiences within the United States as well as abroad. Any learning experience that increases students' knowledge of diverse groups is important to educate nurses to provide care in a sensitive, culturally competent manner.

When developing service learning projects, a plan for educating students prior to the experience about the group's cultural values, norms, family structures, religious beliefs and practices, and their health-related beliefs and practices should be developed and implemented. Without this preparation, students may present themselves as ethnocentric and with a desire to impose their values, beliefs, and behavioral patterns on the recipients of their service.

It is recommended that faculty develop one or more learner objectives for the experience that focus on the provision of culturally competent care. The learner strategies to achieve the objective will vary depending on the curriculum of the nursing program. Students may have done previous academic work focusing on culturally competent care, and the faculty may only need to review those concepts and relate them to the specific culture with which the experience will occur. Or, it may be necessary for extensive work to be done by students, such as completing readings and perhaps even interviewing someone from that culture prior to the experience to be well prepared to provide appropriate care. As the students participate in reflective exercises, questions referring to if and how they provided service in a culturally sensitive manner should be included.

The previously described concepts of service learning projects apply to international experiences as well as experiences designed for implementation in the United States. Coordinated planning between faculty in an institution of higher education and community providers, community service, integration into the academic curriculum through clearly defined learning objectives, student reflection, and reciprocity are still important. Planning for international experiences may be more difficult because of the distance and language barriers. Faculty must be creative and take advantage of all available resources. Becoming acquainted with local individuals who have connections abroad can open doors for the implementation of such projects. Organizations such as churches, health care agencies, service clubs, and government agencies are all appropriate potential resources when attempting to make overseas connections. Individuals in these settings often know of some individual or group who is currently on site abroad who may welcome additional, temporary service providers.

IMPLICATIONS OF SERVICE LEARNING FOR RESEARCH, PRACTICE, AND EDUCATION

There are a large number of studies on service learning in the literature. Eyler (2000) reviewed the research on the impact of service learning on students and found a small but positive effect of service learning on personal qualities such as "efficacy, interpersonal skills, reduced stereotyping, and social responsibility or sense of commitment to future service" (p. 1). As students are prepared to function as care givers in this complex, unpredictable, and turbulent world, it seems logical that learning experiences occurring in that real world setting as opposed to the structured, cognitively oriented classroom would better prepare them with the needed skills. Yet, research has not documented that learning experiences that combine service and academic work actually improve learning and help students develop the needed skills of critical thinking, adaptability, and leadership (Eyler, 2000).

Future research should focus on the impact of service learning on intellectual development to support this apparent intuitive belief of educators that the pedagogy of service learning does result in improved cognitive development. This research also should investigate the outcomes of service learning in terms of competence in the real world, not by testifying to competence in paper and pencil assessments.

Another area of future research should be the assessment of the pedagogy of service learning. Questions to ask might be: (1) How can students be best prepared for a service learning experience? (2) How can the faculty be most effective in guiding the student? and (3) How can reflection be integrated most effectively into the experience? (Eyler, 2000).

As more students have the advantage of service learning experiences, a realistic expectation is that they will develop into a new breed of professional nurses, that is, nurses who are committed to service as an integral part of their practice. As a result of service learning experiences occurring frequently with diverse populations, these new nurses will hopefully have the cultural competence and skills to enable them to work within a global society.

Changes in the health care delivery system and reimbursement policies have resulted in care delivery moving out of acute care facilities and into community-based settings. Practice in these community settings is frequently primary care oriented, which can provide more opportunities for service learning than were previously available in the traditional acute care settings (Cauley et al., 2001). Quality service learning experiences in which students provide preventive, supportive, or restorative care can be designed in consultation with community partners. Community partners frequently welcome students into these settings particularly when faculty involve them in the planning as well as implementing and evaluating the experience.

THE BOLIVIAN EXPERIENCE

The project to be described is one example of an international service learning experience that was designed, planned, and implemented by the author, a nursing faculty member at the University of North Dakota (UND), and a colleague who serves as a campus minister at the same institution. Other significant contributors to this effort included the daughter of the author, who was serving as a Peace Corps Volunteer (PCV) in Bolivia at the time the project was planned and implemented, and other Peace Corps volunteers and health care providers in Bolivia that the PCV had contact with regularly. Planning began ten months prior to the experience. Most of the planning was done via e-mail communication between the project leaders at UND, one student leader of the group, and the PCV. The PCV met with the UND leaders during a vacation visit to North Dakota, her home state, for the initial planning meeting.

The actual project was a three-week service learning experience in Bolivia. Twelve university students, including undergraduate and graduate nursing students plus the two leaders, traveled to Bolivia to learn and provide service. Objectives of the project were to:

1. Gain knowledge and appreciation of the Bolivian culture by living in the culture for three weeks, interacting with Bolivians in work and social settings, and listening and questioning PCVs who had resided in Bolivia for one to two years as they described the culture.

2. Gain an understanding of the process of establishing a sanitary water system by observing a water system at different stages of development, participating in building a water sanitation system in a rural Bolivian community, and following the natural course of a water supply system.

3. Assist in building a greenhouse in a remote community to provide more food throughout the year to indigenous people.
4. Observe different health care delivery settings by visiting a Red Cross "outpost" (primary care setting), a school of nursing, and a clinic funded by USAID.
5. Participate in immunization clinics in rural communities.
6. Provide health education to children in an orphanage through the medium of arts and crafts, and to mothers on the topic of nutrition through the use of PCVs as interpreters.

PLANNING THE TRIP

After the objectives of the trip were identified, a time line was developed that would serve as a guide to the planners until departure. Student involvement was essential for this phase of the project. One student volunteered to be intimately involved in all phases of planning and to serve as a liaison with other students.

A priority during the first months of planning was student recruitment. Since this was not a required course for students in any major, recruitment was an issue. The project was designed to occur at the end of the academic year so recruitment information was distributed at the beginning of the same academic year, or nine months in advance. Project planners believed students needed this much lead time to save money, consult with parents, and plan their activities for the next summer. Recruitment strategies included posting notices about the project around campus, a news article in the September issue of the campus ministry center's newsletter, and announcements in the university's newsletter. Word-of-mouth promotion of the project also proved to be an effective means of recruitment.

The project leaders decided that students would have the option of enrolling in the experience for academic credit or participating for no academic credit. Those that enrolled for academic credit had to meet additional academic requirements. All students were required to participate in the same manner with attainment of project objectives as the goal for all. Participation in reflective activities was required of all students.

Financial concerns were addressed early in the planning process. The need for the most discounted airfare possible was a priority. The student liaison contacted various travel agents and was able to "lock in" a desirable fare months in advance. A grant proposal was written for a local service club that awarded a few hundred dollars to each student. The recipients of the money agreed to participate on their return in a discussion with other university students that would focus on cultural dynamics of the trip. Since Bolivia is a lesser developed country, costs incurred by students once in the country were minimal. For example, lodging in hostels is typically less than two dollars per day. Students sometimes roomed with PCVs. Daily food expenditures were usually less than seven dollars. The opportunity to live so cheaply in countries such as Bolivia makes student travel and learning in them financially desirable.

A critical aspect of preparation for the Bolivian service learning trip was to prepare the students to be culturally sensitive visitors and service providers. The group began meeting monthly about four months prior to departure. Part of each of those meetings was designated as cultural orientation time. Students were assigned required readings prior to the meetings with discussions occurring on those topics at the meetings. On departure, the liaison PCV provided each student with a packet of materials that included information on the food, culture, safety, health, and language in Bolivia.

Because one of the group's objectives was to conduct an immunization clinic, non-nursing students needed instruction on injection procedures; this was optional. Some non-nursing students chose not to learn that skill. Those who wanted to administer injections participated in an injection skills lab conducted in the College of Nursing at UND. Nursing faculty and students conducted the lab using the same procedures as when nursing students are taught to give an injection. Students were required to demonstrate competency to a member of the nursing faculty.

Student health and safety while in Bolivia were dealt with during the planning phase. A nurse from the campus student health center spoke to the students regarding health and potential disease concerns. She worked with the students as a group as they completed the multiple forms that needed to be processed prior to getting their immunizations for travel to Bolivia. The project leaders and the nurse believed that working with students as a group was more efficient than students individually visiting the health center with their questions. Students signed the standard papers releasing the university from liability.

About 1 month prior to departure, riots erupted in Bolivia related to water supply issues. One leader was in contact with personnel at the U.S. embassy in Bolivia. The assurance was offered that no unusual threat to the group's safety was foreseen but that there would be notification prior to departure if there were any changes.

Reciprocity, the concept that the project is of value for the student and the community, was not forgotten. Local agencies that donate to overseas projects were contacted. This resulted in the donation of multiple medical supplies for the affiliating Red Cross outpost in Bolivia. Eleven large boxes were filled with supplies such as bandages, cast materials, splints, stethoscopes, and sphygmomanometers. In order to avoid paying shipping costs of the boxes, each student agreed to bring only one piece of luggage and check the medical supplies box as a second piece of allowed luggage. The boxes were marked with the Red Cross symbol to help ensure safe passage through customs although this was not guaranteed. All boxes did arrive intact and without tampering.

IN BOLIVIA

A detailed itinerary was critical for the success of the trip. The itinerary was developed prior to departure mostly by the in-country PCV as she had access to the community partners and a sense of travel times and community resources. The itinerary included activities for each day, departure and arrival times between sites, sleeping arrangements, and free time. This was distributed to all students immediately prior to departure.

Flexibility was required of the learners and leaders while in Bolivia, which is common with community service learning projects. The business of the community partner does not necessarily progress as planned, and the learning experiences may need to be modified from their original conception. For example, the amount of serum available for the immunization clinic was less than expected, so fewer immunizations were administered than were needed. This was frustrating to the learners as there were many children who did not receive their injections. During the immunization clinics, a different injection protocol was evident between Bolivian Red Cross nurses and students and leaders from America. A decision was made that the American student learners would proceed with the same injection procedures as used in the United States; this was acceptable to the Bolivians.

Cultural adaptations were at times an issue. On arrival in Bolivia, health care personnel were distressed to see that the majority of the students were female. In Bolivia women do not engage in physical labor, and they were concerned that the female students would not be able to do the physical labor demanded in the latrine and greenhouse building projects. Even though the need for conservative dress code had been discussed in the pretrip preparation, the weather became hot and the work exhausting at two of the sites. The students had difficulties understanding the significance of continuing to dress as was required of women in the Bolivian culture. While building the greenhouse, a particularly demanding project, the students began singing. This also is not appropriate in the Bolivian culture, and again it was difficult for the American student visitors to accept this.

On the other hand, positive, unique cultural exchanges occurred frequently throughout the trip. One night American and Bolivian students played basketball together and sang traditional Bolivian and American songs, including the "Star Spangled Banner," even though they did not share the same language. The American learners were invited to drink some "chichi," a traditional Bolivian beverage, with the Bolivians during a marriage celebration. At the orphanage site in Tiraque, Bolivian children taught the American students a traditional dance, and the Americans reciprocated by teaching the children an American country line dance.

In spite of cultural and language barriers, many Bolivians expressed appreciation for service provided. During a traditional Bolivian "barbecue," health care personnel from the Red Cross outpost thanked the Americans and even shed tears of appreciation. It was evident that reciprocity had occurred—both the providers of service and the community partners had benefited from the experience.

A latrine system for a school in a rural community of Primero de Mayo was built through the footings stage. After the group departed, notice was received that the Bolivians were highly motivated about the project and completed it in approximately one month. Trenches and the lower levels of a large greenhouse (90 feet × 30 feet) were dug in the indigenous village of Sacabamba. Health education and entertainment were provided to children in an orphanage in the remote community of Tiraque. The universal language of the music, arts, and dance facilitated this process.

The American PCVs in Bolivia also benefited from participating in this service learning project. The PCVs stated that the energy and work ethic of the students inspired them to accomplish more while in Bolivia; they expressed a feeling of honor to have helped their fellow Americans learn more about the Bolivian culture.

Learners expressed personal benefits during reflective writings and discussions. The cognitive learning of students about this lesser developed country was extensive, particularly in areas related to culture, disease, water sanitation, and health care delivery. This learning was assessed through group discussions and in formal papers written by the students who enrolled in the project for academic credit. Student values had changed and were reflected in comments such as "I've learned that I don't need lots of possessions to be happy," and "One of the things I'm going to miss most is not learning something new each day about a different culture." A greater commitment to a sense of service was evident as three students expressed a desire for future service in the Peace Corps.

RECOMMENDATIONS

When planning a service learning project, if it is to occur with a population different from the majority of the students, preparation for immersion into that culture cannot be stressed enough. The PCV suggested that one strategy that may have helped prevent some of the "culture shock" the students experienced would have been for them to participate in some culture orientation activities on arrival in Bolivia.

Communication among representatives of all involved parties in the learning experience is critical particularly when the experience is overseas. With the Bolivian experience, involved partners included the two leaders at UND, the student leader at UND, the PCV leader in Bolivia as well as other PCVs at each of the work sites, other Peace Corps staff, and Red Cross personnel. Cultural norms in Bolivia had to be considered in that people of different cultures approach the need to plan and address details differently. Respectful communication with all involved is critical during all phases of a project.

CONCLUSIONS

Service learning is a pedagogy that is not new to nursing in the sense that nursing students have been providing service while learning throughout the history of the profession. The current use of this term is somewhat new and refers to a method of learning that is structured around academic objectives, meets the needs of a community partner, and intentionally includes reflection and reciprocity. Cultural sensitivity and the need for culturally competent care are essential components of these experiences. Designing the experiences, whether located within the United States or abroad, may take significant time, energy, and commitment, but the end result is often a learning experience that benefits the students, faculty, and community.

REFERENCES

About Campus Compact. (2002). Retrieved July 22, 2002, from http://www.compact. org/aboutcc/mission.html

Barber, B. R., & Battistoni, R. (1993). A season of service: Introducing service learning into the liberal arts curriculum. *PS: Political Science and Politics, 26,* 235–240, 262.

Bittle, M., Dugglby, W., & Ellison, P. (2002). Implementation of the essential elements of service learning in three nursing courses. *Journal of Nursing Education, 41,* 129–132.

Cauley, K., Canfield, A., Clasen, C., Dobbins, J., Hemphill, S., Jaballas, E., et al. (2001). Service learning: Integrating student learning and community service. *Education for Health, 14,* 173–181.

Cohen, S. S., & Milone-Nuzzo, P. (2001). Advancing health policy in nursing education through service learning. In P. L. Chinn (Ed.), *Advances in Nursing Science* (pp. 28–40). Frederick, MD: Aspen.

Eyler, J. (2000). What do we most need to know about the impact of service learning on student learning? *Michigan Journal of Community Service Learning.* Retrieved July 24, 2002, from http:www.umich.edu/~mjcsl/volumes/researchsample/html

Meek, M. (2000). Implementing service learning at UND. *On Teaching, 10.* Grand Forks, ND: University of North Dakota Office of Instructional Development.

Peterson, S. J., & Schaffer, M. A. (2001). Service learning: Isn't that what nursing education has always been? *Journal of Nursing Education, 40,* 51–52.

Tomey, A. M. (2001). Students learn through service to others. *Sigma Theta Tau Honor Society of Nursing Excellence in Nursing Education, 2,* 1, 4.

Zlotkowski, E. (n.d.). *AAHE Service Learning Project.* Retrieved July 30, 2003, from http://www.aahe.org/service/

Part II

Assessment and Evaluation

Chapter 4

Program Evaluation and Public Accountability

Donna L. Boland

Over the last decade the call for public accountability has helped reshape evaluation within institutions of higher education. Public accountability has drawn educators' attention to issues of program effectiveness and productivity. Outcomes and competencies are becoming the defining characteristics on which evaluation programs are being built. These changes coupled with philosophical shifts from the evaluation of teaching to the assessment of learning have impacted both the process and product of program evaluation. This chapter discusses some of the broad changes in evaluation and how these changes are affecting all higher educational disciplines, including nursing.

EVOLUTION OF PROGRAM EVALUATION

Program evaluation has always been an integral part of program development, implementation, and revision. However, the discipline of program evaluation has evolved over the last century in response to changes external and internal to the institution of higher education. The roots of program evaluation were planted prior to the 20th century (Madaus, Stufflebeam, & Scriven, 1994). Since these early days, evaluation efforts carried out in institutions of higher education have consistently paralleled the economic, social, and political climates of the nation. Early in the 19th century, the industrial revolution "transformed the very structure of society" including the development of a social consciousness that helped shape the placement of higher education within an industrial society (Madaus, Stufflebeam, & Scriven, 1994, pp. 23–25). Systemization, productivity, and efficiency became the driving forces of both the economy and higher education. Institutions of higher education introduced methods of educational measurement based on the three "R's" of reading, writing, and arithmetic (Madaus, Stufflebeam, & Scriven, 1994, pp. 23). The learning indicators measured and the results generated from these measurement activities were more narrowly focused on a particular school system or institution rather than nationally across the educational system at all academic levels.

The pivotal work of Ralph W. Tyler in the mid-20th century transformed both curriculum development and evaluation. Tyler viewed curriculum as "a set of broadly planned school experiences designed and implemented to help students achieve specified behavior outcomes" (Madaus, Stufflebeam, & Scriven, 1994, p. 26). His work became a cornerstone for curriculum and program evaluation for decades to come. The Tylerian approach to curriculum development and evaluation has been a primary force behind the education and evaluation of nursing students for over 50 years.

For nursing faculty, behavioral objectives became the intended learning expectations by which an individual learner's performance was measured. As a result of Tyler's thinking, nursing faculty developed curricula that often involved intricate designs of interwoven, complementary threads of knowledge and structured learning experiences. Student learning experiences were well-defined and orchestrated by faculty. Measurement of students' abilities focused on learning within and at the end of discrete courses. Faculty assumed that students who were successful at each incremental level within the curriculum would meet the program or terminal objectives on completion of the curriculum. Summative evaluation for undergraduate programs rested mainly with graduates' ability to pass the professional nurse licensing examination.

Interestingly, during this same period, graduate nursing education tended to combine the thinking of a tightly structured curriculum with the sense of a "capping" learning experience that would more broadly reflect students' ability to integrate theory, research, and practice into a thesis. The thesis then became an end-of-program measure used to assess student learning. Generally, this summative measure was used as a judge for individual learning and was not viewed as a tool to assess program effectiveness over a cohort of learners.

The years from 1946 through 1972 were defined by the proliferation of educational institutions in response to the postwar emphasis on education. Higher education played a critical role in fueling the postwar society and keeping abreast of the increasing emphasis on technology in a manufacturing driven economy. New models of program evaluation were being proposed that "recognized the need to evaluate goals, look at inputs, examine implementation and delivery of services, as well as measure intended and unintended outcomes of the program" (Madaus, Stufflebeam, & Scriven, 1994, p. 31).

During these postwar years, regional and professional accreditation organizations were requiring documentation of program effectiveness. There also was a proliferation of nursing programs in institutions of higher education where they were required to conform to both regional and professional accreditation standards. In response, nursing faculty focused evaluation primarily on documenting the educational integrity of the teaching process.

CURRENT EVALUATION CLIMATE

Madaus and colleagues (1994) referred to the current developmental cycle as the age of professionalism. During this last decade, the discipline of evaluation has emerged as a legitimate science grounded in theory, theoretical models, research, and testing. This evolutionary growth in the discipline of evaluation has been in response to the public demand for accountability. To meet today's expectations, evaluation must serve multiple purposes. Program evaluation outcomes must assist in determining the quality and productivity of the program under review. Programs of evaluation need to generate information that define, monitor, and refine program direction. Expectations in this current climate are being shaped by the need for evaluation models and plans that respond to increased calls for internal and external program accountability, a shifting paradigm from teaching evaluation to learning outcomes, a renewed emphasis on professional standards to be used as a best-practice guide to building curricula and defining learning outcomes, and an increasing expectation that outcome data will be benchmarked against expected results or outcomes to support quality improvement activities.

Evaluation must be constructed to support faculties' abilities to analyze program outcomes in relation to the mission and goals, and support strategic program planning. Outcomes of evaluation are essential in driving faculty and administrator decision making, including the allocation of scarce resources. Additionally, outcomes of evaluation efforts can identify hallmarks of a program that can be used in marketing and fund-raising efforts.

As a tool, evaluation should not be exclusively tied to accreditation expectations. To view program evaluation solely from the viewpoint of responding to accreditation expectations limits the value of evaluation to program decision makers. This contracted approach to evaluation also curtails the ability of nursing faculty to generate critical information needed to develop and refine effective programming.

COMMON THEORETICAL EVALUATION MODELS

There are a number of theoretical models that have helped to refocus evaluation to serve a broader conceptual focus. It is important that faculty make an informed choice among evaluation models because a particular model or approach being used should fit the characteristics of the educational program and facilitate the attainment of the stated evaluation goals.

If faculty choose to use an existing evaluation model, the model should be based on its ability to generate the desired information considering the identified goals. Generally, the information generated from an effective evaluation program will drive faculty and administrative decisions about:

- Program quality, productivity, and program need and demand
- Program direction and evolution
- Allocation of resources
- Ability of the program to meet the mission, goals, and expected program results
- Strategic planning and complementary budgeting for this planning
- Marketing and recruitment efforts
- Program effectiveness as it relates to internal and external communities of interests (Conrad & Wilson, 1994, p. 183).

There have been a number of evaluation models proposed to deal with one or more of these purposes. Among nurse educators a number of theoretical evaluation models have been found useful in developing a program of evaluation to meet their needs. The stakeholder-focused model has appealed to many nursing educators as the needs and perspectives of stakeholders are at the core of this type of model (Ingersoll & Sauter, 1998).

Another popular program evaluation approach that appeals to nursing faculty has been the goal-free or value-free model proposed by Scriven in 1972. Unlike the stakeholder model, the hallmark of this model presumes that evaluation is free from opinion or individual observations. The appeal of the value-free model is that data collection focuses on actual outcomes, intended or not.

Those nursing faculty who thought that the context in which the program existed was important to the evaluation process developed evaluation plans that were consistent with Stufflebeam's CIPP (context, input, process, and product) model (Stufflebeam, 1985). A more popular contemporary approach to evaluation is to design an evaluation plan that is grounded in the idea of continuous quality improvement. For evaluation to be meaningful within the context of continuous quality improvement the results must be fed back into the program in a framework that is meaningful and has utility for the program.

In the last decade higher education and nursing education have experienced changes in the public's expectations of the higher education system and processes. Faculty need to consider each of these changes when selecting an evaluation model that will produce the desired results. Among nursing educators there appears to be a trend to integrate characteristics from more than one model. For example, an integrated model may borrow the idea of productivity from a continuous quality improvement model, but may wish to look at the concept of productivity within the "context" of the institutional mission and goals.

CHANGES IN EXPECTATIONS

Higher education in the 21st century is not only seen as a process that shapes minds and improves the quality of individual lives, but also as a social infrastructure that produces citizens who can make a significant contribution to the collective process of society (Lovett, 2002, p. 10).

Lovett's view appears to complement the changes being experienced in higher education. The increased pressure for accountability and the refocusing of the educational process to the product of learning have created a philosophical shift in the mission leading to reprioritizing institutional goals for many colleges and universities.

Nurse educators face the same challenge encountered by our colleagues—to design evaluation and assessment plans that are consistent with increasing requests for documentation of accountability. Stakeholders are holding public and private institutions accountable for showing how higher degree programs are adding value to the educational outcomes of their graduates. The voices calling for accountability come not only from the health care system but also from the greater society as a whole. Potential students, parents, health care industry representatives, and consumers of our graduates demand hard evidence that programs demonstrate that they have established clear and obtainable program outcomes and that these outcomes are worth the investment being made by individuals, family members, and funding agencies, including but not limited to local, state, and federal governments.

Fueling the increasing demands for accountability are the increase in competition for static or shrinking funding resources, competition for and rising expense of educational resources, and stakeholders' awareness of the role of the consumer within the higher educational environment. As consumers increasingly exercise their right to question the value obtained on their investment, the traditional view of colleges and universities as observers of society is shifted to being observed by society.

Emphasis on accountability has required faculty teaching in institutions of higher education to produce report cards that can demonstrate institutional and program effectiveness and efficiency. The request for a periodic report card can be befuddling to those who view evaluation only as a tool to measure the success of the curriculum process. Nursing faculty have been faced with the need to align quality with productivity, to determine what information is useful to a diverse group of stakeholders, to resolve differences in effectiveness as defined by educators and learners, to create the role of evaluators in a system that emphasizes change, and to determine how to stimulate change in what is often seen as a fairly static but complex system (Gates et al., 2002, pp. 1–2).

In addition to the increased emphasis on accountability, there has been a shift in the focus of evaluation from the process to the product of learning. As nursing faculty our concern is not only with how well we are doing but also with the degree to which program graduates can demonstrate their ability to use nursing knowledge and skills in advancing practice. As nurse educators, we must pose questions that are critical in shaping the present and future of the discipline. The questions we are asking will continue to be focused on the kinds of knowledge, skills, and attitudes graduates must have to meet today's and tomorrow's demands (known and unknown), and the degree to which nursing programs are accountable for meeting these demands (Davies & Wavering, 1999). Davies and Wavering (1999) argued that the degree to which we, as faculty, are able to meet "the changing nature of knowledge and the demands of the new century" depends on our ability to effectively monitor changing trends and accurately and meaningfully evaluate student learning outcomes (p. 39).

ASSESSMENT OF LEARNING

One of the most important actions that shifted the center of attention of evaluation from teaching to learning was the publishing of the National Institute of Education's 1984 Study Group deliberations. This group was instrumental in placing assessment of learning in the national spotlight by questioning what students were actually learning in their higher education programs. As a result of their deliberations, the group proposed that colleges and universities "set high expectations for student learning, engage students actively in learning, and provide frequent assessment of learning with feedback to students on their performance" (Banta, 2001, p. 7).

The National Institute of Education's report expanded the current focus of program evaluation. By 1988 then Secretary of Education William Bennett issued an executive order requiring that accrediting agencies include in their criteria how they are documenting the educational achievements of their students (Banta, 2001, p. 7). Further, the Department of Education required that this documentation be generated through valid and reliable measures.

The National League for Nursing, not wishing to jeopardize their accreditation status with the Department of Education, moved to define and incorporate learning outcomes into their accreditation standards. This one act has created a cosmic ray that has reverberated off the walls of college and university nursing units for the last decade. The spotlight focused on learning outcomes that would benefit society as a whole. As faculty demonstrate how the knowledge and skills of their graduates contribute to the welfare and economy of today's society, academic administrators can use these outcome data to demonstrate the cost-effectiveness of the educational process for these same graduates.

Focus on Outcomes of Learning

Today's evaluation activities are being redirected in an effort to answer questions about what students are learning. Faculty efforts are aimed at finding ways to approach teaching and learning that will complement this shift in emphasis from teaching to learning. As a result of the shift, nursing faculty are struggling to design program evaluation plans that address what students need to be learning, the level at which this learning needs to occur, the structures that provide the best opportunity for learning to take place, and the assessment environment that best facilitates the students' ability to demonstrate what they have learned.

One may argue that nursing faculty have always thought that student learning was a priority, and they would be right. However, the process of evaluation prior to the 1990s focused primarily on the educational process rather then the outcomes resulting from the educational process. The focus on process appears to have been built on the prevailing thought that if one is willing to trust the process, then the expected outcomes or objectives set forth to guide the process will be achieved. Again, this is not flawed thinking but rather somewhat shortsighted, realizing that each student is a unique learner who brings to and takes from the learning process experiences that can not be entirely be controlled nor formalized within an official curriculum structure.

Assessment and Evaluation

Assessment and evaluation have become closely linked as the focus on student learning has sharpened. Many in higher education have assumed assessment and evaluation to be interchangeable concepts. However, Palomba and Banta (1999) have made a distinction between the two concepts that provides guidance for faculty dealing with assessment and evaluation issues. Assessment, according to these recognized experts, is a "multistep process of examining the quality and productivity of education and professional development activities" whereas evaluation is "one of the steps in the assessment process in which measures of quality and productivity are examined against some standard of the profession" (Gates et al., 2002, p. 3). Evaluation, then, is defined within the broader activities of assessment. The hallmark of evaluation is the act of comparing actual outcomes to expected outcomes. Again, it is important for programs to have well-defined expected outcomes that incorporate identified professional standards or guides.

Current approaches to the development and refinement of evaluation plans tend to blur the distinction between the acts of assessing and evaluating for most nursing faculty. What we should be clear about is that evaluation and assessment activities in the broadest context should incorporate critical examination of students, educational resources, administrative structure, curricula, programs, the academic units, and the institution in which the academic units reside. For those familiar with professional nursing accreditation, these assessment facets are consistent with published accreditation standards.

Assuming that nursing faculty have traditionally anchored evaluation activities within the framework of program quality and productivity of students, faculty, and graduates, recent changes made in evaluation efforts have focused primarily on the incorporation of "benchmarks." Benchmarks have been interpreted as standards or expected results that are consistent with internally or externally defined criteria or goals. Results generated from assessment activities are then held up to the established benchmark, which is often a quantifiable index, to determine the degree to which the expected results have been achieved.

Faculty are required to make a judgment as to the merit of the outcomes achieved based on these documented differences. When discussing quality of learning, we often attempt to determine from our evaluation efforts the "value added" by the educational process and establish benchmarks that reflect this additive effect. Faculties determine the value of their program comparing outcome data to program goals. Program goals reflect the tripartite mission and, for nursing faculty, the addition of the practice mission. A typical evaluation plan may conceptually resemble the layout in Table 4.1.

Measurement is underscored by the desire to generate meaningful information to judge the merit or worth of the educational process. However, as researchers, we recognize how difficult it is to "attribute

TABLE 4.1   Skeleton Evaluation Plan

Evaluation dimensions	Expected results (as defined by benchmarks)	Outcomes (actual results)	Differences (between ideal and actual results)	Decisions and actions (related to quality and productivity based on differences)
Students				
Graduates and alumni				
Faculty				
Baccalaureate curriculum				
Graduate curriculum				

changes to the institution, its students' aptitude or prior achievements, or the quality of students' learning efforts" (Davis, 1994, p. 52). It is a challenge to reliably assess value added when dealing with students who come from diverse educational backgrounds, possess different motivational drivers, and often reflect more nontraditional than traditional student characteristics.

However, it is important that nurse faculty be involved in research activities to develop and test assessment measures that are sensitive to the diverse characteristics of the college student population. Assessment measures must not only be reliable and valid, but must also be able to adequately measure actual outcomes within the context of expected results or outcomes. Expected results must be grounded in standards that reflect the best practices in higher education, nursing education, and nursing practice in response to public accountability.

USE OF PROFESSIONAL STANDARDS AS BENCHMARKS

The call for accountability has increased the emphasis on professional nursing standards and inspired various national nursing organizations to develop new standards or update existing ones. These various professional standards are being incorporated into the evaluation process as a means of identifying program expectations for entry and advanced nursing practice curricula. Standards also are being used to establish outcomes that define the essential competencies an educated person and an educated nurse must possess at the completion of an educational program. Additionally, accrediting bodies are incorporating the idea of professional standards or guidelines into their criteria as a reflection of current and relevant learning expectations.

It is the responsibility of nursing faculty to choose professional standards that are consistent with the goals of their department, college, or school. Standards also need to represent the range of degree programs and specialties being offered, and must be obtainable by the student body admitted to these degree programs. Professional standards can be used to inform curricular decisions related to identifying program expectations, competencies, structure, and learning experiences, and to determining the appropriate measures to be used in evaluating program achievements. As faculty adopt specific professional standards, they must integrate these standards into all programmatic elements including evaluation so that the chosen standards form the foundation of the whole program. The integration of standards should be apparent in developing self-studies for accreditation purposes, in compiling a "report card" for external and internal stakeholders, and in presenting arguments for retaining, sustaining, or increasing program resources.

Connecting program goals with professional nursing standards creates a synergistic effect that is more supportable to external stakeholders than the generation of goals based singularly on a philosophical belief or theoretical models that are more difficult to defend outside the discipline. By way of example, Table 4.2 maps a professional competency for a baccalaureate program and Table 4.3 examines how a master's level professional competency might look for a program that has a clinical nurse specialist focus.

EMPHASIS ON STUDENT LEARNING

Student learning has received the majority of press in the nursing literature this last decade as faculty have attempted to respond primarily to changes in professional accreditation standards. Learning outcomes,

TABLE 4.2   Professional Competency for a Baccalaureate Program

Professional competency: Uses critical thinking as a basis
for independent and interdependent decision making

Associated behaviors or expected results	Supporting knowledge and skills	Learning experiences	Assessment outcomes
Use appropriate theories and models in framing problems or issues	Scientific theories Humanistic models Physiologic models	Case studies Grand round presentation Issue-resolution paper	Grading rubrics Peer evaluation Portfolio
Applies scientifically based knowledge and principles as foundation in shaping care practices	Research utilization skills Evidence-based practice	Patient problem paper Case studies Research utilization project	Portfolio Grade based on ability to implement practice

Adapted from American Association of Colleges of Nursing (AACN). (1998). *The essentials of baccalaureate education for professional nursing practice.* Washington. DC: Author.

which include the concepts of critical thinking, communication, cultural understanding, and competency in the delivery of care, have set the stage for the evaluation of student learning for both undergraduate and graduate programs. Although nurse educators have been involved in conversations about what should constitute learning for nursing students, there is still minimal agreement as to the learning expectations that should drive assessment and evaluation. This lack of agreement can be attributed to regional differences in the health care system, philosophical differences among faculty, differences in educational emphasis among private and public colleges and universities, and diversity of program resources and student populations.

The identification and definition of expected learning outcomes must resonate with the:

1. Undergraduate and graduate learning missions and goals of the parent institution
2. Strategic goals of the nursing unit
3. Professional standards adopted by the faculty

TABLE 4.3   Professional Competency for a Master's Program

Professional competency: Implements population-based programs of care
by integrating nursing interventions and medical treatments, as appropriate,
to enhance patient outcomes cost-effectively

Associated behaviors or expected results	Supporting knowledge and skills	Learning experiences	Assessment outcomes
Design an intervention plan for a population-based program for implementation Analyze the cost-benefit of the proposed plan	Theoretical models and assumptions underlying a population-based program Cost–benefit analysis Appropriate nursing interventions by needs Standard medical treatments	Needs assessment of a particular patient population Critique of existing programs to meet needs Discussions with developers of existing programs Plan a population based program within a given structured budget	Expert critique of proposed plan Portfolio assessment Grading rubrics

Adapted from the National Association of Clinical Nurse Specialists (NACNS). (1998). *Statement on clinical nurse specialist practice and education.* Harrisburg, PA: Author.

4. Outcomes that employers of graduates expect to see in graduates hired
5. Expertise and skills of the faculty (current and future)
6. Expertise and skills available in the community to support the attainment of identified results
7. Availability of learning experiences to facilitate accomplishments of results
8. Potential of the population of learners from which the student body will be drawn.

Integrated Approach to Program Evaluation

The learning mission, as defined by the expected outcomes for the degree programs offered by the school of nursing, must be integrated into, at least in part, or complement the research, service, and practice missions of the nursing unit and the parent institution. For example, it is not enough to examine exclusively the numbers or practice expertise of faculty teaching in the curriculum when designing a comprehensive integrative evaluation model. Although sufficient numbers and an array of expertise within the faculty body are critical in carrying out the teaching mission, it is important to examine the contribution of faculty research, scholarship, service, and practice efforts in meeting the teaching mission. This integrative approach enriches the ability to speak to program effectiveness in a more comprehensive and meaningful fashion.

An integrative approach to evaluation ties all assessment to expected outcomes. A program that emphasizes learning develops an evaluation plan in which the concept of learning becomes the bond by which all factions of the evaluation plan are held together. The marriage of the faculty tripartite mission (teaching, research, and service/clinical practice) to assessment is particularly critical in higher education, which has educational excellence as an institutional mission priority. Within the context of educational excellence, assessment plans must collect, interpret, and evaluate faculty contributions inside and outside the classroom against benchmarks that recognize faculty impact on learning through teaching, research/scholarship, service, and practice outcomes. In this model it is expected that faculty productivity significantly contributes to overall program quality and effectiveness.

Relationship of Evaluation to Faculty Goals

In playing out this expectation, faculty identify annual goals that complement and advance the mission and goals of the academic unit. Faculty goals are written to reflect the level of learning dictated by the type of degree programs being offered. Annually, faculty analyze their accomplishments in relation to their established goals. They also examine program resources that facilitated or inhibited the obtainment of their goals. Faculty accomplishments are aggregated around unit and institutional goals and become part of the unit and institutional "report card."

The obstacles and enhancements to faculty productivity are considered in the allocation of program resources. An informed approach to resource allocation is critical to continuous quality improvement of program faculty and administrators. Additionally, faculty searches are based on the perceived ability of candidates to make significant contributions to the expectations of the nursing unit and the parent institution. However, within the reality of today's faculty shortage, it is easier to value this goal-oriented approach to hiring, retaining, promoting, recognizing, and rewarding faculty for their contributions to the mission and goals of the program than it is to implement it.

Angelo (1999) argued that faculty should approach assessment from the perspective that learning matters the most. He outlined ten guidelines that should shape our approach to assessing student learning. From his perspective, the educational process should prepare students with knowledge, competencies, and values needed to:

- Actively engage intellectually and emotionally in their studies.
- Set meaningful goals that can be realistically obtained but stretch abilities.
- Use feedback that has been given in a timely fashion to expand abilities.
- Become aware of personal values and their impact on learning.
- Expand personal learning capacities that are consistent with learning styles and preferences.
- Synthesize knowledge by making connections with prior knowledge and learning experiences.
- Actively participate in assessment and evaluation and value this process.
- Collaborate with faculty in producing works that are meaningful.
- Use peer resources in producing works that reflect knowledge and skills.
- Invest time and energy in producing high-quality work that best represents abilities (p. 34).

ASSESSMENT APPROACHES

There are a number of assessment approaches that have been gaining in popularity as faculty focus on learning outcomes. Prior to choosing the assessment approaches that are most meaningful in determining program quality and effectiveness, it is important to know the nature of the learning expected from students throughout and at the end of the curriculum. According to Gagne, there are five categories of learning outcomes: (1) intellectual skills, (2) verbal information, (3) cognitive strategies, (4) attitudes, and (5) motor skills (Gagne & Driscoll, 1998). The challenges in assessing learning are linked with the ability of faculty to clearly and adequately define what students need to learn, to help students understand what learning expectations faculty have for students, and to make the links between the acquisition of knowledge and skills to the demonstration of the knowledge and skills through identified assessment approaches.

Competency Statements

In defining what learning is expected to take place, faculty must state learning in such a way that it ultimately can be measured. Competency statements have gained in popularity among nurse faculty as a means of stating learning in measurable terms. Competency statements or learning objectives must then be "unpacked." The process of "unpacking" requires that the faculty identify the knowledge, skills, attitudes, and values incorporated within each competency or learning objective. It is these learning particulars that guide assessment of learning efforts. Faculty must be able to clearly articulate what is to be learned or assessment becomes a meaningless exercise. Davies and Wavering (1999) stated that "teaching and assessment are inextricably intertwined" and that the approach we use in assessing student learning "drives both what and how we teach" (p. 39).

Types of Assessment Approaches

As noted earlier there has been an increasing emphasis on student involvement in the learning process. The desire to more actively involve students in the learning process has prompted the development of assessment approaches that require more student engagement. Many of the newer assessment approaches place the learner at the center of an interactive process. This type of engagement requires students to take more responsibility for the integrity of the assessment process. At the same time, the learner is able to collect, analyze, and respond to assessment feedback in a more immediate time frame.

A number of newer approaches being used in the assessment of learning outcomes include the use of objective structured clinical examinations (OSCE), portfolios, exhibitions, and problem-based learning. A few universities are setting up assessment and learning centers that provide support to faculty as they identify and use various assessment methods to measure learning outcomes. These centers employ experts in evaluation and learning who support faculty in designing and implementing effective assessment plans.

Objective Structured Clinical Examinations

One of the more popular learning assessment strategies, most frequently employed in medicine and dentistry programs, is the use of objective structured clinical examinations (OSCE). This assessment tool complements problem-based learning approaches and has appeal to professional programs in which the learning outcomes are imbedded not in what the student knows but in what the student is able to do with the knowledge.

The OSCE assessment strategy often employs the use of trained patients to simulate specific clinical problems. In these evaluation scenarios, students must demonstrate intellectual skills, verbal abilities, problem-solving strategies, clinical reasoning, and assessment and intervention skills. As the interactions between the student and trained patient-player unfold, student attitudes often are evident. Evaluation of learning is rich as the patient-player is an evaluator, along with a designated "expert" evaluator, who may or may not be the course instructor, and the student.

These examinations can be taped for reference and reviewed as a feedback mechanism for the learner. The ability to review performances increases students' ability to reflect on their learning and note areas of knowledge and/or skill deficiency or expertise. Taping also is a tool for training new patient-players. The use of the OSCE requires that the evaluation standards be clearly articulated and relate directly to the stated objectives. Inter-rater reliability is addressed by using multiple evaluators including the student.

Portfolio

The portfolio concept has become another popular method for assessing student learning. The portfolio is attractive in that it can be structured to include examples of student learning in any or all of the five areas in which learning occurs. Faculty using the portfolio as an assessment mechanism must clearly articulate what experiences are appropriate and adequate to effectively measure the expected learning results.

The portfolio mechanism is a tool by which students are able to exhibit their ability to meet learning outcomes through a series of accomplishments. These accomplishments can take the form of papers, projects, and other creative expressions of learning. These experiences must be purposely interwoven into the curriculum so there is opportunity to generate outcome information that will become part of a student's portfolio. It is important to establish the criteria or benchmarks by which the individual learning experiences that will make up the portfolio will be judged. Along with the criteria for judging the quality and quantity of each learning experience, there needs to be criteria for evaluating the overall portfolio experience across all students at the completion of the program. The portfolio is often evaluated at specified times during the program to validate that students possess the knowledge and skills to advance to the next level of expected performance.

The portfolio process is particularly helpful in assessing synthesis of learning. As nursing faculty modify undergraduate curricula to include a "capping" or "synthesizing" experience, the portfolio can be an effective assessment tool for documenting the achievement of learning outcomes and program effectiveness. The portfolio is appealing because it can be maintained electronically or in hard copy. For those programs offered primarily or exclusively through distributive educational means (e.g., Web-based, televised, and packaged course materials), the portfolio is an efficient way of noting student achievement. The portfolio also can be used by students and graduates as they seek employment opportunities and pursue additional educational experiences.

Exhibitions

Burke (1994) discussed the use of exhibitions as an effective end-of-program assessment tool. The three evaluation components of the exhibition assessment method proposed by Burke are (1) a public presentation forum, (2) an opportunity to demonstrate the integration of knowledge and skills for a specified purpose, and (3) the ability to demonstrate behaviors that are consistent with learning outcomes. This three-pronged approach is complex and is time and resource intensive. It does allow, however, for assessment at the levels of comprehension, application, and synthesis. It also provides students with the opportunity to demonstrate integration of knowledge and skills into their behaviors or actions.

Problem-Based Learning

Problem-based learning is an effective nonlinear learning tool, but one of the sometimes overlooked values of problem-based learning is the ability to incorporate assessment into the learning process. Problem-based learning provides an opportunity to critique learning and provide feedback to the student. In this method students analyze case studies or simulations of real and potential problems and receive feedback on their proposed actions from peers and faculty. The challenge in problem-based learning is to identify clearly the expected results and outcome measures that enable the faculty to assess learning in the aggregate in addition to one student at a time.

Students also must be comfortable with critique as both a learning and assessment tool. The ability to effectively critique the thinking of others may require explicit guidelines that will facilitate meaningful feedback among learners. Again, students must commit to sharing the responsibility for self-learning as well as the learning of others.

Other approaches for the assessment of learning outcomes are cooperative learning groups, exit cards, journals, simulations, and observations (Davies & Wavering, 1999, p. 39). Journals have gained in popularity as a mechanism for students to assess overall learning or learning within a specified context or situation. The use of observations and simulations are traditional assessment tools and used extensively by nursing faculty in evaluating clinical performance.

DISTANCE LEARNING AND EVALUATION

The ability to expand the boundaries of the classroom is increasing in colleges and universities across the nation (Ryan, Carlton, & Ali, 1999). A variety of technology has been used in extending or removing the traditional classroom walls that have served to contain the art and science of teaching and student learning. In the early 1990s, two-way video was a popular mechanism for expanding instruction beyond the traditional classroom. Early technology was limiting for those faculty wishing to implement teaching strategies that would actively engage the students in the learning process. Today, the Internet is the technology of choice. As the Internet becomes the primary mode for distributing courses and programs to students locally and nationally, there is an increasing need to develop valid mechanisms to assess the learning outcomes within the e-learning environment.

To date, the majority of the research conducted on distance education has focused on the participants' perceptions of the quality of the educational experience, issues related to the technology, and the pros and cons of distance versus classroom encounters (Ryan, Carlton, & Ali, 1999; Thyer, Polk, & Gaudin, 1997; Truell, 2001). It is obvious that any distributive educational method improves access to learning. What is less obvious, however, but more important for the long-term investment in distributive education, is the use of technology to design new pedagogies to facilitate learning among a diverse student population (Weigel, 2000). The ability to create new teaching pedagogies with the use of technology challenges faculty to design evaluation tools that will best capture learning outcomes expected from these different teaching approaches.

A critical aspect of an evaluation plan for schools using e-learning technology is the engagement in data collection that will provide ongoing cost-benefit analyses. It is critical in the evaluation of student learning to include not only performance in a course but also to examine performance from the broader aspects of program effectiveness and quality. Dominguez and Ridley (2001) argued that "a focus on student-level data does not provide institutions with practical information for program improvement or refinement [nor] does the information help individual faculty in improving distance education students' performance" (p. 15). They proposed that the learning by distance education students must be evaluated over a program of coursework for an aggregate of students. Improvements or refinements made to a curriculum should not be generalized from data collected on an individual student's experience or on one isolated learning experience.

Weigel (2000) questioned the rationality of evaluating e-learning by using the same benchmarks and measurements as we currently use in our traditional classroom approaches. He suggested that if we only view the Internet as an alternative to the classroom to which we import in-class lecture content, reading assignments, testing, lecture notes, and so forth, there is no reason for evaluating if there are differences between these approaches because they are essentially the same course.

The evaluation of online courses and programs should be sensitive enough to assess the degree to which learner characteristics affect the e-learning environment and the knowledge and skills learned within that environment. To date, there is little research to guide us in counseling students into a particular course delivery format or in determining those courses or teaching modalities that are most effective and efficient in the e-learning context.

As distributive educational activities increase, there is a related need to find reliable assessment tools. The Academic Computing Assessment Data Repository (ACADR) developed at Seton Hall University is one such resource. The ACADR is a Web-based tool for developing reliable, customizable survey instruments for collecting program assessment data, evaluating results, and submitting assessments (Santovec, 2002). This repository is available to faculty with the understanding that results will be shared with the larger higher education community.

There are few evaluation tools that have broad application for use in a comprehensive examination of distributive educational activities. The majority of tools are institution-specific, and therefore the ability to generalize results to a broader population is limited. The Teaching, Learning, and Technology Group (TLTG) (2002) has been working on an assessment model that identifies both benchmarks and assessment tools for use with courses taught in an online format. The national Flashlight Program, developed by this group, offers faculty the ability to tailor assessment tools for use with online courses, examine cost-effectiveness, use benchmarking in facilitating program decision making, and use rubrics for judging student experiences.

SUMMARY

The issues of accountability and productivity will continue to play a significant role in the future of higher education evaluation. In addition to evaluation and assessment focusing on the effectiveness of the educational process, other factors in the productivity equation will be efficiency, as defined by rising educational costs and decreasing resources. For the immediate future, external and internal stakeholders will continue to define educational effectiveness from the perspective of the learners' abilities. Nurse educators' primary challenge in maintaining contemporary evaluation and assessment programs will be keeping abreast of changes in knowledge and skills demanded by tomorrow's professionals. As nurse educators we must assume that the infrastructures of higher education and health care will redefine who we prepare as students, how we prepare them, and what we prepare them to do.

For evaluation programs to play an integral role in providing a rich and continually refreshing data source, nurse educators need to embrace change as an opportunity. Embracing change is not always easy because it requires giving up rigid routines, comfortable excuses, and traditional views. Evaluation and assessment of learning provide educators with exciting options for examining the contributions that we make to the education of one or more generations of learners—learners who possess the knowledge and skills to make a difference (Clark, 1993).

REFERENCES

Angelo, T. A. (1999). Doing assessment as if learning matters most. *AAHE Bulletin, 51*(9), 3–6.

Banta, T. W. (2001). Assessing competence in higher education. In C. A. Palomba & T. W. Banta (Eds.), *Assessing student competence in accredited disciplines— pioneering approaches to assessment in higher education* (pp. 1–12). Sterling, VA: Stylus Publishing.

Burke, K. (1994). *How to assess authentic learning.* Arlington Heights, IL: IRI/Sky-light Publishing.

Clark, K. K. (1993). *Life is change, growth is optional.* St. Paul, MN: Center for Executive Planning.

Conrad, C. F., & Wilson, R. F. (1994). Academic program reviews: Institutional approaches, expectations, and controversies. In J. S. Stark & A. Thomas (Eds.), *Assessment and program evaluation* (pp. 183–198). Needham Heights, MA: Simon & Schuster.

Davies, M. A., & Wavering, M. (1999). Alternative assessment: New directions in teaching and learning. *Contemporary Education, 71*(1), 39–45.

Davis, B. G. (1994). Demystifying assessment: Learning from the field of evaluation. In J. S.Stark & A. Thomas (Eds.), *Assessment and program evaluation* (pp. 45–57). Needham Heights, MA: Simon & Schuster.

Dominguez, P. S., & Ridley, D. R. (2001). Assessing distance education courses and discipline differences in their effectiveness. *Journal of Instructional Psychology, 28*(1), 15–19.

Gagne, R. M., & Driscoll, M. P. (1988). *Essential of learning for instruction.* Boston, MA: Allyn & Bacon.

Gates, S. M., Augustine, C. H., Benjamin, R., Bikson, T. K., Kaganoff, T., Levy, D. G., et al. (2002). Ensuring quality and productivity in higher education: An analysis of assessment practices. *ASHE-ERIC Higher Education Reports, 29*(1), 1–171.

Ingersoll, G. L., & Sauter, M. (1998). Integrating accreditation criteria into educational program evaluation. *Nursing & Health Care Perspectives, 19*(5), 224–229.

Lovett, C. M. (2002). Cracks in the bedrock: Can U.S. higher education remain number one? *Change, 34*(2), 10–15.

Madaus, G. F., Stufflebeam, D., & Scriven, M. S. (1994). Program evaluation: A historical overview. In J. S. Stark & A. Thomas (Eds.), *Assessment and program evaluation* (pp. 23–38). Needham Heights, MA: Simon & Schuster Custom Publishing.

National Institute of Education Study Group. (1984). *Involvement in learning: Realizing the potential of American higher education.* Washington, DC: Author.

Palomba, C. A., & Banta, T. W. (1999). *Assessment essentials: Planning, implementing and improving assessment in higher education.* San Francisco: Jossey Bass.

Ryan, M., Carlton, K. H., & Ali, N. S. (1999). Evaluation of traditional classroom teaching methods versus course delivery via the World Wide Web. *Journal of Nursing Education, 38,* 272–277.

Santovec, M. L. (2002). Seton Hall's state of the art assessment tool. *Distance Education Report, 6*(12), 8.

Scriven, M. S. (1972). Pros and cons about goal-free evaluation. *Evaluation Comment, The Journal of Educational Evaluation, 3*(4), 1–4.

Stufflebeam, D. L. (1985). *Conducting educational assessments.* Boston, MA: Kluwer-Nijhoff.

The Teaching, Learning, and Technology Group (TLTG). (2002). TLTG Home Page. Retrieved February 22, 2003, from http://www.tltgroup.org/default.htm

Thyer, B. A., Polk, G., & Gaudin, J. G. (1997). Distance learning in social work education: A preliminary evaluation. *Journal of Social Work Education, 33,* 363–367.

Truell, A. D. (2001). Student attitudes toward and evaluation of Internet-assisted instruction. *Delta Pi Epsilon Journal, 43*(1), 40–49.

Weigel, V. (2000). E-Learning and the tradeoff between richness and reach in higher education. *Change, 33*(5), 10–15.

Chapter 5

Assessing the Ineffable: A Creative Challenge for Nurse Educators and Students

Kathleen T. Heinrich and M. Ruth Neese

> Meaning is invisible, but the invisible is not contradictory of
> the visible: the visible itself has an invisible inner framework,
> and the invisible is the secret counterpart of the visible.
> —M. Merleau-Ponty

At a conference session on assessing ineffable phenomena, a female educator shared this dilemma:

> My experience tells me that the Chinese view the mind–body connection
> differently from Westerners, I just don't know how to get at that difference.
> For the last 5 years, I've been asking Chinese healers to describe how
> they understand the connection between the mind and the body. Not
> one has been able to put words around it.

Fellow participants suggested that she ask healers to use images from Chinese art, iconic characters from the Chinese alphabet, or scales from Chinese music as metaphorical representations of the mind–body link. Excitement replaced frustration as this woman intuited the range of creative possibilities opened by assessing the mind-body connection as an ineffable phenomenon.

Like many educators, nursing faculty often greet the idea of assessment with a disdain that masks feelings of inadequacy. While there are good reasons for this almost unanimous aversion to assessment, the best one is rarely recognized. Consider the "kinds of understandings, dispositions, habits of mind, ways of thinking, knowing, and problem solving" (Maki, 2002, p. 3) that students are promised on graduation. Since these attributes and competencies inhabit the realm of the ineffable, nurse educators are being challenged to measure phenomena that are, in essence, unmeasurable (Heinrich, Chiffer, McKelvey, & Zraunig, 2002).

Real, but not tangible, an ineffable is too overwhelming to be described in words. Synonyms for ineffable include the words indescribable, incredible, unspeakable, taboo, invisible, transcendent, and nameless. What Merleau-Ponty (1964/1968, p. 215) calls the "invisible inner framework," ineffable phenomena form the secret counterpart to the visible. Just as maps represent geographical territory, metaphors bridge the invisible and visible worlds. When ineffables are assessed using strategies drawn from aesthetic-expressive, and qualitative as well as quantitative, strategies, assessment becomes a creative act that requires an alchemy of art and science, serendipity and synchronicity.

Although the opening vignette amplifies the complexity of exploring a single ineffable phenomenon, nurse educators are being challenged to creatively assess the achievement of ineffable phenomena in and across courses, curricula, and programs. No wonder they feel inadequate before the task.

BACKGROUND

Inadequate does not begin to describe how I (Kathleen) felt when our accreditation report advised us to have an effective assessment program in place by the next accreditation visit. While the University of Hartford (UH) nursing faculty agreed that our assessment program generated mountains of unused quantitative data, we knew of no alternatives. Recognizing the limits of paper-and-pencil inventories alone to assess the richness and diversity of lived experience, we began our search for alternative assessment strategies and expanded our definition of assessment to include faculty and students. A phenomenological researcher used to being in a state of "not knowing," it was natural for me to turn to my faculty and student colleagues in search of a new approach to program assessment. The vision of creating a curriculum grounded in our lived experiences led us to replace the traditional definition of curriculum—the sequence of courses in a program—with a definition that emerged from Nancy Diekelmann's (1991) research: "a living and dynamic phenomena that involves students' relationships with faculty as well as teaching strategies, coursework, and clinical practicums" (p. 102). Although the traditional definition of program assessment "focuses on the impact of a curriculum on the knowledge, skills, and values attained by groups of students" (Palomba, 2002, p. 205), this new assessment program needed to be a "collaborative activity that yields a rich understanding of what and how faculty and students learn during their educational careers" (American Association for Higher Education (AAHE), 2002, p. 1).

An internal grant enabled me to train master's students to facilitate focus groups with graduating students that explored their lived experience in the program and catalogued their recommendations for changes. That graduating class told us, "If you want to graduate master's students who are scholars, you must prepare us to become scholars" (Heinrich, Cote, Mathews, & Varholak, 2002). After this program assessment project surfaced scholarly identity development as the most salient theme, an NLN Nursing Education 2001 Research grant funded the assessment of an evidence-based course designed to foster master's students' development of scholarly identity (Heinrich, Bona, McKelvey, & Solernou, 2002). This course marked the initiation of an evidence-based curriculum and scholarly identity became a program outcome.

After we completed teaching this evidence-based course, I came across the concept of "assessing the achievement of the ineffable" (AAHE, 2002, p. 1). In that instant I found an apt description of my activities as a teacher-scholar. Over the last 25 years, I have assessed assignments and teaching innovations that give form to ineffable phenomena using assessment strategies combining qualitative, aesthetic-expressive, and quantitative methods. Now that I knew about assessing ineffables, I suspected that what frightened our faculty group most about finding a new assessment program was the specter of measuring the unmeasurable.

After participating in the NLN-funded, course assessment project, Ruth agreed to conduct a literature search on the state of the art in the domain of assessing ineffables for this chapter. Ruth's comprehensive review of the literature describes the ways that educational researchers across disciplines are moving beyond traditional, objectivist/utilitarian approaches to include assessment strategies emerging from the subjectivist/intuitionist camp that explore students' and faculty's lived experiences (Banta, 2002). It is clear from this review that although nurse educators often assess ineffable phenomena in classroom and clinical settings, nothing in the nursing literature explicitly addresses this process. To show how this process unfolds in a nursing education setting, this chapter describes how we use a dialogue journal as a writing assignment to assess the ineffable phenomenon of scholarly identity development. A three-step process is introduced that guides nurse educators in identifying an ineffable phenomenon they wish to explore, translating that ineffable into a form that can be assessed, and designing ways to assess the ineffable using an alchemy of strategies.

REVIEW OF THE LITERATURE

Why attempt to assess something as nebulous as an ineffable phenomenon? Surely competency checklists, NCLEX passage rates, and Likert-scale summative course evaluations are adequate. Though important, these rational-empirical tools are reductionistic, limiting assessment to tightly defined, didactic learning outcomes. Assessment is as much about how individuals learn as it is about outcomes (Krechevsky & Stork, 2000). The process and context of learning are just as important as products and outcomes, and acknowledging the ineffable encourages teachers to attend to process and embed learning in context (Eisner, 1997; Krechevsky & Stork, 2002).

Why should educators acknowledge the ineffable in assessment? Focusing on making the invisible visible adds a richness of meaning to educational interactions (Krechevsky & Stork, 2000; Starr-Glass, 2002). Investigating the lived experience of students allows educators access to other world views and meaning systems (Eisner, 1997; Krechevsky & Stork, 2002; Starr-Glass, 2002). Contextual influences from outside the classroom—social, cultural, ethical, and political—can be acknowledged and incorporated into learning (Krechevsky & Stork, 2002). Grounding educational experiences in context enlarges understanding and clarifies the message (Eisner, 1997).

One means of aiding clarity is developing a shared language describing the ineffable phenomenon of interest. This is accomplished through dialogue, where educator and student become colearners as they negotiate mutual understanding (Krechevsky & Stork, 2000; Starr-Glass,

2002). Starr-Glass states that this negotiation prevents fragmentation of experience and allows meaning to be created through the use of pre-existing ideas and concepts. Through dialogue, educators and students rearrange these ideas and concepts until they are sure they are speaking the same language. Shared language and meaning bring a sense of particularity to assessment (Eisner, 1997). Even when a phenomenon is invisible, coming to know its distinctive qualities and attributes makes it more real. If it can be named and described, it can be researched.

If the process of assessing the ineffable is beginning to sound messy, it should. Eisner (1997) refers to this as "productive ambiguity" (p. 8) and states that it is the result of acknowledging multiple perspectives. These ambiguities and perspectives are there to be explored and make investigating the phenomenon of interest more complex. This increased attention to complexity avoids reductionistic thinking and generates new insights (Eisner, 1997; Starr-Glass, 2002).

Focusing on the ineffable, with its attendant ambiguities, complexities, and insights, allows educators to ask new questions about teaching and learning (Eisner, 1997). Educators interested in examining the ineffable contend that affective, aesthetic, and moral forms of knowing are worthy of inquiry (Krechevsky & Stork, 2000; Maki, 2002; Miller & Morgan, 2000). Exploring these forms of knowing requires new questions and methods capable of providing answers. Research into which methods provide the best answers has begun in the health and social sciences. Writing and dialogue have received the most attention as assessment methods. Other strategies of interest include drawing, collage, and role play.

WRITING AS ASSESSMENT

Interest in writing as an assessment method has focused on the use of metaphor and narrative. Metaphor serves as a way to give form to the ineffable, a linguistic symbol representing the unknowable. Naming a phenomenon through metaphor produces actions that create the reality and give it identity (Akin & Palmer, 2000). Metaphors communicate meaning and enable us to make sense of complex or novel situations by applying familiar terms and concepts. Using metaphors in new ways could provide new understanding of experience (Kemp, 1999).

Kemp (1999) used metaphor to evaluate personal and professional development in social work students during clinical rotations. Each clinical group had to choose a metaphor to represent their initial clinical experience and revise this metaphor to reflect development over time. Metaphors were recorded in students' own words without input from clinical preceptors or the investigator. Over a 1-year time period, metaphor use was found to strengthen students' ability to highlight positive and negative clinical experiences and foster development as reflective practitioners. Metaphor revisions effectively tracked personal and professional growth and reflected transformation of student perspectives. These findings were used to enrich quantitative course and program evaluation data, resulting in some revisions.

NARRATIVE

Another form of writing being investigated is narrative or storytelling. Human beings construct meaning and individual versions of reality constantly through the interpretation of lived experiences. Constructing narratives, or stories, is one means of defining the self and tracking changes in perspective (Harrison, 1999). "The very act of storytelling is an act of evaluation" (Harrison, 1999, p. 132). To tell a story, an individual must decide which experiences to own and which to discard through reflection on the experiences. New knowledge and insight are constructed through the interaction of the writer and the process of writing (Diekelmann & Ironside, 1998; Harrison, 1999).

Harrison (1999) examined the use of narrative as a course evaluation method by using storytelling to track student personal development and perspective transformation in an English class. Their narratives reflected personal growth, but students were not the only ones making meaning from the stories. Narrative construction became a formative evaluation strategy that prompted the investigator to reflect on educational practices and modify them to accommodate variations in student learning styles.

Sims and Swenson (2001) described the use of narrative to frame the curriculum of a family nurse practitioner program. They revised a problem-based learning format to one called narrative-based learning. Learning was facilitated by giving students access to a complex clinical story without telling them what they were supposed to learn from it. The stories came from actual clinical practice, which increased student motivation to learn. Stories were shared and meaning sought across stories. Evaluation was based on verbal and written narrative self-reflection. The authors acknowledged that this method is more suited for graduate students, but also believe that teaching with stories would enrich all levels of nursing education.

DIALOGUE—WRITTEN AND VERBAL

Dialogue is another evaluation method that can touch the ineffable and has been described in written and verbal applications. Writing as dialogue is a method used in reflective journaling that encourages students to explore personal knowledge and compare these beliefs to issues in the literature and practice (Bilinski, 2002; Heinrich, 1992; Hodges, 1996). Sensitive faculty feedback is then used to guide students in examining these beliefs and assumptions in light of the literature. This type of faculty-student dialogue encourages growth and fosters higher-level thinking. The journal is used to track student development and transformation across time.

Writing as dialogue has also been described in conjunction with creating a scholarly identity (Diekelmann & Ironside, 1998). Writing allows a budding scholar to dialogue with texts and self, permitting a synthesis of new knowledge and a different way of knowing (Diekelmann & Ironside, 1998; Hofmeyer, 2002). It is this "different way of knowing" that transforms a student and marks scholarly identity.

Verbal dialogue has been described in the context of face-to-face interviews and focus groups. Personal interviews allow educators to hear the language students use to describe lived experience (Starr-Glass, 2002). This unique language should be honored and explored to allow the creation of shared meaning. Focus groups allow students to dialogue with each other about their learning and provide educators with student interpretations of learning experiences (Heinrich & Witt, 1998; Maki, 2002). Each method of dialogue encourages the development of shared meaning and adds richness and context to quantitative evaluation methods.

OTHER METHODS

There have been some studies investigating the use of other assessment methods. Krueger and Irvine (2001) had undergraduate sociology students provide a written description of sociologists and a drawing of a sociologist. The drawings revealed stereotypes held by the students that did not appear in the written descriptions. Using drawings permitted different perceptions and understandings to emerge. Nurse-architect Keddy (2002) had a group of nurses construct experiential collages based on their lived body experiences in practice settings. These collages were created to foster the development of a shared language with architects, thereby allowing the architects to better understand nurses' needs in the design of practice settings.

Kennedy (2001), exploring the use of role play in teaching communication skills to medical students, made a serendipitous discovery. Some students found playing the patient role to be embarrassing and expressed resentment at having to undress for a physical examination. This simple role play uncovered previously unknown attitudes that became a focus for educational intervention. It is unlikely that pencil and paper assessment methods would have illuminated any of these findings. The insights were gained by entering the aesthetic-expressive realm.

Though illuminating, the aesthetic-expressive realm cannot provide precise data as defined by the quantitative realm (Eisner, 1997). The ineffable can be difficult to nail down. Miller and Morgan (2000) remind educational researchers that assessing the ineffable is an interpretive, inductive process. Therefore, the framework used for data analysis must be explicit and open to scrutiny (Eisner, 1997; Kemp, 1999; Krechevsky & Stork, 2000; Miller & Morgan, 2000). An explicit framework allows exploration of possibilities and limitations surrounding the chosen assessment method. Results from innovative methods should be compared with more traditional methods to guard against misinterpretation (Kemp, 1999; Miller & Morgan, 2000).

CAVEATS

Regardless of the chosen assessment method, the literature contained three caveats: (1) students should be informed of any alternative assessment methods and how these will be used, (2) an atmosphere of safety and trust is essential, and (3) student responses must be accepted "as is." Since most students are unfamiliar with alternative assessment strategies, fully informing them of the what, where, why, and how reduces confusion and increases trust in the learning environment (Harrison, 1999; Kemp, 1999; Sims & Swenson, 2001). An atmosphere of safety and trust is essential if educators are engaging affective, aesthetic, or moral forms of knowing to prevent distressing learning experiences and to encourage risk taking and critical thinking (Bilinski, 2002; Brooker & MacDonald, 1999; Harrison, 1999; Heinrich, 1992; Kemp, 1999; Krechevsky & Stork, 2000). Finally, student responses must be accepted "as is," without a predetermined filter of what constitutes an acceptable or "correct" answer. Imposition of what the investigator or institution considers "right" blocks true dialogue, stifles student voice, and strips alternative assessment of the context and richness of meaning it was designed to capture (Bilinski, 2002; Brooker & MacDonald, 1999; Harrison, 1999; Heinrich, 1992; Kemp, 1999; Krechevsky & Stork, 2000; McGillion & Nelson, 2002; Starr-Glass, 2002).

In spite of the ambiguity and sense of feeling lost when engaging the ineffable, this invisible realm can be a rich source of curricular and pedagogical innovation. When educators and students become cocreators of meaning, new possibilities linking personal experience and academic learning become visible (Brooker & MacDonald, 1999; Krechevsky & Stork, 2000; Starr-Glass, 2002). Educators investigating ineffable phenomena can become generators of educational theory, curricular innovation, and site-specific pedagogy, in other words, scholars. These teacher-scholars then become role models and mentors for others whose passion is investigating the ineffable, motivating learning and spurring additional innovations.

DIALOGUE JOURNAL ASSESSES THE ACHIEVEMENT OF PERSPECTIVE TRANSFORMATION

There are those who liken attempts to measure ineffables to strangling the goose that laid the golden egg. Although the intrepid educators assessing ineffables readily admit this is a messy and ambiguous process, taken together their scholarly work outlines steps to follow. To be assessed, ineffables must first be given a visible form through metaphor, for example, artwork or narrative constructions. The assessment of such metaphorical representations is an interpretive, inductive process. To guard against misinterpretation, this process requires the development of an explicit framework or rubric that can be shared and assessed using a combination of strategies. The dialogue journal is an exemplar of an ineffable given the form of an academic assignment that was assessed as both a course requirement and a data source.

When graduates in the focus group program assessment project told our faculty that we needed to purposefully prepare students to become scholars, we designed and assessed an evidence-based course to do just that. Our working definition of scholarly identity was a developmental process that enables nurses to articulate, verbally and in writing, ideas grounded in the literature. Based on his research with midlife women returning to school, Mezirow (1991) describes this developmental process as a "perspective transformation."

Perspective transformation is the process of becoming critically aware of how and why our assumptions have come to constrain the way we perceive, understand, and feel about our world; changing these structures of habitual expectation to make possible a more inclusive, discriminating, and integrative perspective; and finally making choices or otherwise acting on these new understandings (p. 167). Mezirow (1991) used the term "transformative learning" to describe the "social process of constructing and appropriating a new or revised interpretation of the meaning of one's experiences as a guide to action" (p. 222). In adapting this concept to nursing, Maltby and Andrusyszyn (1997) suggested that registered nurses experience a transformation in their perspective "of nursing, nursing roles, and themselves" while pursuing higher education (p. 9).

During the evidence-based course we called "Perspective Transformation: Socialization into Scholarly Identity," we hoped that newly matriculated, students' perspectives would transform from seasoned clinicians and managers into budding scholars (Heinrich, Bona, McKelvey, & Solernou, 2001). Designed to foster students' scholarly identity development, this course required us to deconstruct scholarly practices into learning episodes and assignments like the dialogue journals that were then evaluated as course assignments and assessed as data.

At the orientation program prior to the first class, I explained that students were entering an introductory course that was also an educational research project. To receive academic credit, students must complete all assignments including the dialogue journal. Only those students who volunteered to participate in the research project would submit their dialogue journal at the end of the semester to be included in the data set. The dialogue journal assignment as described in the course syllabus is excerpted as follows:

Feminist educators are bringing the passion back into classrooms by honoring ideas and feelings equally. One of the most effective techniques for reconnecting head and heart is journal writing. Journal writing is an introspective exercise in which students record their thoughts, feelings, and experiences. While journals are written mainly for the self, the fact that they are shared with a teacher creates an intimate link between inner dialogue and dialogue with another person. Since the instructor reads student journals for meaning rather than mechanics, the student-teacher dialogue is noncritical. Journaling is a powerful medium through which students give words to their inner dialogue and share their precious memories, reflections, and insights with one other person—the instructor. This supportive dialogue empowers students to risk sharing ideas in the classroom.

A journal is neither a diary nor class notes but borrows features from both. Like diaries, journals are written in the first person about issues that you as a student care about; like class notes, journals are concerned with the content of a particular course. General principles for being successful with journal writing include: (1) remember you are writing for an audience—flesh out your ideas so readers can understand your ideas easily; (2) support your ideas with examples from your personal/professional experiences and the readings; and (3) when you do quote or cite an idea from the literature make sure that you tell the reader what the idea means to you. Journal entries are reviewed weekly for completeness by how well you address each of the three areas.

For the final class, entitle your journal and each entry; design a cover that gives creative form to your experience over the semester; write a Table of Contents; and an evaluative conclusion that tells what it has been like for you to journal over this semester.

DIALOGUE JOURNAL: COURSE ASSIGNMENT AND ASSESSMENT DATA

Assessing aesthetic-expressive, scholarly products like dialogue journals presents a challenge for nurse educators and educational researchers alike. As an academic assignment, 5% of the final grade was allocated to the creativity reflected in students' dialogue journal covers and entry titles (Table 5.1). Not artists, we were unsure how to establish criteria to judge the quality of students' creativity. So whenever dialogue journals included a cover page with a descriptive title for the journal and for each entry title, students were awarded the full 5%.

When faced with the challenge of assessing 41 students' dialogue journals as a data set, we used an inductive approach to create a rubric that traced students' perspective transformation over the semester as documented in their journal. Each of us individually reviewed one

TABLE 5.1   Grading for Dialogue Journal Project

Criteria	Percentage
• Creativity of cover and entry titles	5
• Personal/professional life experiences	20
• Class	20
• Readings	20
• Synthesis	20
• Evaluative conclusion	15

journal agreed to be an exemplar of excellence. When we convened as a group, we surfaced the themes from our review of the four exemplar journals and created an assessment rubric from the emergent themes (Table 5.2).

To ensure that we did not misinterpret the findings about students' perspective transformation from these dialogue journals, the project used an integrated, assessment design. This alchemy of assessment strategies included a quantitative instrument we developed from Diekelmann and Ironsides' (1998) description of "scholarly practices." Students completed this instrument called the "Scholarly Skills Self-Assessment Inventory" at the beginning, at mid-semester, and at the end of the semester. Transcriptions of students' responses to questions posed in focus groups the first evening and the last evening of class are being analyzed as qualitative data. Posters giving creative form to students' perspective transformation into scholarly identity is an assessment strategy drawn from the aesthetic-expressive realm.

Based on our assessment of the qualitative and aesthetic-expressive data thus far, we believe that this course achieved the ineffable of perspective transformation given that dialogue journals, transcripts from the final focus groups, and posters indicated that they began to see themselves in the words of one student, as "budding scholars." As the quantitative data have not yet been analyzed, it remains to be seen if those findings support the findings from qualitative, and aesthetic expressive, assessment strategies.

LESSONS LEARNED ABOUT ASSESSING INEFFABLES

Although challenging, we found the process of giving form to the ineffable phenomenon of perspective transformation into scholarly identity

TABLE 5.2   Rubric for Analyzing Dialogue Journals as Aesthetic/Expressive Data

Creative presentation/metaphors and symbols used:
  Journal title:
  Cover:
  Cover pages for journal entries:
  Congruency of artwork & text:

Presence:
  How does student make self known to me in this journal?

Catalytic event(s) described in journal:

Lifeline over semester (line-drawing of pattern reflected in students' narrative):

Perspective transformation:
  Difference in the way student looks at self
  Difference in the way student sees the profession
  Difference in the range of professional opportunities student sees for self
  Difference in student's perception of a master's degree
  Where is student in seeing self moving beyond the identity of seasoned practitioner to seeing self as budding scholar—scholarly identity development?

Supportive relationships:
  Self
  Co-workers
  Classmates
  Student/Graduate Presenters
  Family
  Friends

a creative and intellectually stimulating exercise. From this experience, we discovered that assessing the achievement of the ineffable involves three steps: (1) listen to your students and your own experience as an educator to identify ineffable phenomena; (2) transform this ineffable phenomenon into a form that can be assessed; and (3) assess the achievement of the ineffable using an alchemy of assessment strategies.

While the foregoing review of the literature was conducted after we completed data gathering, our experience with assessing ineffables supports the caveats surfaced in the literature review. Specifically, we informed students before class began that an alchemy of quantitative and qualitative assessments tools would be used to explore students' perspective transformation over the semester. To create a sense of safety and trust in this classroom, *Peace and Power: Building Communities for* the Future (Chinn, 2001) was assigned as a required text. Peggy Chinn's (2001) techniques for fostering dialogue and negotiating conflict were used throughout the course. We strove always to accept and to understand students' response "as is." For example, when three students in the management track said that they could not relate to the course because most readings were drawn from nursing education, master's students in their final year of the program were consulted for suggestions for pertinent readings from the management literature. These suggested articles were immediately added to the course readings to the delight of the management students.

Last, we learned not to be afraid when we felt lost. There were many times that we felt overwhelmed by the process of translating ineffable phenomena into learning episodes, assignments, or assessment tools. When faced with operationalizing scholarly practices, for example, we had to translate a phenomenon like "thinking in a scholarly way" into a teaching/learning episode. Feeling lost did not end with creating these teaching/learning episodes; it has continued into the assessment phase. We spent one day sitting in my living room surrounded by piles of dialogue journals clueless about how we were going to analyze the hundreds of pages of narrative and artwork as assessment data. We were overjoyed when the rubric we designed that day effectively surfaced themes and patterns that are elucidating this cohort's perspective transformation into scholarly identity (Table 5.2).

HOW CAN YOU ASSESS THE INEFFABLE IN YOUR SETTING?

The worksheet in Table 5.3 outlines the three steps we used to name, transform, and assess the ineffable phenomenon of "perspective transformation into scholarly identity." You can adapt this process in your own program.

SUMMARY

Schools of nursing across the country are searching for meaningful ways to assess courses, curricula, and programs. When nurse educators appreciate that measuring the unmeasurable is the true challenge of

TABLE 5.3   Faculty Worksheet: Naming, Transforming, and Assessing Ineffables

Step #1. *Listen* to your students' lived experiences and your own wisdom as an educator. Choose an ineffable phenomenon that you would like to explore further based on what you have learned from listening to students, from your own experiences of teaching, from reviewing mid-semester and final course evaluations, or from the literature.

> The ineffable phenomenon we chose to study was "perspective transformation into scholarly identity."
>
> *The ineffable phenomenon I wish to study is* _____.

Step #2. *Transform* this ineffable phenomenon into a form that can be assessed, e.g., a teaching/learning episode or a course assignment. Remember that ineffable phenomena take the form of metaphors that you can then transform into a learning episode or a class assignment.

> Our ineffable phenomenon took the form of a dialogue journal that traced students' transformation into "budding scholars" in entries submitted weekly over the semester.
>
> *This ineffable phenomenon I wish to study will take the form of* _____.

Step #3. *Assess* the achievement of the ineffable using an alchemy of assessment strategies. Assessing the ineffable integrates qualitative and quantitative measures, as well as aesthetic-expressive approaches.

> The achievement of the ineffable of perspective transformation into scholarly identity was an integrated design that included focus groups, a Scholarly Skills Assessment Inventory, and a "Perspective Transformation" poster to assess the phenomenon we identified.
>
> *I will assess the achievement of this ineffable by* _____.

assessment, they are likely to extend assessment beyond the purely quantitative and engage both faculty and students in the process. Rather than suggesting that alternative assessment strategies "stand in opposition" to traditional methods, this chapter proposed that nurse educators take a "both/and" approach to assessment design that integrates qualitative and aesthetic-expressive, in addition to, quantitative methods. To support nurse educators to think creatively and collaboratively about assessment, this chapter introduced a three-step assessment approach in which faculty and students identify ineffable phenomena, translate phenomena into forms that can be assessed, and use a plethora of assessment strategies to evaluate the phenomena.

When students' and faculty's lived experiences are translated into evidence-based learning episodes, assignments, and curricula that are assessed for the achievement of the ineffable, "curriculum as relationship" will be actualized in communities of scholarly caring made up of faculty and students. On the basis of iterative and innovative assessment programs, nurse educators will be able to demonstrate that they are preparing nurse clinicians, leaders, entrepreneurs, educators, scholars, and researchers for the challenges of the new millennium.

ACKNOWLEDGMENT

With gratitude to Dale Chiffer for her editorial comments grounded in her participation in the focus group assessment projects and our conference presentation on assessing ineffables that served as the basis for this chapter.

REFERENCES

American Association for Higher Education (AAHE). (2002, June). *2002 Assessment Conference: A Shared Commitment*. Boston, MA: Author.

Akin, G., & Palmer, I. (2000, Winter). Putting metaphor to work for change in organizations [Electronic version]. *Organizational Dynamics*, 67–77.

Banta, T. W. (2002). *Building a scholarship of assessment*. San Francisco: Jossey-Bass.

Bilinski, H. (2002). The mentored journal. *Nurse Educator, 27*, 37–41.

Brooker, R., & MacDonald, D. (1999). Did we hear you? Issues of student voice in a curricular innovation [Electronic version]. *Journal of Curriculum Studies, 31*(1), 83–97.

Chinn, P. L. (2001). *Peace & power: Building communities for the future*. New York: National League for Nursing (NLN) Press.

Diekelmann, N. (1991). The nursing curriculum: Lived experiences of students. *The curriculum revolution*. New York: National League for Nursing Press.

Diekelmann, N., & Ironside, P. M. (1998). Preserving writing in doctoral education: Exploring the concernful practices of schooling learning teaching. *Journal of Advanced Nursing, 28*, 1347–1355.

Eisner, E. W. (1997). The promise and perils of alternative forms of data representation. *Educational Researcher, 26*(6), 4–10.

Harrison, M. D. (1999). *Writing and being: The transformational power of storytelling reported through narrative based evaluation* (UMI No. 9923935). Retrieved November 1, 2002, from Dissertation Abstracts database.

Heinrich, K. T. (1992). The intimate dialogue: Journal writing by students. *Nurse Educator, 17*(6), 17–20.

Heinrich, K. T., Bona, G., McKelvey, M., & Solernou, S. (2001, September). Is scholarly identity development an outcome of a transformative learning environment? Initiating a research-based curriculum. NLN Nursing Education Grant.

Heinrich, K. T., Chiffer, D., McKelvey, M. M., & Zraunig, M. (2002, June 22). Assessing the Ineffable: An Alchemy of Science, Art & Synchronicity. *2002 Assessment Conference: A Shared Commitment.* Boston, MA: AAHE.

Heinrich, K. T., Cote, J. A., Mathews, M. B., & Varholak, D. (2002, March 21–23). Faculty-student program evaluation research project grounds a curriculum revision. Fourteenth Annual Scientific Session of the Eastern Nursing Research Society. University Park, PA: The Pennsylvania State University.

Heinrich, K. T., & Witt, B. (1998). Serendipity: A focus group turned hermeneutic evaluation. *Nurse Educator, 23*(4), 40–44.

Hodges, H. F. (1996). Journal writing as a mode of thinking for RN-BSN students: A leveled approach to learning to listen to self and others. *Journal of Nursing Education, 35,* 137–141.

Hofmeyer, A. (2002). Using text as data and writing as the method of inquiry and discovery. *Nursing Inquiry, 9,* 215–217.

Keddy, K. (2002, November). Socio-spatial characteristics of nursing activities: A poststructuralist feminist research framework. Paper presented at the Twelfth Annual International Conference on Critical and Feminist Perspectives in Nursing, Portland, ME.

Kemp, E. (1999). Metaphor as a tool for evaluation [Electronic version]. *Assessment and Evaluation in Higher Education, 24,* 81–90.

Kennedy, M. (2001). Teaching communication skills to medical students: Unexpected attitudes and outcomes [Electronic version]. *Teaching in Higher Education, 6*(1), 119–123.

Krechevsky, M., & Stork, J. (2000). Challenging educational assumptions: Lessons from an Italian-American collaboration [Electronic version]. *Cambridge Journal of Education, 30*(1), 57–74.

Krueger, P. M., & Irvine, L. (2001). Visualizing the ineffable: Using drawn and written representations to assess students' stereotypes of sociologists. *Sociological Imagination, 38.* Retrieved November 1, 2002, from EBSCO host database.

Maki, P. (2002, January 15). Using multiple assessment methods to explore student learning and development inside and outside of the classroom. Retrieved October 31, 2002, from the National Association of Student Personnel Administrators Web site: http://www.naspa.org/NetResults/

Maltby, H. J., & Andrusyszyn, M. A. (1997). Perspective transformation: Challenging the resocialization concept of degree-seeking registered nurses. *Nurse Educator, 22*(2), 9–11.

McGillion, M., & Nelson, S. (2002, November). Expertise or performance? Calling into question the rhetoric of contemporary narrative use in nursing. Paper presented at the Twelfth Annual International Conference on Critical and Feminist Perspectives in Nursing, Portland, ME.

Merleau-Ponty, M. (1968). *The visible and the invisible: Followed by working notes.* (C. Lefort, Ed. & A. Lingis, Trans.). Evanston, IL: Northwestern University Press. (Original work published 1964)

Mezirow, J. (1991). A critical theory of adult learning and education. *Adult Education, 32*(1), 3–24.

Miller, S. I., & Morgan, R. R. (2000). Establishing credibility of alternative forms of data representation [Electronic version]. *Educational Studies, 31,* 119–131.

Palomba, C. A. (2002). Scholarly assessment of student learning in the major and general education. In T. W. Banta & Associates (Eds.), *Building a scholarship of assessment* (pp. 201–222). San Francisco: Jossey-Bass.

Sims, S. L., & Swenson, M. M. (2001). Preparing teachers and students for narrative learning [Electronic version]. *Journal of Scholarship of Teaching and Learning, 1*(2). Retrieved August 8, 2002, from Indiana University South Bend Web site http://www.iusb.edu/~josotl/

Starr-Glass, D. (2002). Metaphor and totem: Exploring and evaluating prior experiential learning [Electronic version]. *Assessment and Evaluation in Higher Education, 27,* 221–231.

Chapter 6

A Praxis for Grading

Peggy L. Chinn

"I hate grading."

"If it weren't for having to grade students, I would love teaching."

"Maybe if we used a pass/fail system, we could focus more on learning."

"All students think about are their grades, not what and how they are learning."

"I manage to create a really good collegial atmosphere in the classroom, until it comes to grading. Then it all falls apart."

"Students seem to expect to get 'A' grades, so the pressure is really terrible."

"I am worried about grade inflation, but I don't know what we can do about it."

These kinds of comments ring throughout the hallways of higher education, and many readers of this volume may have uttered very similar words. I have struggled with all of the issues suggested in these comments for many years, and although I have not arrived at a solution that suits all situations, I have formed some underlying thoughts and responses that have helped me to deal with the difficult issue of grades and grading.

The purposes of this chapter are to discuss issues related to traditional practices of grading, and to suggest practices that are consistent with values that are generally claimed in nursing about human interactions. Grading practices are so engrained in the culture of academics that any attempt to even discuss alternatives is met with great resistance and skepticism. Pollio and Beck (2000) point out that grades and grading procedures retain their unmovable hold in education despite consistent evidence that they are flawed psychometric indices, and that they have a persistently negative influence on genuine learning. Pollio and Beck speculate that the persistence of grades and grading procedures has to do in part with two prevailing social attitudes—a belief in the value of numbers regardless of how they are produced, and the significance of competition in the western world.

Despite the intransigence of grades and grading practices, many faculty sincerely wish to change their practices in the classroom but have great difficulty implementing the desired changes. The prospect of making change is overwhelming not because of lack of will to change, nor because of inadequate intelligence or creativity. The fact is that we teach in institutions that are created to impart the values of the larger culture and that serve to perpetuate the dominant practices of the culture. The very act of grading accomplishes these subtle, unwritten, and unstated reasons for institutional existence. Nonetheless, even in these contexts, the sense of longing for a better way to deal with grades and grading persists, just as many faculty long for better ways to teach; for more interesting, challenging, and stimulating modes of delivery; or for more efficient ways to present the increasing volume of material that needs to be covered.

My own perspectives on grades and grading are based on several assumptions: Teachers and students alike are socialized within institutions to act in prescribed, role-defined ways. To change these expectations, and the realities, is exceedingly difficulty no matter how much we wish to change. This is because the context typically remains the same.

Total elimination of grading in some form may be possible, but not probable in our currently structured institutions. There are prestigious colleges that have abolished grades, but the processes of evaluation by faculty remain intact in the form of narrative transcripts. I personally favor this approach, but it is unlikely to be widely adopted, and more fundamentally, it still retains the fundamental institutional role of "teacher as evaluator." In my own career I have contemplated the issues and considered alternatives but remain situated in grade-oriented institutions. Therefore, I have chosen to address grades and grading issues as a practical reality.

A well-articulated and deeply integrated personal philosophy and value system is essential if one wishes to change a practice that is as fully institutionalized as is grading. A deeply integrated value system provides the anchor from which various practices emerge and evolve over time, and with shifting circumstances.

WHY CHANGE?

Aside from a desire to change grading practices because the traditional practices seem uncomfortable and inadequate, there are important reasons to seriously examine traditional practices and to consider alternatives.

First, our philosophies of nursing do not match our traditional practices. There are several philosophical points that could be addressed in this regard. The most important with respect to grading practices is the fundamental value that appears frequently in the philosophies of schools of nursing that each individual is unique. Traditional grading practices ignore students as unique individuals, and are designed to mold everyone into the same rigid set of expectations. If we hold as true that humans are unique individuals (not just patients), then grading practices need to be tailored to consistently reflect this belief. This does not mean that we just accept everyone and everything without regard to the professional standards and expectations of the curriculum. But it does mean that we reconsider how we treat people in groups, while maintaining respect for the uniqueness of individuals. Take for example the issue of "equal treatment," which often enters into a discussion of grading practices. If "equal" is taken to mean that everyone is treated the same, particularly when rigid rules of grading are used, grading practices of necessity disregard the uniqueness of individuals. "Equal," in the context of respect for individuals, is better conceptualized as "equity," where each individual has what he or she needs in order to have an "equal" opportunity to succeed.

Another philosophic tenet common to many schools of nursing is the value of growth and development toward high-level wellness or optimum potential. If grading is emphasized in the context of traditional grading practices, very little, if any, growth occurs. Students in a grade-intensive environment use the most efficient way to get the grade regardless of what this implies in terms of personal and professional growth and development. Students should be congratulated for their cleverness in doing so, not criticized. Faculty bear the responsibility for recognizing what our practices prompt in terms of student response, and create practices that bring forth instead the kinds of growth and development that we seek (Svinicki, 1998).

The ideal of seeking growth and development is closely related to another common value in nursing school philosophies—that of "caring." Caring is defined and viewed in different ways, but the core of caring, which focuses on a genuine response to human needs, implies moving away from practices that alienate and diminish, as traditional grading practices often do, to practices that respond to student needs. Student needs include, but are not limited to, that which students state that they need. Students also need that which is defined by the profession in terms of professional standards, faculty-defined values for learning and growth, and that which society expects from professional nurses. Students also deserve the fundamental human needs that are common in all relationships, such as clear and open communication, respect for human dignity, and ethical integrity. Traditional grading practices tend to mystify rather than clarify, promote power-over interactions that dehumanize and disempower, and engender manipulation between teacher and student rather than mutual respect and negotiation.

UNDERLYING ISSUES

There are many underlying issues that enter into any discussion of grades and grading practice. The three issues that I will discuss briefly are not meant to be exhaustive of all of the issues involved. They illustrate shifts in thinking that are required in order to move beyond issues, to clarify one's underlying philosophy and values, and to come to a reasonable construction of alternative practices that more fully expresses your values as a teacher.

GRADE INFLATION

The notion of grade inflation can only make sense in a context in which competition, standardization, and norm-based, statistical, bell-curve grading is considered to be the ideal. Norm-based grading by definition assigns a mean around which all other scores are distributed above and below. The distribution is assumed to apply to scores that actually have a very narrow range (as in 90 to 100), just as they would apply to a wide range of scores (as in 0 to 100) consistent with the assumptions on which normative grading is based. The term "grade inflation" is a misnomer if all students earn high scores and truly deserve high grades. If teachers use a norm-based standardized bell curve to assign grades in a situation in which all students are highly qualified and have achieved high marks, then many students are unfairly assigned low, even failing grades, when they in fact deserve to be assigned a good grade.

The term "grade inflation" has been the object of several articles reflecting many points of view, debating whether or not such as thing exists, and if so, why it exists (Basinger, 1997; Edwards, 2000; Lawler, 2001; Loustau & O'Connor, 1999; McSpirit, Chapman, Kopacz, & Jones, 2000; Shoemaker & DeVox, 1999). There is little research that addresses the various speculations about grade inflation, but there is consensus that in many colleges, students in general are better prepared to handle college material than in the past, that admission standards are more rigorous, and that these factors alone can account for higher grade profiles. Some believe that faculty feel pressured to assign higher grades because of more aggressive student attitudes and expectations, but many deny that faculty are tending to acquiesce to student pressures, and there is no research evidence either way. The most thoughtful authors advocate turning our attention away from the ubiquitous notion of grade inflation to the quality of instruction, the underlying issues involved in various grading practices, how students respond to alternative grading practices, and sound methods of assessment of real learning achievement (Basinger, 1997; Edwards, 2000; Loustau & O'Connor, 1999).

Many teachers have turned to criterion-based approaches to grading (which in fact are part of the practices that I advocate), whereby all students who demonstrate competency are assigned grades based on the standards or criteria established for the course. In such a model, all students can potentially be assigned high grades, representing either uniform excellence for all students or gross teacher negligence in estimating the actual competencies of students. The latter situation could be called a form of "grade inflation." However, the term obscures the real problem, if there is one, and is too readily used as a rhetorical tool that diverts attention away from serious examination of the real issues involved.

PASS/FAIL GRADING

Pass/fail grading has been adopted by a number of schools, colleges, or programs in an effort to address some of the difficult aspects of grades and to avoid perpetuating the inadequacies of the grade point average (GPA) as a measure of achievement. Pass/fail grades do eliminate the GPA, for better or worse, but they accomplish little else. The underlying assumptions that typically accompany traditional grading practices persist, meaning that the teacher is assumed to be "right" in making subjective judgments of achievement, students are assumed to be passive recipients of the pass or fail grade, and the methods for assessing learning typically do not change in any appreciable way. In some pass/fail systems, students are still awarded "grades" that distinguish levels of competence, such as "high pass," "pass," or "low pass," which is fact is not very different from assigning grades of A, B, or C. Teachers can still mystify grading expectations and processes, with the expectations for passing or failing remaining unstated and poorly defined until a problem arises. And, of course, the teacher is the one who has the ability to identify "a problem."

Being essentially situated within a paradigm that assumes that students require or deserve recognition from the teacher for levels of performance, pass/fail grading carries the disadvantage of not being able to distinguish and reward excellent performance, which leads to the shift to "high" and "low" passing marks. Rewarding or recognizing outstanding or excellent performance in itself is not the issue, and in fact the practices that I present below include ways to do so. However, when the promise of a reward (a high grade) is assumed to be the motivator for learning and is structured into the teaching plan as a motivator, the "lesson" conveyed is the importance of external rewards as motivators. This is a problem if as a teacher you would prefer to promote the intrinsic value of learning, of achieving one's potential, and stretching to reach toward excellence.

POWER/RELATIONSHIP ISSUES

Unlike the issues of grade inflation and pass/fail grading, the issue of inherent power imbalances inherent in traditional grading practices is seldom addressed in discussions of grading practices. Power dynamics in the classroom are hegemonic and fully institutionalized; they are so inherently "the way it is" that both teachers and students find it very difficult to deconstruct and examine the situation, even when we wish to do so.

To change power relationships in the classroom does not mean that the teacher abdicates power (as I tended to do early in my teaching career), nor does it mean that students take over what has traditionally been assumed to be the teacher's role (Espeland & Shanta, 2001). Power is not a property to be acquired and exchanged; it is a human quality that can be expressed to various degrees, given the context, the confidence, the knowledge, and the will to do so. Traditional grading practices perpetuate power-over dynamics, whereby the teacher holds the power to render judgment, to grant favors, or withholds. The student is assumed to have little to say about what the teacher renders in judgment, favors, or withholds. The student who does speak up and advocate for him- or herself is often viewed as "difficult," and the teacher who shifts toward a more open and sharing interaction is viewed from the traditional perspective as easy, soft, or irresponsible.

In fact, these typical assumptions and views of the situation are grounded in a dualistic, competitively-oriented, and often paternalistic world view. In order to shift, a fundamental shift in world view is required. In order to shift grading practices, all of these assumptions and viewpoints must be recognized as part of the problem. Recognizing power relationships in the classroom as part of the problem does not prescribe a solution; rather, the next step is to thoughtfully consider the ethic that will undergird classroom relationships, the meaning of power in the classroom, the ideal expressions of power, and what conditions can be created to open the way for power relationships to take on new forms. In short, this is the first step toward a praxis for grading.

PRAXIS

Praxis is thoughtful reflection and action that occurs in synchrony, directed toward transforming the world (Chinn, 2001). There is no single starting point, but for many teachers, the process begins with a realization that something about their practices of grading (action) is not satisfactory, and they begin to reflect on what they might do differently. When teachers begin to reflect on not only how things might change, but why, and what ideal they seek, they are entering the realm of praxis. Their grading practices change in deliberate, well-founded directions. As new practices take shape, the practices and the underlying values and ideals are again called into question and reframed in light of the experience in the world of action. The sections that follow outline the fundamental building blocks of my philosophical foundation for teaching, specifically in relation to grading practices. These are offered as examples along with an invitation to consider the elements that you might adopt or adapt for your own practices.

NODDINGS' FEMINIST PHILOSOPHY OF EDUCATION

My own teaching and grading practices are grounded in Nel Noddings' philosophy of education (Noddings, 1989, 1995). The fundamental premise underlying this philosophy is that all people can call forth their highest good. Given this premise, educational practices aim to provide a context in which this is not only possible, but probable.

Noddings acknowledges that all people (students and teachers) have the capacity for both good and evil, and that how "good" a person can be depends at least in part on how well he or she is treated. Traditional pedagogies and grading practices tend to be implicitly based on the premise that teachers are right and good, whereas students are prone to being wrong, lazy, cheaters, or otherwise "evil." When the assumption is that students are prone to evil, then grading practices must be designed to police all students, expecting that they will be found wanting or guilty of wrongdoing. Grades are given with the underlying assumption that they serve as punishments for not achieving or for not accomplishing something.

Noddings' philosophy shifts to practices that call forth the best in everyone, including teachers. The focus is on celebrating accomplishments, with clearly defined standards and expectations that convey for everyone what is expected. One of the most important aspects of the philosophy in practice is the shift toward reducing the opportunities and temptations for "evil," instead of policing to prevent wrongdoing. When teachers state that students cannot share their work with one another and must keep their work to themselves, for example, an entire structure must be set up to police this expectation, conveying to students that the teacher views any sharing as "cheating." If, instead, the teacher encourages students to share their work, and integrates the process of collegial critique into the learning and grading process, then "cheating" is no longer an issue.

There are four dimensions of Noddings' approach to caring education. They are modeling, dialogue, practice, and confirmation.

Modeling is showing what it means to care. In terms of grading practices, modeling includes keeping promises by giving students clearly defined expectations and criteria for performance, and being consistent (not rigid) with those expectations in all evaluation and grading practices. The difference between consistency and rigidity is like the difference between water and ice. Both are composed of the same elements—clearly stated expectations. However, consistency means that you can flow with circumstances in applying and using the criteria. You give specific feedback and encourage students to learn from mistakes or "less-than" early attempts, with suggestions for the next step tailored to meet the needs of each situation. Positive encouragement every step of the way includes helping students to make realistic choices about what they are doing and what they might accomplish.

Dialogue is the ongoing process of discussing what you are doing and why. Where grading practices are concerned, this means shifting from a power-over mode of interaction to an interactive process. Teachers are responsible to assure that students meet certain professional standards of performance. Students are responsible to invest time and effort in attaining the standards. Grades can be conceptually defined in terms of the standards. Early discussion of the standards helps everyone (including the teacher) better understand how this class, and the expectations for grades, contribute to each student's competence in the profession. In the early discussions, teachers and students enter into a mutual dialogue that might include negotiating some of the details of the grading plan and expectations without compromising the professional standards that guide sound nursing practice.

For example, students might have an idea for an activity that is different from the activities planned by the teacher, but that is equally well suited to meeting the expectations of the course. The teacher brings up issues or concerns from their perspective (perhaps the time lines involved) and other students also contribute their perspectives. Everyone considers if this activity is adequate to address the underlying standards of the profession. Everyone comes to an agreement about the activity. In this way, the teacher is not the sole "broker" deciding whether or not an alternative can be pursued, and all students have the benefit of considering the possibility of an alternative, not just a few.

Practice in caring includes the processes of cooperation and sharing. In grading practices, this can mean engaging broad "audiences" as witnesses of what students are accomplishing. Sharing drafts of writing with one another, and giving one another constructive feedback, helps students to learn the practice of giving and taking constructive criticism. Presentations of their work to a group of nurses or fellow students provide the opportunity to receive recognition and feedback for what they have accomplished. Witnesses provide a context in which one another's talents and perspectives are respected. Knowing that your work is unique, special, or creative only happens when others see it, and when grading practices include others as observers, witnesses, and evaluators, the teacher's voice becomes one of many rather than a single (power-over) judge.

Confirmation is the process of affirming the best for all. Grades are defined conceptually so that they are linked to a meaningful idea that connects what is happening in the classroom with what is happening in the larger professional world. Confirmation implies criterion-based assessment, wherein the standards of performance are clearly set forth in advance, and all students know what is required to achieve the standards. In this approach to grading, all students can reach the best levels of performance in terms of the standards, but even more important, all students can reach their best level of performance given their personal abilities and circumstances. All students are responsible for engaging in ongoing reflections about what they are doing and why, to make decisions about their learning experience, and to demonstrate what they have accomplished. When these shifts occur, then the focus moves away from grades for the sake of getting grades. Even in grade-oriented systems, when the teacher builds in various ways to give and receive confirmation, and engages everyone in the process, students learn how to become self-reflective practitioners and how to give and receive constructive feedback.

FEMINIST VALUE-BASED IDEALS

One of the most important insights that comes from feminist thought is expressed in the phrase "the personal is political." This powerful phrase has many dimensions of meaning including the idea that one's personal values inevitably become expressed in public actions, words and deeds. In western cultures, people are accustomed in the public realm to words that say one thing and actions that convey another. In fact, words can easily belie one's underlying values; actions are more often consistent with the real underlying values. This same dynamic is all too often characteristic of grading practices in a classroom, where a teacher states that the grading practices are just, fair, and responsive to student concerns, but in actual practice, being structured within the traditions of patriarchal institutions, the practices are far from the stated ideal. The typical outcomes of most traditional grading practices are alienation, advantage for some, disadvantage for others, and individual dissatisfaction.

From a feminist perspective, the ideal would be a world where words and actions are consistent, with both grounded in a system of explicit values that benefit all members of a community. One of the first steps toward reaching this ideal is to clarify and make explicit the values on which your words and actions rest. The next step is to design grading practices that match these values as closely as possible. In *Peace and Power: Building Communities for the Future* (Chinn, 2001), I discussed a number of personal powers that can form a solid value-based foundation from which to design alternative grading practices. These powers, and how they translate into grading practices, are:

Power of consciousness. This is a fundamental power on which alternative grading practices are based. Traditional grading practices are planned and implemented without consciousness; very few teachers consider why they are administering a test, or assigning a paper, why they are grading in a certain way, much less examining the underlying assumptions and values on which their assignments and tests are based. In shifting to conscious grading practices, you may or may not administer a test, or assign a written paper. If you do include these traditional bases for grades, you will do so with conscious rationale, conscious intention, and a consciously constructed approach to how the work is used in the grading process.

Power of responsibility. This is another fundamental power on which alternative grading practices are based. Responsibility from a feminist standpoint means making your own values and your intentions transparent and keeping everyone informed so that nothing is mystified. Most traditional grading practices are shrouded in mystery, so much so that even the teacher may not be sure as to what underlies a particular grading practice (for example, what is the rationale for an "A" grade being a score of 95–100?). Teachers are responsible for demystifying their grading practices and for providing a rich supply of learning tools to enhance growth and achievement. Students (and teachers) are responsible for investing their time and energy into the activities that nurture and call forth their growth and development.

Power of process. This means setting aside time in the classroom for everyone to discuss the grading practices and the value basis from which the practices have been designed. It means that the practices include a process-orientation, meaning that students have time and opportunities to develop their work in stages, receiving feedback along the way to encourage their development.

Power of letting go. For teachers, this means letting go of old practices in order to embrace the alternatives, and continually reflecting on your words and actions to increase your awareness of ways in which old habits are creeping back into your interactions. It also can mean letting go of the exclusive power to judge student work.

Powers of the whole and of collectivity. These powers mean taking into the account the interests of the group as a whole, and bringing everyone's concern into discussions of grading practices. Instead of students coming to the teacher to request a "grace period" for a due date on an assignment, for example, the emphasis shifts to everyone bringing any ideas they have for altering the grading plan to the whole class so that everyone can consider the alternative. The outcome might be that everyone (including the teacher) agrees to a new due date, or everyone agrees that those who need it can have a different due date from others in the class.

Power of solidarity. Solidarity means openly addressing conflict and difference. It does not mean passive agreement or consensus. When grading practices are at issue, the issues are brought into the open, and all concerns are considered in coming to a resolution.

Powers of sharing, integration, and nurturing. These powers, taken together, mean that everyone treats everyone else in the group with respect. Everyone contributes to assisting one another to grow and develop, with constructive feedback exchanged freely. As students receive feedback on their work from several different other people in the class (including the teacher), they realize that different people perceive their work differently. Everyone learns to value the integration of different perspectives, and learns to discern those perspectives that are the most beneficial in promoting their own growth and development.

Power of distribution. This means taking steps to overcome imbalances in resources among members of the group, and assuring that everyone has what they need to accomplish their best. Unless it is essential to an accomplishment that something be done within a set period of time, then if some students need more time to accomplish a task, the extra time is actually equalizing the resource that they need to succeed relative to those students who do not require the same amount of time.

Power of intuition. Drawing on the power of intuition means taking the time to think, feel and experience what is unfolding as your grading practices are put into effect. If you begin to feel uncomfortable with what is happening, or if others are feeling uncomfortable, then it is time to acknowledge the "dis-ease," discuss it with those who are most directly affected, and take the risks involved in shifting what is happening if this is indicated.

Power of diversity. In order to embrace the anticipated needs and concerns of different students, grading practices are designed with options and alternatives that can accommodate different needs and circumstances. You will not be able to anticipate each and every need or concern, but if your grading practices reflect the value that your intention is to be responsive to individual needs, then students learn this value and learn to accommodate and embrace a wider diversity of response from others as well. If your expectation is the best from everyone, then most often students respond with appreciation for your efforts to acknowledge their needs and are, in turn, more able to respond to your needs as a teacher.

EXAMPLES

The grading practices that I have designed and used vary widely, and can be quite different for undergraduate, master's, or doctoral students. However, there also are many similarities based on the consistent underlying values. One fundamental tool for demystification of grading is to conceptually define the grades that are to be earned in the course. This practice guides the development of a criterion-based grading plan and helps students and teacher remain focused on the "why" of what happens in the class, rather than the "what" of getting things done. Students are encouraged to work toward a professional standard, not a score. For example, in an undergraduate clinical course, conceptual definitions for grades might be:

- C: a passing grade that represents accomplishment of the course objectives, and achieving fundamental safety in one's own nursing practice.
- B: above competencies, plus ability to influence the quality of care for a group of patients.
- A: above competencies, plus ability to influence nursing care standards.

These conceptual definitions then guide learning activities and a grading plan that encourages students to anticipate and decide what level of effort and accomplishment they can and will invest in the learning experience. Students who earn a grade of "A," for example, might present at a meeting of a professional organization a case study that examines the quality of care in a clinical situation and proposes ways in which the standard might be strengthened. The feedback that they receive from those who attend the presentation can be incorporated into their learning portfolio. In this type of clinical course, multiple-choice exams can be viewed similarly to the NCLEX. All students must achieve a passing score (indicating fundamental safety) in order to pass the course (typically a grade of C or better), but high scores do not contribute to higher grades. Many students earn higher grades, which has intrinsic value as confirmation of how well the student knows and understands factual material. When grades are not linked to exam scores, the energy shifts toward learning the material and toward activities that demonstrate achievements other than comprehension of facts.

Being explicit about expectations in making assignments is fundamental to sound, value-based grading. Table 6.1 shows an example of a group project assignment from a course designed for first-year nursing majors, and open to all students in the university. The course is entitled "Introduction to Health." The section that I taught had a total of 78 students enrolled on five campuses. It was delivered synchronously using a televised interactive system. There also was a WebCT component. All course materials were available on WebCT, and all assignments and quizzes were completed on WebCT. I rotated my presence on each campus so that I interacted in person with each group of students several times during the semester.

The group project was designed to meet the course objective: Explore avenues for responsible participation in sociopolitical action to influence the health of communities worldwide. The assignment was

TABLE 6.1   Example of Group Project Assignment for Freshman Course

Guidelines for community resource project groups

Purpose

To identify and assess the adequacy of the resources on your campus, in the surrounding community, and on the Web that are available for students and related to your assigned topic. Each group will be assigned a topic, and will be responsible for presenting its findings on the date identified in the course syllabus. Specifically, you will:

1. Find out what resources and services are available for information, prevention, recovery, and emergency assistance related to your topic
2. Identify how to access each resource or service
3. Assess how adequate each resource is and how it could be improved
4. Identify what is missing and propose what needs to be implemented to adequately serve the campus community

Suggested Ways to Gather Information

- Contact the student health service, campus security, logically related administrative offices or organizations on campus and in your community. If they have an office or physical location, visit the location and talk with people about what you are doing. Obtain literature or information that they would hand out to any "walk-in" student.
- Set up interviews with key informants who can give you more information about their services. Use the information in the text that is related to your topic to form questions about the kinds of services they offer. Ask the informant their own assessment of how adequate their service is, how it could be improved, and what is needed to make the changes.
- Surf the Web to find out what is available on the Web if a student needs information or assistance. Identify one or two sample sources that are not helpful (to demonstrate to the class) and those sources that you think are very helpful.
- In your group meetings, share what you are finding and suggest any other ideas for follow-up.

Group Members and Responsibilities

Each group will have between 4 and 7 members. Every member of the group will conduct at least one interview (with one or two other group members if possible). Every member of the group will collect ideas for resources from the Web. In addition, depending on your group size, select members to accomplish your task. Here is a suggested outline of roles that you can consider:

1. Community Liaison (contact person for keeping track of interviews and for coordinating the contacts between group members and people in the community)

(continued)

TABLE 6.1 *(continued)*

---

2. Community Scout (in charge of collecting all the leads for places to explore on campus and in the community)
    # 1 and 2 can be combined into one role
3. Convener (coordinates group meetings and organizes agendas to discuss what the group is finding and how to bring it all together)
4. Recorder (keeps track of who is doing what and takes minutes of the group meetings)
    # 3 and 4 can be combined
5. Web organizer (collects leads on the Web and does an initial assessment of how useful the sites are)
6. Presentation producer (makes sure that all the materials are ready for the presentation, e.g., handouts, Power Point, leaflets, etc.)
7. Presentation director (develops the plan for the presentation and makes sure everyone knows what to do)
    # 6 and 7 can be combined.

Process Guidelines

- Plan on meeting as often as you need in order to get your work done. Any member of the group can request a meeting. The Convener will gather all the agenda items and coordinate the time and place for group meetings.
- The class period on October 10 (the day the midterm exam is due) will be devoted to group meetings. There also will be 15 to 20 minutes at the end of selected class sessions that can be used for group meetings.
- Contact the instructor by class e-mail at any time that you need assistance.
- Take the "letter of introduction" from the instructor to every site you visit, and to every interview, and be sure that the people you speak to know you are doing this as a class assignment.
- At least 2 members should attend every interview with a community resource person.

---

also intended to enhance personal interaction and involvement among members of the class on each campus, as well as to provide an opportunity for students to display their accomplishments for the entire group on all campuses in a final presentation. The initial description sets the stage for what is expected, suggestions on how to go about accomplishing the task, and sets the groundwork for what is expected of each student.

Grades for this assignment were based on three narrative "progress reports" completed by each student. Students were evaluated based on their own work and their personal reflections as to what they were accomplishing, and on what they were learning about how to work effectively in a group. Effective group process guidelines were presented and discussed in class, and the information also was available on WebCT for review and discussion.

Each narrative assignment asked for the student's reflections concerning how they were progressing in their group, the issues or challenges of the group, the strengths of the group, and what they needed to be able to complete their part of the group work. Each assignment was preceded by an explanation as to how their responses would be graded. The second progress report, for example, had the following explanation:

> By the time you complete this progress report, you should know what your group responsibilities are, who else is in your group and what they are going to do, and have a schedule of group meetings. Complete the items below with an emphasis on your own reflections and ideas. Your grade is based on the cohesiveness of your plan for your own work in the group, your insights related to the group process, and your understanding of the link between your role and the purposes of the group project. This report is worth 10 points toward your course grade.

The grading of essay responses (as in this example) is clearly a subjective judgment, and yet guidelines can be developed and shared to demystify how you are viewing narrative assignments and what you value in a response. Here is an example of the guidelines I used in providing feedback, and grades, for narrative assignments in the "Introduction to Health" course:

- GOOD—full credit. Response is well focused on the assignment, thoughtful, reflects depth of insight, and reflects application of the principles and theories covered in class and in readings
- MODERATE—partial credit. Response is pertinent to the assignment, including some necessary reflection, insight, and application of principles.
- POOR—lowest credit. Response is pertinent to the assignment but lacks specific reflection and insight.
- INADEQUATE—no credit. Response is not related to the assignment or is missing.

For a doctoral class of 6–12 students, the approach I use for grading is quite different. My grading practices shift to a more interactive and collegial style. The most influential factor is the group size, not necessarily the level of student; I tend to use this type of style in any class that is smaller than about 15 students. However, for doctoral students I anticipate that they will welcome the opportunity to self-design specific projects that fit the overall scholarly agenda that they are developing. The approach outlines an initial set of activities that I plan in advance as a basis for accomplishing the course objectives, and subsequently for grading. The initial activities are discussed during the first class. At any time during the semester, students (or the teacher) can suggest alternatives to the initial plan as long as the alternatives are presented to the group as a whole. In fact, this does not happen often, but when it does, it is always to the benefit of everyone involved. Each student prepares a portfolio demonstrating their accomplishments, and includes a self-evaluation narrative that includes a self-assigned grade.

As I indicate in the course syllabus, my role is to "bear witness" and affirm their accomplishments. If I cannot do this in good conscious, then we discuss the issues involved. In about 20 years of using this approach to graduate-level grading, I have had very few occasions when I have had to address issues with a student. In several instances, I felt that the student had underestimated their accomplishments and deserved a better grade than they self-assigned. Contrary to the expectation that many might have concerning such an approach, not all the self-assigned grades have been "A" grades. Many self-assigned grades are "A minus" or "B plus." A few students have even self-assigned "B minus" or "C," with which I typically have concurred. But in fact, I do not expect this kind of grade to surface often, given the very high level of competence that graduate students have demonstrated in order to even enter a graduate program. In almost every instance, I have been satisfied that the accomplishments justify the student's self-assigned grade.

Table 6.2 shows the "grades" section of a syllabus from a recent doctoral course. The basic components of the grading plan could apply to almost any course in which students are engaging in independently defined assignments and projects. The plan is deliberately general and not specific to the actual "assignments" because the group may design alternatives to the outline of activities that I provide in the syllabus. In the course from which this table is extracted, students typically complete one project that is presented to everyone in the class, and one scholarly writing project. They typically have participated in providing feedback

TABLE 6.2   Example of a Grading Plan for a Doctoral-Level Course

Grades

Grades in this course are an expression of the quality of your scholarly achievements. Grades are earned, not given, and are derived through a process of mutual reflection. The learning activities that are suggested provide guidance in developing your scholarship, but you are the primary architect of your learning experience, and you shape your achievements according to your personal goals and interests. Early in the course, reflect on the course objectives and the planned learning activities. Reflect on what you want to learn and accomplish in this class, and draft a plan to guide your experiences. Keep this plan and revise it frequently, and use it as a basis for your self-evaluation at the end of the course.

The process for deriving your grade begins with the development of your scholarly portfolio. The portfolio includes, but is not limited to, your:

- Personal learning goals for this class.
- Written self-evaluation of your achievements.
- Statement of the grade you earned through these achievements.
- Material providing evidence of your self-evaluation (scholarly writing, notes or outlines used for class discussions/presentations, etc.)

Your self-evaluation can be based on your own ideas about what you personally hoped to accomplish in this class, as well as reflections on your personal growth and learning. Also reflect on the quality of your achievements in terms of the following questions:

- Has my work been consistent with the course objectives?
- Did I also accomplish my personal goals for the course?
- Is my written work readable, concise, clearly written, and attractively presented?
- Have my group presentations been clear and interesting?
- Have my written and verbal presentations included my own original ideas?
- Have I frequently considered more than one point of view?
- Have I thought about and presented possibilities for future directions in nursing?
- Have I accurately credited other authors where I have drawn on their work?

Generally, if you can answer "yes" to each of these questions, you have met the essential expectations of the course and certainly have earned a grade of "B." If your answers to several of these questions is not only "yes" but an enthusiastic "YES," and you also were able to exercise creativity and accomplishments beyond your expectations, be confident and proud that you have earned an "A" grade.

These questions also will be considered by faculty in verifying your statement of the grade earned through your achievements. If the faculty has reservations about your self-evaluation, we will discuss these reservations until we agree on a grade that you have earned

Incomplete grades will not be used, except in the case of extenuating circumstances that emerge after the last date for withdrawal.

for one another as they develop their work, and have discussed one another's work in class at length, the processes and outcomes of which can be integrated into their portfolio.

CONCLUSIONS

Grading is one of the most difficult challenges for teachers who wish to move toward interactions that are more consistent with nursing philosophies and values than are the traditional approaches. The tensions and conflicts that teachers experience in this process are inherent in the contradictions of living and working in systems that rest on a set of values that stand in sharp contrast to the human values upon which nursing rests, and that many teachers prefer to embrace. The tensions also reflect internal conflicts between how we have been socialized into the academic community, and our desire to shift to preferred practices that are not as comfortable or familiar. The efforts to make that shift are often fraught with difficulty. I have offered some suggestions and insights based on my experiences, and examples that might be useful. However, the best teacher and guide in making the shift is, I believe, an internal awareness of the self that emerges as one opens to the journey, experiencing and following one's own feelings and responses along the way.

REFERENCES

Basinger, D. (1997). Fighting grade inflation: A misguided effort? *College Teaching,* 45(3), 88–91.

Chinn, P. L. (2001). *Peace & power: Building communities for the future* (5th ed.). Sudbury, MA: Jones & Bartlett.

Edwards, C. H. (2000). Grade inflation: The effects on educational quality and personal well being. *Education, 120,* 538–546.

Espeland, K., & Shanta, L. (2001). Empowering versus enabling in academia. *Journal of Nursing Education, 40,* 343–346.

Lawler, P. A. (2001). Grade inflation, democracy, and the Ivy League. *Perspectives on Political Science, 30,* 133–136.

Loustau, A., & O'Connor, A. B. (1999). Commentary. *Journal of Nursing Education, 38,* 398–399.

McSpirit, S., Chapman, A., Kopacz, P., & Jones, K. (2000). Faculty ironies on grade inflation. *Journal of Instructional Psychology, 27,* 104–109.

Noddings, N. (1989). *Women and evil*. Berkeley, CA: University of California Press.

Noddings, N. (1995). *Philosophy of education*. Boulder, CO: Westview Press.

Pollio, H. R., & Beck, H. P. (2000). When the tail wags the dog. *Journal of Higher Education, 71*(1), 84–102.

Shoemaker, J. K., & DeVox, M. (1999). Are we a gift shop? A perspective on grade inflation. *Journal of Nursing Education, 38*, 394–398.

Svinicki, M. D. (1998). Helping students understand grades. *College Teaching, 46*, 101–105.

Chapter 7

Computers and Testing

Marilyn Blau Klainberg

Although computers have been around for a considerable time, the use of computers in health care and health care education, specifically nursing and nursing education, has only been notable within the past ten years. Initially, because of the cost and cumbersome size of computers, they were used mainly for data collection and analysis. The introduction of desktop and laptop computers, personal digital assistants (PDAs), the Internet, and the World Wide Web has forever changed the use of computers in health care and health care education. Rapid expansion of computers and the Internet in the home and in education has affected how we present information, analyze data, and measure knowledge. The focus of this chapter is computer testing in nursing education. The chapter examines available computer testing software, discusses the benefits and drawbacks for faculty and students of computer testing, and provides an overview of available technology for computer testing.

NCLEX-RN EXAMINATION

In 1986, the decision-making body of the National Council of the State Boards of Nursing voted to attempt to improve the method of testing new graduates by exploring and developing computerized testing. It was determined that Computerized Adaptive Testing (CAT) software would be used to assess nurses' competence for safe practice (Julian, Wendt, Way, & Zara, 2001).

Prior to using the computer for the National Council Licensing Examination for Registered Nurses (NCLEX-RN), testing new nursing school graduates took two days and consisted of 372 questions. Between 1990 and 1992, the National Council of the State Boards of Nursing conducted two field tests using the NCLEX-RN CAT format. Volunteer students were recruited for these field tests. The volunteers took the NCLEX-RN test with paper and pencil, either followed or preceded by the NCLEX-RN CAT. The outcome of this testing was that in 1994, the National Council of State Boards of Nursing changed from a paper-and-pencil test format to the CAT method of testing (Julian, Wendt, Way, & Zara, 2001).

COMPUTERIZED ADAPTIVE TESTING

Computer-Adaptive Testing uses item response theory, which is different from classical test theory in that it decreases test length and improves reliability (Gershon & Bergstrom, 1991). The examination for each test taker is compared with a passing standard to determine whether the individual passed or failed the examination (Julian, Wendt, Way, & Zara, 2001). A CAT is designed to measure mastery of a subject by the test taker and may vary in length for each test taker. It adapts to the demands of the test provider and to the knowledge of the test taker. A CAT utilizes a pool of questions at incremental levels. As the test taker correctly responds to a question, the level of difficulty of the examination increases (Bushweller, 2000). With each correct response, the number of questions needed to be answered by the test taker decreases.

According to the Northwest Evaluation Association, a nonprofit educational research organization, as the CAT adjusts the questions given, based on a test taker's responses, it is not only tailoring the examination to discover the information known but also is assessing the student's knowledge more quickly (Bushweller, 2000). This also reduces considerably the amount of time that is required for the test taker to complete the examination. For example, NCLEX-RN CAT can take a maximum of four hours and a minimum of one hour to complete as opposed to two days of testing using a paper-and-pencil method (Bloom & Trice, 1997). If the test taker answers a question incorrectly, the difficulty of the questions initially decreases, and more questions are used to determine the test taker's knowledge of the subject matter.

Therefore, on the CAT, not all question difficulty is the same, nor do all test takers have the same number of questions to answer. The examination is personalized to assess each individual test taker's knowledge (Bushweller, 2000).

Although CAT software is available for classroom testing, at this moment the technology for this type of test construction is cumbersome and not cost effective. FastTest and FastTEST Professional, available from Assessment Systems Corporation (2002a), are examples of adaptive testing. These programs use item response theory and audio and visual graphics for specific types of testing. They create a hierarchical item bank that can be used to generate paper and pencil examinations with an optional delivery on a personal computer. However, the software is expensive and complicated to use. As technology advances, less expensive and complicated software is not far behind.

For now, there are testing software packages, which provide examinations for students to take on the computer, that are readily available, cost effective, and easy to use. Despite this, and the fact that the NCLEX-RN is offered exclusively on the computer, computer testing of nursing students in the classroom remains comparatively underutilized in nursing education. There is concern that the lack of testing by computer might affect the success of nursing students who are not exposed to computerized testing prior to taking the NCLEX-RN. As students become more familiar with reading and answering questions from a computer screen, they increase their comfort level and skill related to this method of testing.

OTHER SOFTWARE FOR COMPUTER TESTING

Computer technology for the actual development of examinations for assessment of classroom knowledge, or other areas of testing, is available with diverse software at varying levels of sophistication. This technology can be used to create examinations that can be given on the computer itself, or using the traditional paper-and-pencil method. It has the ability to develop tests using traditional multiple choice, multiple response, matching (selection/association), true/false, fill-in, and simulation questions. These are simple to score via the computer, provide the test taker with immediate electronic feedback, and provide faculty with immediate information about test outcomes. These programs include tests or testing programs that are provided on an internal network, a disk, or a CD-ROM, or are available at a Web site that offers computer testing programs.

There also are some essay testing programs in which questions are posed and students answer these in composition or essay form. Although these are offered by computer, they require faculty to read and grade each paper individually (Valenti, Cucchiarelli, & Panti, 2002).

Examinations may be provided using either an Internet testing provider or by placing the test on a computer disk or CD-ROM. Internet programs permit the instructor to place an examination online, and then students can access the test via the Internet, either in a particular place and/or at a specific time. These programs may stand alone or be part of a total Internet package to which the educational institution subscribes. For example, Blackboard and WebCT offer ExamView (FSCreations, Inc., 2002) computer examination software, as part of their online delivery systems. Computer examinations may be given to individual students or groups of students. These software packages also provide the opportunity for faculty to develop test banks from which to generate tests for the group or prepare individual multiple question examinations.

Platform and system requirements of the computers must be considered when purchasing computer software or using available testing freeware. Schools or departments of nursing must work closely with their technology departments to find programs that will not only meet the needs of the faculty and students but also will meet the hardware requirements of the computers.

Underutilization of online testing and other software programs that provide computer testing may be due to a variety of reasons. These include:

- Insufficient availability of computers on which students may be tested
- Inability to monitor students using the computer for testing
- Faculty or support staff unfamiliar or uncomfortable with the methodology of transferring the examination to the computer (which initially may be time consuming)
- Discomfort of faculty in using the computer software

However, the benefits of using computer testing, discussed later in the chapter, far outweigh the difficulty with adjusting to using the computer for testing.

OTHER USES OF COMPUTER TECHNOLOGY FOR TESTING IN NURSING

Associate technology has long been available to grade paper-and-pencil examinations. While schools of nursing may not use computer technology for classroom testing of students, many schools use some form of technology to analyze and grade multiple choice, multiple response, matching, and true/false paper-and-pencil examinations. An example of this would be the use of an optical scanner for the grading of answer sheets that are completed by the students after reading questions from a paper-and-pencil examination. These answer sheets are then put through a computer that has an optical scanner. The results provide a score for each student and analyze the data for the total number of students. This is considered an associate program. It is different from other computer software programs that provide actual testing of the student using a computer testing program, which provides the examination and response availability on the computer itself.

The simplest software for these computer programs grades examinations, and the more advanced software analyzes the data generated from the examinations themselves. The advanced software provides the faculty member with information about the item analysis of each question, information concerning the deviation from the standard of the mean of individual students, and aggregate data.

Products such as Examiner (Assessment Systems Corporation, 2002b) create paper-and-pencil or computer-based multimedia tests that improve the teacher's ability to use visuals as part of the testing package. Computerized tests using Examiner allow the teacher to add graphics, sound, video and CD-ROMs for questions for which graphics would be required. There are many other test software packages available.

As simulation programs grow more available on the computer, they may become the next wave of computerized testing. An example of this is programs that provide laboratory testing for online chemistry courses in distance education programs.

Another area in nursing that already uses computer technology to provide testing is Computer Assisted Instruction (CAI). Computer Assisted Instruction technology has been available for many years. With CAI, students take multiple choice, matching, true/false, or fill-in questions at the end of the program on the computer. This gives immediate feedback to the students about what information they have or have not acquired from the CAI. The test outcomes may provide additional grades to the faculty member or simply may be used to provide information to the student.

CAI programs are available on computer disks, CD ROM, and most recently the Internet. Additionally, desktop and Internet computer programs are available that provide NCLEX-RN test preparation courses and mock examinations. These may be purchased at bookstores or through online providers. Companies such as Educational Resources, Inc. (2002) provide diagnostic testing online or via a disk or CD ROM at a desktop computer for individual courses throughout a nursing program or as part of a total testing preparation and NCLEX-RN review. Additionally, nursing courses offered for distance education use computer testing to assess learning. These may include continuing education courses as well as distance education courses that are part of a nursing curriculum. Courses offered and tested by computer may either be hybrid courses, which include both face-to-face and online components, or distance education courses offered entirely on the computer. Computerized testing is often used in distance education courses for feedback. Whether distance education courses are for continuing education or as part of the curriculum, computerized testing is a quick and efficient way to monitor what students are learning and assess their individual needs. Computerized testing provides immediate feedback for the student as well as the faculty member who is teaching the course.

BENEFITS OF COMPUTERIZED TESTING FOR FACULTY AND STUDENTS

An advantage for faculty and students using a computerized test is the time saved. There may be little or no need for a posttest review in the classroom following the examination. Students taking an examination using either a computer testing program on a disk, the network, or the Internet can get immediate feedback and the rationale for the correct or incorrect responses after submitting their examination. Classroom time is often limited, and computer testing frees up classroom time for additional learning opportunities (Bloom & Trice, 1997). Paper-and-pencil tests are more time consuming than computer testing, and reviewing the test during class wastes valuable class and faculty time that is better used for teaching. Research indicates that computer testing takes from one-quarter to one-half the amount of time as a paper-and-pencil test (Bloom & Trice, 1997).

Most computer testing programs provide immediate feedback for the student following the submission of the examination. Furthermore, they grade the examination and provide immediate information to the instructor. Faculty calibrate the computer software to accommodate how the computer will score the examination and provide feedback to the students. Examples of this might include the value of each question and whether the correct answer is provided to the student with an explanation. Some faculty also might include the rationale for incorrect answers. In addition, these programs interpret the raw score and do an item analysis for the faculty, making weak test questions easily identifiable.

Another advantage to developing computerized tests is that test bank item pools can be easily created so that student examinations can be individualized. Changes can be made to the examination up to minutes before actual testing, and there is no more need to send an examination for printing several weeks in advance. As this is a paper-free environment, the examination can be frequently changed or added to by the faculty. If test items seem too easy or hard, or no longer meet the objectives of the course, the flexibility in adjusting the test items even moments before an examination is rapid and simple. There also is flexibility in scheduling examinations and benefits to the environment by using less paper for testing.

If CAT formats are used in the preparation of an examination, time is saved in administration of the examination itself, since the testing process adapts to the correct or incorrect answers of the student. Whether a CAT or a standard computerized examination that is not adaptive is used, research indicates that students using the computer for testing take less time to complete examinations.

Despite some anxiety on the part of the student to using the computer for testing, computerized testing is efficient and saves time. There is little difference between the outcomes of paper-and-pencil and computer testing (DeAngelis, 2000). Faculty can feel secure that an examination offered on the computer will not affect or diminish the student's grade. However, simply placing a poorly constructed test into a computer-based testing program will not improve the examination or its intended outcomes. Preparing for the NCLEX-RN by taking examinations using a computer assists nursing students in developing skills such as reading and answering test questions on the computer.

When the issue of insufficient computers is the rationale for not providing computerized testing, then scheduling examinations may be the solution to the problem. Many educators schedule several examination periods during which students are tested. The student signs up for a specific time in the computer laboratory that is convenient for them. Students may be proctored by laboratory personnel, which saves classroom time and further frees up faculty. The cost of a proctor is minimal compared with the cost of faculty time.

To accommodate students, examinations may need to be scheduled over several time periods during the day or week. Some schools of nursing use the honor code for individual testing in a laboratory situation or if the student is taking the examination by computer at home. Other methods of controlling cheating on computerized tests may be scrambling questions on the examination, placing questions in a different order; choosing questions from a pool of items that would make each test different; and limiting the time of entry to and exit from the examination, which also limits the time per question. These would be a deterrent for student cheating if there is no proctor at the testing site.

A benefit for students is that they may be able to take the test at a time that best suits them. This further frees up class time and may eliminate the need for make-up examinations. Students also benefit from immediate feedback and are being prepared to take the NCLEX-RN on a computer (McEntee, 2002).

Faculty developing an examination to be given on the computer have the option to use either a self-designed examination or a commercially designed, computer-driven test bank. Most commercial test banks are available to accompany the textbook used in a course. Faculty, however, need to review the quality of items in these commercial test banks.

Faculty designed tests can be placed into a test bank that can be easily controlled to generate several tests that can then be retrieved and adjusted to a particular curriculum or testing site. Tests can be easily improved from semester to semester by using the item analysis, and faculty can build a pool of valid test questions.

SECURITY ISSUES RELATED TO COMPUTERIZED TESTING

Issues of security are a concern for many faculty. Several levels of security can be included in the development and implementation of the examination. These can range from minimal security, such as a pass code provided each test taker, to extremely secure test environments.

Examples of security for computer examinations might include photo identification on entering the computer testing area, further checking the photo identification with the class roster, a proctor or computer laboratory monitor to observe during testing periods, and restricting items such as books, paper, and book bags from the testing area. If paper is required for the test, such as scrap paper for calculations, paper should be provided to the test taker and retrieved at the end of the examination.

Whether an examination uses a proctor and photo identification or not, a pass code for access to take the examination should be provided to each student, with a specific time during which the test can be taken. Test taking protocols should include a beginning and an ending time after which the examination on the computer automatically ends.

Limited time access to a computerized test also is suggested for individual test takers whether the student takes the examination at home or on at the campus. Limiting the time the student has to read and respond to a question decreases the ability to look up answers. It is recommended that when using computer testing for large student groups, the faculty should arrange the same security and monitoring of the computer examinations as during any classroom examinations. Timed computer program software prohibits students from opening the program on the computer before a specific time and ends the examination at a specific time, which is determined by the faculty or institution.

RESEARCH: COMPUTER VERSUS PAPER-AND-PENCIL TESTING

Research by Bloom and Trice (1997) indicated that students who were given a test on a computer performed as well as students taking the paper-and-pencil form of the examination. The students included in this research were seniors in obstetrics/women's health and had been previous tested by computer in health assessment as beginning students. The outcome of the study indicated that senior students had significantly higher scores on their final examination than students in year two of the nursing program. Although this study did not explore previous experiences that students had with computers, it did strongly suggested that student familiarity with taking any format of an examination decreases anxiety. Bloom and Trice (1997) in their research recommended that nurse educators attempt to decrease anxiety in test taking by making students more familiar with computers and increasing computer literacy.

Indications are that familiarity with computer testing procedures increases the student's sense of security in using the computer for testing. Furthermore, examinations given by computer compared with those given by paper and pencil did not affect or bias student progress in the course (Bloom & Trice, 1997).

DeAngelis (2000) examined computer versus paper-based versions of an examination. Thirty senior dental hygiene students were randomly divided into two groups. Each group was tested, one using the computer for testing and one using a paper-and-pencil test for the first examination. The groups were then switched and took a second examination. Each student completed a survey that explored attitude, perception, and experience with computer testing. There were no significant differences between the scores of the students surveyed. Benefits expressed by the students about the computer examination included reduced time taking the examination and preference for immediate feedback. A major benefit identified by faculty was ease of item analysis for the group (DeAngelis, 2000).

A pilot study by Klainberg, Mottola, Trolman, Quigley, and Mawhirter (2000) sampled 48 senior nursing students. All students received a minimum of 45 minutes of training to prepare them for computer testing. CyberExam (Math Medics, LLC., 2002), a free, secure Internet computer testing program, was used. Two examinations were administered. The first was a midterm examination, the second a final examination. Students were randomly divided into two groups. Students in group one took the midterm examination using the computer, and students in group two took the same examination using the paper-and-pencil version. The groups were rotated for the final examination. There was no significant difference in test scores between students taking the computerized versus paper-and-pencil examination. Although there was a high level of anxiety among students taking the computerized examination, neither anxiety nor testing method had a statistically significant impact on test scores.

Rossignol and Scollin's (2001) study explored the use of computerized practice tests for students in an undergraduate nursing course. Two computerized practice tests were available for students prior to a paper-and-pencil unit examination. Scores were generally higher on the classroom test for those students who took the practice examination prior to the actual test. However, there was no significant difference between the scores of the students who did and did not take the practice test prior to the classroom test. A questionnaire provided the students following the classroom examination on the computer indicated that they enjoyed taking the practice exam and felt particularly that the immediate feedback and summary printouts were helpful. Students also expressed that they were better prepared to take the NCLEX-RN.

Attitudes toward computer testing were explored in the study done by Ogilvie, Trusk, and Blue (1999). Their study tested medical students using multiple-choice or matching image-based questions on computer examinations as well as extra credit quizzes. Two hundred and two students were tested in 1996 and 1997. The outcomes indicated overall satisfaction with computer testing. Students reported that they enjoyed taking both quizzes and examinations on the computer and that test taking was less time consuming.

Bushweller (2000) discussed concerns with computerized testing. He indicated that there are critics of computerized testing who believe that educators are accepting the trend toward computer testing, particularly in national standardized testing programs, without sufficient evaluation of its impact. In his study with eighth grade students, Bushweller compared students accustomed to writing on a computer with those who were not. He found that students familiar with writing on a computer did better on electronic testing than those who were not used to writing on the computer (Bushweller, 2000). If this is accurate, by not using computers for testing before taking the NCLEX-RN, are we placing our students at a disadvantage?

In a survey of 29 nursing programs, only 11 schools used computers for testing as part of the classroom experience. Students in 11 programs completed computer testing with their CAIs. Only 6 schools were using computers for test development and 10 to analyze test outcomes (Klainberg, unpublished data, 2002).

SUMMARY

Although schools of nursing may use computer programs to meet a variety of programmatic needs, such as developing test banks, creating tests, test scoring, item analysis, as part of CAIs, and for NCLEX-RN review, most still do not offer examinations on the computer to test classroom learning. Faculty continue to rely on paper-and-pencil testing.

Nursing faculty must meet the challenges of the 21st century. Computers are here to stay, and if we wish to prepare students to take the NCLEX-RN examination, we need to administer computerized tests. This will help reduce student test anxiety, help them to read efficiently from a computer screen, and enhance their ability to take the NCLEX-RN and other standardized computerized examinations. Clearly computer testing is here until the next bit of technology arrives to improve it in the future.

USEFUL WEB SITES FOR COMPUTER-TESTING SOFTWARE

Item Banking and Computerized Testing, see Assessment Systems Corporation at http://www.assess.com/Software/sSumTest.htm and http://www.assess.com/home.htm

CQuest Computerized Testing at http://www.cqtest.com/cqadmin.htm

ExamView at http://www.examview.com

REFERENCES

Assessment Systems Corporation. (2002a). *FastTEST Professional Makes Adaptive Testing Simple!* Retrieved November 16, 2002, from http://www.assess.com/Software/FTP16CAT.htm

Assessment Systems Corporation. (2002b). *The Examiner*. Retrieved November 16, 2002, from http://www.assess.com/

Bloom, K. C., & Trice, L. B. (1997). The efficacy of individualized computerized testing in nursing education. *Computers in Nursing, 15*, 82–88.

Bushweller, K. (2000). *Throw away the No. 2 pencils—Here comes computerized testing*. The School Technology Authority. Retrieved December 11, 2002, from www.electronic-school.com/2000/06/0600f1.html

DeAngelis, S. (2000). Equivalency of computer-based and paper-and-pencil testing. *Journal of Allied Health, 29*, 161–164.

Educational Resources, Inc. (2002). *Total Testing®*. Retrieved December 11, 2002, from http://www.eriworld.com/

FSCreations, Inc. (2002). *ExamView*. Retrieved November 16, 2002, from http://www.examview.com/

Gershon, R. C., & Bergstrom, B. (1991). *Individual differences In computer adaptive testing: Anxiety, computer literacy and satisfaction*. Paper presented at the Annual

Meeting of the National Council on Measurements in Education, San Francisco, CA.

Julian, E., Wendt, A., Way, D., & Zara, A. (2001). Moving a national licensure examination to computer. *Nurse Educator, 26,* 264–267.

Klainberg, M. (2002).

Klainberg, M., Mottola, C., Trolman, A., Quigley, M., & Mawhirter, D. (2000). The relationship of anxiety and testing method to test scores among senior student nurses. Unpublished paper.

Math Medics, LLC. (2002). *CyberExam.* Retrieved December 11, 2002, from http://www.sosmath.com/cyberexam/cyber.html

McEntee, S. (2002). Computerized testing not for every student: Online exams growing in popularity. *Columbia Chronicle Online.* Retrieved December 11, 2002, from http://www.ccchronicle.com/back/2002-03-04/campus5.html

Ogilvie, R. W., Trusk, T. C., & Blue, A. V. (1999). Students' attitudes towards computer testing in a basic science course. *Medical Education, 33,* 828–832.

Rossignol, M., & Scollin, P. (2001). Piloting use of computerized practice tests. *Computers in Nursing, 19,* 206–212.

Valenti, S., Cucchiarelli, A., & Panti, M. (2001, May 17). A framework for the evaluation of test management systems. *Current Issues in Education* [Online], 4(6). Available at: http://cie.ed.asu.edu/volume4/number6/.

Chapter 8

Usability Testing for Online Nursing Education: Thinking Aloud and Heuristic Evaluation

Dee McGonigle, Kathleen Mastrian, and Nedra Farcus

Online learning, electronic learning, or e-learning is an educational delivery tool being adopted by many nurse educators. The reasons for this are varied and include pressure from administrators who view online learning as a way to compete in a global market, from students who want the flexibility afforded by online learning, and from educators themselves who recognize the potential of e-learning. Educators involved in the design of e-learning episodes (subdivisions of learning such as a lesson, class, course, or program of study) span the continuum from novice to expert in technological integration skills. The extreme gap in the breadth and depth of skills may result in the design of online learning episodes that do not meet intended instructional goals. We believe that usability testing can help to ensure the quality of online learning materials.

You may be asking yourself, "Why should I be concerned with usability in online nursing education? Isn't usability a tool for software designers?" In this chapter we illustrate the adaptation of usability testing techniques, explain the reasons behind the need for this important validity check, and suggest a simple way to conduct two usability tests.

Educators who are developing e-learning episodes need a solid understanding of instructional design techniques and an indepth knowledge of online capabilities in order to develop dynamic learning materials. Often the online materials are only face-to-face materials placed in an electronic format. Instructors type in their syllabus and materials, and voilà, they proclaim an online course! This is one of the worst case examples. With even the best intentioned instructor, the result is anything but useful for learners. We must step back and realize that the medium itself has a critical impact on learning. How have we harnessed the potential of this medium to support our materials or course projection? Have we thought about the needs of our users/learners? Is our site intuitive? Did we provide a site map? These questions led us to adapt Nielsen's (1994) simplified thinking aloud and heuristics evaluation for the online nursing education environment.

THE E-LEARNING ENVIRONMENT

Online or e-learning is typically situated within course management systems (CMS) or course development shells. The wide variety of e-learning products such as CMS and development tools, as well as instructor-made or home-grown materials, creates a concern over the quality of the resulting educational episode. The learner must be able to easily access and use the course or educational materials to meet the learning goals. Initially, the usability issues must address the interface or the CMS. The various CMS environments on the market are similar enough in design and require minimal learning to move from one system to another. As learners become more familiar with the CMS environments, they will master the system technology, and it should eventually fade and become transparent.

As a learner-centered approach to education gains momentum, we recognize that the system is not what makes the most powerful impact on learning—it is the quality of learning materials or course content housed in the system. We must create a learning environment that enhances our learners' experience and fully engages them in the learning process. At times, our students learn in spite of the quality of our materials. However, we must commit to the critical evaluation of our materials to ensure that the learners have a quality educational experience.

All too often nurse educators are mired in the record keeping required by state boards of nursing, accrediting agencies, and curricular redesigns, without using basic tools to increase the usability of the educational materials. We evaluate what we teach but not how the critical content is made available to the learner. Evaluations typically do not address the fundamental usability of information or course work. With the addition of Internet-based or e-learning materials, usability assessments are even more critical.

USABILITY TESTING

"Usability" is how intuitive and easy it is for individuals to learn how to use and to interact with educational materials and products (Preece, 2001, p. 5). According to Bohmann (2001), "User interfaces have high levels of usability when users can achieve their goals" (p. 1). Programmers have applied usability testing techniques to the design of CMS interfaces and other tools that house course content. Usability testing, however, has not been systematically applied to educational materials or the actual content of online learning. Usability studies have focused primarily on the human-computer interaction side of technology development and implementation.

We believe that nurse educators must concern themselves with the usability of educational materials similar to programmers concerning themselves with the usability of the software, interfaces, and systems they develop. How do learners use our materials to learn in electronic educational episodes? An electronic educational episode can be a lesson, class, seminar, workshop, course, or program of study. We should verify and validate that the instructional intent is clear and that the goals of learning can be met given our instructional approach. These goals of learning, which can be cognitive, affective, or psychomotor, refer to the learners' definitions of what they are trying to accomplish by enrolling in our electronic educational episode. The situational use to which the learner is putting the e-learning content/materials at any given time during the learning episode is important. Usability testing also examines the way content is presented to the learner and how the learner potentially interacts with the content/materials, teacher, other learners, and experts in the field.

Online learning must be learner-centered. Brodsky (2003) stated, "Designing effective e-learning that keeps learners' needs in mind requires that any infatuation with technology, in and of itself, be put aside. The real focus must be on the practical execution of basic, sound instructional design and development principles" (p. 14). New adopters of technology may become enamored with the technology at the expense of learning goals. As educators, we should strive to meet the needs of the learners by creating useful materials that facilitate the instructional intent.

Learning is the intent of instruction. The authors define learning as a process used by students to integrate new skills, data, and information into their existing knowledge and skill base, resulting in enduring changes in knowledge, behavior, attitude, and/or capability. The framework for this process is developed at an early age and is continually refined. The question we must ask as educators is, "From the learner's perspective, how usable are my materials?" In other words, are we facilitating the student's learning process?

INNOVATION

Comprehensive usability studies used by software or product designers are expensive and time-intensive. The current university and nursing budget climate creates a barrier to the use of this comprehensive testing. Nevertheless, nurse educators must recognize what is essential to the creation of quality online learning experiences. Therefore, we must devise cost-effective ways of addressing usability issues. This challenge led us to explore Nielsen's (1994) discount usability techniques.

Usability testing can be daunting to those who do not understand Nielsen's (1994) concept or strategy. According to him, discount usability engineering can save money and time. The method is based on the use of three techniques: scenarios, simplified thinking aloud, and heuristic evaluation. Each of these techniques can be adapted to test the usability of our educational materials. This is an important first step for nursing educators. The marketplace is highly competitive, and we must ensure that our materials meet the goals of learning. Usability testing helps verify that our materials meet the instructional intent. Once usability problems are identified, they can be corrected, and our online materials will become more robust for the learners.

We have selected two of Nielsen's techniques, simplified thinking aloud and heuristic evaluation, for adaptation to nursing education usability testing. Simplified thinking aloud refers to bringing in real users, giving them typical instructional tasks, and asking them to think out loud while they perform them (Nielsen, 1994). We can ask students to explore and use portions of our materials, have them state out loud what they are doing, and take notes for review. This is a relatively simple, yet powerful and inexpensive way to assess the ease with which future learners can use the materials. Nielsen recommended asking three to five test users for each usability test.

Heuristic evaluation is what it implies—using standards to assess the usability of our materials. As shown in Table 8.1, a mnemonic has been created using the letters in the word usability (McGonigle, 2002). This guide for usability in e-learning helps us remember the usability issues. The "U" refers to the user or learner when the usability testing is applied to the educational milieu. The remaining letters refer to the system, attributes, basics, interface, learning engagement, interaction, target, and yield. Walking through this mnemonic provides a quick overview on usability and helps us focus on the usability issues. The criteria reflect what we should be looking for in relation to our e-learning educational materials.

McGonigle (2003) has suggested a preliminary set of educational attributes important to usability testing. These nine attributes cover the standards or principles that should be assessed during the heuristic evaluation of online or e-learning materials (Table 8.2). The attributes range from number one, relating to the purpose of the e-learning episode, to number nine, dealing with user/learner satisfaction.

APPLICATION

Know thy learner! Usability is the key to the development of a learner-centered perspective. Application of the e-learning simplified thinking aloud and heuristic techniques can provide insights for educators as to how they may strengthen their learner-centered approaches and interactive learning experiences in the materials they develop.

To implement usability testing, we suggest that you select small sections of your materials and conduct a simplified thinking aloud evaluation. For each section, observe three to five learners using your materials. The learners should be representative of your end users. The typical time frame for this type of testing ranges from 1 to 2 hours. Choose a learning episode that the learners can work through in your allotted time frame, for example, working through an assignment or one lesson in your course.

TABLE 8.1   Usability for Online Learning

Usability issue	Criteria
USER/Learner	Characteristics Capabilities • Cognitive • Affective • Psychomotor • Computer savvy • E-learning savvy Impairments Educational level Gender Age Socioeconomic status Learning style

SYSTEM	System technology
	• Access
	  • Browser requirements
	  • Diverse users
	  • Users with disabilities
	• Download time
	• Navigation
	• Ease of use
	• Support/help desk
	• Display
	• Layout/look and feel
	• Input devices
	• Output devices
	• Error handling/feedback

ATTRIBUTES	See Table 8.2
BASICS	Purpose of content of materials and learning goal Objectives clear and measurable Orientation to content Guidance prior to beginning Help available online (tutorials)/ offline (out of the course management system)

TABLE 8.1 *(continued)*

Usability issue	Criteria
INTERFACE	Input and output—interacting with system Interfacing with content • Access • Ease of use • Intuitive • Navigation • Error handling • Ability to download materials
LEARNING ENGAGEMENT	Challenging Motivating Satisfying
INTERACTION	Learning community Collaboration: Instructor Collaboration: Other learners Collaboration: Experts Synchronous/Asynchronous E-mail usage Text-based Audio-based Video-based Combination (text, audio, and video) Interaction initiation (who initiates, who can initiate) Feedback
TARGET	Goal of learning Instructional intent Knowledge • Acquisition—gains new knowledge • Integration—integrates into knowledge base and long-term memory (enduring) • Generation—generates knowledge and builds existing knowledge base

(continued)

TABLE 8.1   (*continued*)

Usability issue	Criteria
	Skills • Acquisition—gains new skills • Integration—integrates into knowledge/skill base and long-term memory (enduring) • Generation—generates new skills and builds existing knowledge/skill base Affective (attitude) • Acquisition—gains new attitude/affect • Integration—integrates into attitudinal/affective/knowledge base and long-term memory (enduring) • Generation—generates new attitudes or affective responses and builds existing attitudinal/affective/knowledge base
YIELD	Meets targets or goal(s)

Adapted with permission from Educational Advancement Associates, Kittanning, Pennsylvania, March 2003.

Next, you should prepare the learners participating in your testing as you would your actual learners. Ask them to begin by opening the CMS, locate the selected assignment, follow the directions, complete the assignment, and then submit it appropriately. Each learner should think aloud through this process, communicating approaches they used in completing the selected assignment and their thoughts and feelings about it. Learners might need to be reminded to think aloud because it is easy to forget to say out loud what they are thinking.

The educator or developer of the materials should observe and record the learners' comments during the simplified thinking aloud session. The observer/recorder only interacts with the learners to remind them to think out loud but does not assist them in answering questions related to the task. After the five learners have worked through the assignment and submitted it, the notes made by the observer/recorder

TABLE 8.2   Attributes for Heuristic Evaluation of Online Learning

Attributes	Criteria
Attribute I—Purpose	The purpose of the educational episode must be clear to the learner. Are objectives present and clearly stated? Are the objectives measurable?
Attribute II—Introduction/orientation	Orientation to content Guidance prior to beginning Help available online (tutorials)/offline (out of the course management system)
Attribute III—Instructor control	Instructional design Information dissemination/chunking/ access Calendar Evaluative methods Critical thinking episodes Motivation Engaging the learner Preparation
Attribute IV—Learner control	Learning style Interaction Information retrieval (timing and amount) Time management (when access materials, complete work) Location of access (home, work, library) Motivation Becoming engaged Preparation
Attribute V—Information	Dynamic/static Structured/nonstructured Level of information—geared to learner Amount of information appropriate Timeliness of information (current) Availability (enabled or disabled) Dissemination schedule (when available) Access Navigation Location markers (do learners know where they are in the materials?)

(continued)

TABLE 8.2 *(continued)*

Attributes	Criteria
Attribute VI—Interaction	Structured/nonstructured (Java hut, Open Group areas)
	Interaction initiation (who initiates, who can initiate)
	Synchronous/asynchronous
	Collaboration
	Learner/professor(s)
	Learner/learner(s)
	Learner/expert(s)
	E-mail usage
	Text-based
	Audio-based
	Video-based
	Combination (text, audio, and video)
	Efficient
	Effective
	Internal course interaction
	External course interaction
	Access
	Navigation
	Ease of use/interacting
Attribute VII—Evaluation	Objectives—present/measurable
	Cognitive, affective, psychomotor
	Assignments
	Assessment (self-checks, quizzes, examinations)
	Objective/subjective
Attribute VIII—Feedback	How feedback provided (e-mail, audio, video)
	Timeliness of feedback
	Amount of feedback
Attribute IX—Satisfaction	Learner satisfied with online learning episode
	Content
	Perceived applicability of materials/ content
	Was it fun/enjoyable?
	Why satisfied?
	Why not satisfied?

Adapted with permission from Educational Advancement Associates, Kittanning, Pennsylvania, March 2003.

can be analyzed and synthesized to identify usability problems. The submitted assignments also should be assessed for quality and graded, comparing them to the instructor's expectations. This simple technique provides a wealth of information that can be used to enhance the online materials and identify areas for revision.

Using the nine attributes listed in Table 8.2, you can conduct the heuristic evaluation of your online course materials. This should be a methodical examination of the online materials to identify any usability problems that exist based on the heuristics. You might decide to hire usability consultants or have several different people conduct the heuristic evaluation. The choices you make will depend on your financial resources and the amount of time you have to devote to usability testing. It is important to identify usability problems early to avoid frustrating or losing students.

An example of a heuristic evaluation would begin with the selection of the evaluators. Other nursing instructors or a hired usability consultant could serve as evaluators. We suggest selecting three evaluators, possibly two educators and one usability consultant. The evaluators would assess the e-learning content in relation to each of the nine attributes and their criteria identified in Table 8.2. A report would be developed from the evaluator's perspective relating to the presence/absence and strength/weakness of the attributes' criteria in the content. The heuristic evaluation is conducted with the intent of uncovering usability problems. For this reason, the report should be scrutinized to gain insights into the reasons for the identified usability problems. The information contained in the report also provides a basis for revision of the materials.

In addition to written reports, the evaluators should discuss their evaluation with the developers of the materials. This gives the developers a chance to clarify any ambiguities in the reports. The discussion also provides an opportunity for the developers to review the changes they plan to make on the basis of the evaluation.

According to van Dijck (2000), "The best way to get started in usability is getting your hands dirty. Yes, people, that means testing" (p. 1). Usability testing should begin during the development of the materials and continue through iterations and revisions. The resultant e-learning materials will be learner-centered and useful to your learners. E-learning materials that have been thoroughly tested for usability and refined allow learners to concentrate on learning, and avoid the distractions and frustrations associated with poorly designed materials.

REFERENCES

Bohmann, K. (2001). *Usability defined.* Retrieved March 5, 2003, from http://www.bohmann.dk/observations/2001jun27.html

Brodsky, M. (2003). *Designing e-learning from the outside-in.* Retrieved March 5, 2003, from http://www.elearningmag.com/elearning/article/articleDetail.jsp?id=48117

McGonigle, D. (2002). *Usability for online learning.* Retrieved March 5, 2003, from http://eaa-knowledge.com/eaa/usability.htm

McGonigle, D. (2003). *Usability attributes—Heuristics for online learning.* Retrieved March 5, 2003, from http://eaa-knowledge.com/eaa/attributes.htm

Nielsen, J. (1994). *Guerilla HCI: Using discount usability engineering to penetrate the intimidation barrier.* Retrieved March 5, 2003, from http://www.useit.com/papers/guerrilla_hci.html

Preece, J. (2001). *Sociability and usability in online communities: Determining and measuring success.* Retrieved March 5, 2003, from http://www.ifsm.umbc.edu/~preece/paper/4%20BIT%20Twenty%20years.pdf

van Dijck, P. (2000). *Getting started with usability testing.* Retrieved March 5, 2003, from http://www.evolt.org/article/Getting_Started_with_Usability_Testing/4090/1604/

Part III

Simulation Labs
in Nursing Education

Chapter 9

Using Simulation in Nursing Education: The University of Maryland and Georgetown University Experiences

Patricia Gonce Morton and Carol A. Rauen

The turmoil of the health care system offers numerous challenges to nurse educators. Advances in knowledge about diseases and their treatment, coupled with the development of complex technologies, have allowed patients to live longer. As a result, acute care hospitals, outpatient clinics, and home care agencies are dealing with high acuity patients with complex needs. Society expects health care providers to meet these needs by offering accessible, quality, error free, and affordable health care. Yet, we are challenged to address these demands in an era of decreased economic and human resources.

In addition to the difficulties we confront with the health care system, nurse educators face unparalleled challenges in nursing education. Nursing students are an increasingly diverse population who are often technologically savvy and discontent with the overuse of traditional lecture methods of teaching. While struggling to meet students' complex learning needs, schools of nursing are dealing with a dramatic decline in the number of faculty. This decline has often resulted in increased student to faculty ratios that can be problematic, particularly in the clinical setting. In the midst of these dilemmas, educators are faced with pressure from multiple nursing specialties to increase content about that specialty in an already demanding nursing curriculum. In addition, our colleagues from the service sector tell us that nursing graduates often do not have the requisite competencies to meet the challenges of the work environment. Employers warn us that they no longer have the human or economic resources to provide lengthy orientation programs and that our graduates must "hit the ground running."

To address these challenges, educators have turned to simulation as an integral teaching method in the nursing curriculum. This chapter describes the experience of two schools of nursing in developing and implementing clinical simulation for nursing education.

SIMULATION

Simulation is a teaching strategy that seeks to "replicate some or nearly all of the essential aspects of a clinical situation so that the situation may be more easily understood and managed when it occurs for real in clinical practice" (Alspach, 1995, p. 85). Simulated experiences offer the student risk-free learning opportunities in the cognitive, psychomotor, and affective domains. Within a controlled environment, the student is able to focus on critical thinking, problem solving, and psychomotor skill acquisition while receiving immediate feedback and reinforcement. Table 9.1 lists additional advantages and disadvantages of simulation as a teaching method.

REVIEW OF THE LITERATURE ON SIMULATION

The use of deliberate practice or simulation in nursing education probably dates back as far as Florence Nightingale's training school for nurses. As our skill requirements became more complex and our training tools more sophisticated, psychomotor skill training became an integral part of the nursing education process. Like many aspects of nursing anthropology, what seemed logical is what became reality. Unfortunately many of our traditional practices evolved without supportive research. This lack of research is certainly found today with the practice of simulation and the use of high fidelity human patient simulators. Logic and anecdotal evidence suggest this teaching strategy is a wonderful method for learning (Eaves & Flagg, 2001; Gordon, Wilkerson, Shaffer, & Armstrong, 2001; Morton, 1997; Rauen, 2001), but there is little nursing education research to support these claims (Miracle, 1999; Rauen, 2001).

Simulation is an event or situation made to resemble clinical practice as closely as possible to teach theory, assessment, technology, pharma-

TABLE 9.1   Advantages and Disadvantages of Simulation as Teaching Method

Advantages of simulations

- Can approximate the reality of clinical situation more closely than classroom teaching methods
- Simplify reality by focusing on aspects intended for learning and by removing extraneous environmental factors that might interfere with learning
- Reduce the time required for learning by compressing into single learning experience what might have taken days or weeks to obtain in clinical setting
- May afford learning experiences that otherwise would not be available in classroom or clinical settings
- Engage learners more directly and actively in learning process than purely didactic or observational learning experiences
- Provide for novelty and variety in teaching methods
- Afford immediate feedback and reinforcement of learning
- Can be used without incurring risk of adverse effects (of elements related to safety, comfort, privacy, and learner inexperience) on patients
- Provide learners with opportunity for self-paced learning and practicing of skills in controlled setting and at times convenient to learner
- Allow learners time to make mistakes and refine skills in atmosphere free of danger, anxiety, censure, and embarrassment
- May enable proficient nurse to attain learning outcomes in less time than by conventional classroom teaching methods
- Offer a means for teaching in cognitive, affective, and psychomotor domains
- Use learner and instructor time more efficiently than in clinical setting since increased educator-to-learner ratio can be used
- Offer hands-on and socially engaging learning experiences for learners whose learning style preferences are in this category
- Provide an alternative learning setting if clinical facilities are crowded with too many students

Disadvantages of simulations

- Offer learning experience that to varying degrees does not approximate reality
- Cost too much to be affordable for some schools or agencies
- Require considerable amount of time to store, maintain, and clean the equipment
- Necessitate frequent replacement or upgrade of equipment
- Can be limited by lack of availability of certain equipment
- Does not assure that student will translate learning gained from simulation to clinical setting

From Alspach, J. (1995). *The educational process in nursing staff development* (p. 86). St. Louis: C. V. Mosby. Reprinted with permission from Elsevier.

cology, and skills (Rauen, 2001). There is evidence throughout the research, education, and critical care literature documenting that this method of teaching and evaluating learners is more realistic, enhances both acquisition and retention of knowledge, sharpens critical thinking and psychomotor skills, and is more enjoyable than traditional methods (Done & Parr 2002; Eaves & Flagg, 2001; Gaba, 2002; Gordon, Wilkerson, Shaffer, Armstrong, 2001; Issenberg et al., 1999; Jeffries, Rew, & Cramer, 2002; Morgan, Cleave-Hogg, McIlroy, & Devitt, 2002; Morton, 1997; Naik et al., 2001; Rauen, 2001; Rogers, Jacob, Rashwan, & Pinsky, 2001; Rowles & Brigham, 1998; Traver, 1999; Wik, Myklebust, Auestad, & Steen, 2002). Simulation also affords learners the opportunity to apply their knowledge, participate in their learning, and witness the outcomes of their actions, all key elements in adult learning (Bandman & Bandman, 1995; Benner, 2000; Benner, Hooper-Kyriakidis, & Stannard, 1999; Daly, 1998, 2001).

Dr. David Gaba, a pioneer in the use of simulation in medical training, said, "No industry in which human lives depend on skilled performance of responsible operators has waited for unequivocal proof of the benefit of simulation before embracing it" (Gaba, 1992, p. 491). Many educators and clinicians support this claim and have embraced simulation as a teaching strategy using a variety of methods and simulators. With the sophistication of simulators and their ability to almost replicate reality, questions arise as to whether simulation can be used as a substitute for clinical education. There also is a movement underway in anesthesia training to require simulation as part of board certification exams. Before we can adapt these major academic philosophical changes, however, we need evidence of the effectiveness of simulation.

The new high-technology human simulators are light-years more advanced than the rubber mannequins that have been used for decades to teach and practice many clinical skills. These first training models were used for physical assessment, catheter insertions, dressing applications, and about any other skill that could be practiced on a body part. There is no question that this type of practice is helpful for nursing students to learn many aspects of clinical care. In addition to allowing for specific psychomotor skill practice, the new high-tech and computer driven, interactive simulators allow for dynamic assessment. They also require critical thinking skills and are useful in the development and implementation of a plan of care. The learner can witness the outcome of that plan and can evaluate its effectiveness. The entire nursing process can be simulated, rehearsed, and analyzed.

There are research-based and descriptive summaries in the nursing, medical, and educational literature to support simulation as an excellent teaching method. Friedrich (2002), in an editorial in the *Journal of the American Medical Association*, reported on his interviews of several simulation center directors (school- and hospital-based) around the country. The center directors verified that the simulation method of training allowed for risk-free practice and that practice frequently increased the skills and confidence of the novice. Issenberg and colleagues .(1999), in another survey, determined that simulation improved acquisition and retention of knowledge compared with traditional lectures. In their summary the authors suggested that the "key element in the successful use of simulation" was for it to "become integrated throughout the entire curriculum" (p. 865).

Rodgers, Jacob, Rashwan, and Pinsky (2001) studied fourth-year medical students in their critical care rotation. The students were evaluated using a written test, skill station, and simulation with an interactive high-tech simulator. Although the pretests, given at the beginning of the rotation, showed similar results across these three methods, disparity existed in the posttest results between the written and simulator testing. The students performed much better on the written exam than in the simulation-testing model. This suggested that although theory had been learned during the clinical rotation, the students still lacked the ability to apply this knowledge in a "real" patient care setting.

Eaves and Flagg (2001), using live actors, full-body simulators, and other specialized mannequins, developed a ten-bed Simulated Medical Unit (SMU). The SMU was utilized during nursing orientation. The orientees actually worked full shifts on the unit where realistic case scenarios were acted out and technical skills practiced. Problem solving, critical thinking, communication, and delegation challenges were incorporated into the scenarios, and the actions/responses were videotaped. The SMU training received positive evaluations from the orientees, preceptors, and educators. Unfortunately, this was a demonstration project, and a control group was not used.

Simulation as a teaching method and an adjunct to both theory and clinical education will undoubtedly continue to expand in both sophistication and application. With this growth and integration of simulation into nursing curricula will come an even greater need for nursing education research. It is possible that simulation can increase retention of knowledge, sharpen critical thinking skills, build confidence, and decrease clinical practice requirements in a nursing curriculum. The changing health care and educational environments are soon likely to require simulation exercises (Miracle, 1999). Nursing research should be undertaken to offer evidence as to whether this is an appropriate direction in which to move.

THE UNIVERSITY OF MARYLAND SCHOOL OF NURSING EXPERIENCE

In the late 1980s, I was teaching adult health nursing and critical care nursing and found the lecture method inadequate to meet the objectives of the courses. I wanted to create a critical care patient simulation laboratory (CCPSL) where students could have opportunities for learning in the cognitive, psychomotor, and affective domains. Creating a laboratory that could meet the needs of our student population was a challenge because of our size. At that time, our school of nursing enrolled about 750 upper division baccalaureate students, 650 master's students, and about 100 doctoral students.

Development of Patient-Simulation Laboratories

To launch our vision of teaching through simulation, we sought funding for our project. With the help of two faculty colleagues, we obtained a $138,035 grant from the Helene Fuld Foundation in 1989 to create a three-bed CCPSL. To supplement the equipment purchased through the grant, we obtained a pulse oximeter and an infusion pump through an educational partnership for schools sponsored by the American Association of Critical-Care Nurses and the vendors. I also approached the biomedical department at our hospital and received donations of equipment that was being taken out of service. Often hospitals purchase new models of equipment but are unable to return the current equipment to the manufacturer for a refund. In addition, one of our clinical sites, the occupational health department of the telephone company in Maryland, was renovating its center and made a donation of hospital beds and various equipment to our growing CCPSL. In 1991, we obtained a second grant of $53,852 from the Helene Fuld Foundation that allowed us to purchase audiovisual and computer-assisted instructional materials to supplement students' learning in the CCPSL.

Our CCPSL laboratory was an overwhelming success, but we needed more space and equipment to meet the needs of our large student body. In addition, faculty from other specialties wanted to create laboratories for students in their courses. To meet our desire to teach through clinical simulation, the dean and the administrative team requested that a new addition be built to the existing school of nursing building. This process required extensive documentation of evidence of need to the University and the State of Maryland, and years of planning. Finally groundbreaking for a new seven-story $38 million addition occurred in 1996, and we moved into the new addition in January of 1999.

The new facility houses 24 state-of-the-art patient-simulation laboratories (PSLs), comprising a 128-bed hospital in the school building (Figure 9.1A, 9.1B). These PSLs include health assessment laboratories, a basic hospital unit, a 10-bed adult critical care unit, a pediatric unit, a neonatal intensive care unit, a labor and delivery unit, and an operating room. Each lab contains a variety of mannequins from stagnate body parts to fully automated, high-fidelity human simulators. A computer is at each bedside in most laboratories so that the student can review computer-assisted instruction as part of the learning experience. To simulate a home environment, the facility houses an apartment with a living room, eat-in kitchen, bedroom, and two baths.

The new building also contains a Clinical Education and Evaluation Center where students work with trained professional actors (known as standardized patients) who portray a patient based on a predetermined script. This joint venture with the School of Medicine provides students with opportunities to learn assessment skills, communication skills, and diagnostic reasoning through the use of six patient examination rooms equipped with video cameras and two-way audio response capability. The main control room houses six observation stations, a computer control panel for video projection and videotape recording, and audio announcement capability.

The construction phase of the project allowed us ample time to obtain equipment for the 24 PSLs, although our efforts to solicit gifts and donations were focused on the critical care laboratory because of the high cost to equip it. We solicited funds from private foundations, alumni, and friends of the school of nursing. Our greatest success was our partnership with corporations who gave generous gifts of equipment to the critical care laboratory. Before approaching these corporations, I worked closely with the School of Nursing's development and public

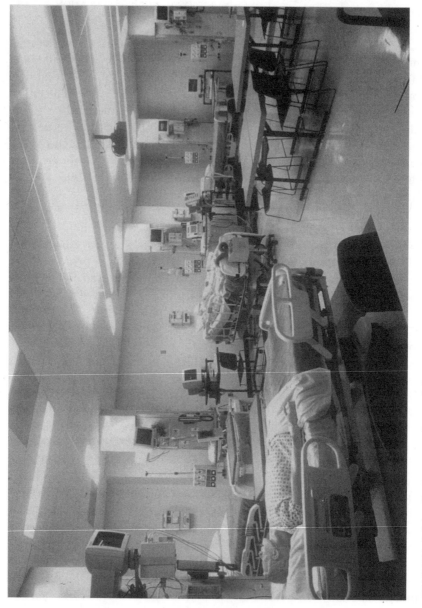

FIGURE 9.1A Patient-simulation laboratories, University of Maryland.

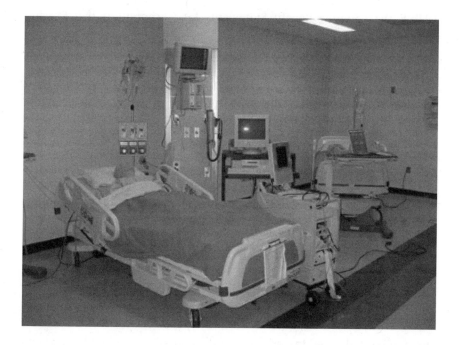

FIGURE 9.1B   Patient-simulation laboratories, University of Maryland.

relations offices to obtain essential information about the corporations, their funding priorities, and their history of giving to the university. Through several years of concerted effort we were able to obtain $3.2 million worth of donated equipment including cardiac monitors, infusion pumps, defibrillators, intra-aortic balloon pumps, pulse oximeters, warming blankets, pulmonary artery catheters, central line insertion kits, airway equipment, and disposable products. A key ingredient in the success of working with the vendors was establishing a win-win partnership. Benefits of the partnership were discussed with each vendor, and examples of these benefit statements are listed in Table 9.2.

Use of Patient-Simulation Laboratories in Undergraduate and Graduate Programs

Undergraduate and graduate students use the PSLs extensively. At the undergraduate level each specialty includes simulated learning experi-

TABLE 9.2   Sample Benefit Statements for Corporations that Provide Equipment

- The corporation will have access to the simulation laboratories to photograph its equipment for marketing materials.
- The corporation will have access to the simulation laboratories to train sales representatives on the operation of the equipment.
- The corporation's equipment will be seen and used by nurses and other staff members who are (or will be) key decision makers in purchasing equipment.
- The corporation will receive feedback on features of its equipment that may need to be redesigned to make the equipment more user-friendly and cost-effective.
- The corporation will be provided with consultation on the development of educational materials to accompany its equipment.
- The corporation will be recognized as a donor; its name will be listed on a plaque hanging in the simulation laboratory and in the lobby of the School of Nursing.
- The corporation will be recognized in newsletters and other publications from the School of Nursing.

From Morton, P. (1996). Creating a laboratory that simulates the critical care environment. *Critical Care Nurse, 16*(6), p. 80. Reprinted with permission of American Association of Critical-Care Nurses, Aliso Viejo, California.

ences in the PSL as an integral part of the course. For example, students learn fundamental skills in the basic PSL, care of the neonate and child in the pediatric and neonatal intensive care PSLs, management of the patient in cardiac arrest in the critical care PSL, and care of the mother giving birth in the labor and delivery PSL. Students also have opportunities to role play a home visit in the simulated apartment before their community health rotation. Simulated experiences are also an integral part of elective courses such as critical care and peri-operative nursing.

At the master's level, the University of Maryland School of Nursing offers twenty specialties, many of which prepare students as nurse practitioners. The PSLs and the Clinical Education and Evaluation Center have been ideal sites for master's students to learn health assessment, and psychomotor skills such as suturing, central lines insertion, and intubation. Doctoral students have used the PSLs or equipment from the PSLs for their dissertation research since the PSLs offer a wealth of resources for measuring physiologic phenomenon.

Sharing of Simulation Laboratories with Other Facilities

In addition to our students, nurses from other facilities have used the PSLs for orientation classes, competency validation, and continuing education courses. Sharing our PSLs with other agencies has been a way to reciprocate the valuable time preceptors spend with our students. At other times, opening the PSLs to outsiders has been a way to generate revenue so that we can continue to purchase necessary materials for the PSLs.

After four years in our new building and extensive use of simulation as an integral part of our teaching, we are more committed than ever to this teaching method for nurses at all levels. We have received excellent evaluations from our students and from their employers regarding their level of preparation to enter the workforce. In addition, we have had nurses and physicians from throughout the United States and around the world visit our PSLs, and they are now implementing our model of simulation into their curricula.

THE GEORGETOWN UNIVERSITY EXPERIENCE

The School of Nursing and Health Studies at Georgetown University launched its commitment to learning with simulation by acquiring its first high-fidelity patient simulator in 1997. The desire arose for the simulator when we opened our Nurse Anesthesia Program (NAP) because of the demonstrated benefit of this teaching modality in anesthesia training. The NAP faculty lobbied both their fellow undergraduate faculty and the parents' council for funding. The latter actually donated the $106,000 needed to buy a MedSim (the company name at the time was Eagle) simulator that was named GUS, meaning the Georgetown University Simulator. This first-generation interactive simulator had many physiological features including a gas analyzer and a drug recognition unit.

Simulator Coordinator Role

A member of the NAP faculty became the simulator coordinator. Through his hard work, he integrated simulation into the NAP program very quickly and with great success. The simulator remains a significant part of the clinical education program and a strong recruitment tool for the NAP. Anesthesia training programs (medical and nursing) have historically been heavy users of patient simulators and prospective students are aware of this fact when they look at graduate programs. We have actually heard new students say, "I selected Georgetown because you have and use a simulator."

There was little use of the GUS by other programs in the school during the first few years. The simulator coordinator offered training workshops and open lab time when any faculty or student could come and work with the simulator. The coordinator typically would be alone during these times, and he eventually just pinned a note to GUS's chest saying anyone wanting help could come and get him from his office.

When meeting simulation coordinators around the country, I discovered that our early experience was not uncommon. The "if you build it (or in this case buy it), they will come" theory does not seem to apply to high-fidelity simulators and nursing education, or at least it did not in the late 1990s. Our experience changed significantly when the simulation coordinator role (CR) was transferred to an undergraduate faculty member with critical care and technical experience. The dean also directed me to increase our use of the simulator in the undergraduate program because by this time the parents' council had started asking why their children were not using the expensive piece of equipment they had purchased.

I welcomed this role and began reading everything in the literature (which was not much) about human simulators as teaching tools. I was excited by the many benefits to this mode of instruction and possibilities for clinical education (Table 9.1), and I can say we lived them all at Georgetown.

Full-time coordinators now run most simulation centers, but at the time, our program was small and our use of the simulator limited. It seemed that a faculty member with a full-time teaching workload could handle the coordination role without difficulty. In retrospect, that was a mistake and probably cost us two years of development.

As a critical care clinical nurse specialist, I had worked with basic critical care simulators and therefore quickly became comfortable using GUS. I also had only recently left the practice environment and was accustomed to small group training that had to be repeated multiple times. I was running the simulator while teaching and often repeated a 2-hour session five to eight times a week or every 2 weeks. I then tried, with limited success, to have my colleagues teaching in the other clinical courses follow this model.

The integration of simulation would have been more successful had we allocated someone full-time to the coordination role. A dedicated person would have been able to offer the faculty more support, both technically and methodologically. I had learned a great deal about this teaching method, which is vastly different from traditional methods, yet I was not there to assist my colleagues in the transition. I taught them how to turn on the simulator and perform some basic functions, and then they were on their own. They did not have technical support should something go wrong (I was in class or clinic), and it was frustrating for both the faculty and students. After two semesters, we realized that this method was not benefiting anyone. Even the GUS suffered because the novice/infrequent users were apt to use the equipment incorrectly.

A technician would be appropriate for faculty support if the faculty were well versed in the pedagogy of simulation as a teaching method. However, most faculty members currently are not. Recently we changed our approach, and I was able to hire a teaching assistant to "drive" the simulator for faculty and also troubleshoot any problems. I worked with my colleagues on integration of the teaching method, development of simulation sessions, and evaluation of outcomes, but was not responsible for the day-to-day running of the simulator or its routine maintenance.

Current Experiences with Simulator

Today, our use of the simulator is frequent enough that we are considering hiring someone to be a full-time simulation coordinator. Currently, every undergraduate clinical course has simulation sessions throughout the four years of the baccalaureate program, beginning with the first semester. All of our clinical graduate programs also use simulation. The NAP remains the most frequent user with more than six hours of simulation a week. Table 9.3 provides a summary of our simulation sessions.

New Simulation Center and Use

In August 2002, the School of Nursing and Health Studies at Georgetown University moved into a newly renovated building. We now have a modern simulation center (Figure 9.2) and also purchased a second patient simulator (Figures 9.3A–9.3C). Thanks to a generous donation from an alumni family, we were able to build what we needed to meet our

TABLE 9.3   Simulation Sessions Offered at Georgetown University

Course and program level	Simulation session	Major objectives	Evaluation/ comments
First-year students Introduction to nursing course	Critically ill patient on every type of technology. Patient is withdrawn from life support and allowed to die. More observation than interaction.	Introduction to technology. Introduction to therapeutic communication with families in crisis. Introduction to end of life experience.	Overwhelmingly positive evaluations from students. Welcome getting into simulation lab first semester. Major comment is "unaware that nurses do things like that."
First-year students Physical assessment course	General physical assessment. Interactive sessions.	Practice general physical assessment skills. Identify and compare normal and abnormal findings. Heart sounds, breath sounds, pulses, blood pressure, pupils, etc.	Good to assess abnormal findings before assessing them on "real patients." Can talk about findings as a group and learn from each other.
First-year students Human biology course	Patient on ECG monitor. Review of lead placement and basic rhythms. Observational more than interaction.	Practical application of cardiac electro-physiology theory. Identification of axis vectors compared to ECG tracing.	Helps students to identify early clinical application of science content.

TABLE 9.3 *(continued)*

Course and program level	Simulation session	Major objectives	Evaluation/ comments
Sophomore students Assessment II, pharmacology, and pathophysiology courses	Clinic patient with hypertension and peripheral vascular disease. Treated with antihypertensive agent, becomes hypotensive needing treatment. Discharged after receiving patient education for drugs and disease.	Use assessment skills. Identification of treatment needed. Assessment of drug actions and proper treatments given. Identification of patient needs, development and implementation of appropriate patient education plan.	Helps students see integration of three courses that are typically taught separately. Helps them to identify how this content "comes together" in development of nursing plan of care, including patient education.
Junior students Medical/surgical, pediatrics, women's health, and advanced skill courses	Eight different interactive cases presented throughout year for medical/surgical nursing and pediatric nursing courses (taught together). Skills include airway management, suctioning, chest tubes, assessment of critical events.	Identification of abnormal assessment findings. Focused patient assessment. Treatment of critical events and evaluation of treatments.	Low-frequency, high-acuity events can be reviewed/assessed and practiced. Student might not witness these events in clinical practice. Controlled learning environment. Simulation can be paused for discussion.

(continued)

TABLE 9.3 *(continued)*

Course and program level	Simulation session	Major objectives	Evaluation/comments
	Disease management of acute states related to DKA, increased ICP, seizures, and post op hemorrhage. Women's health clinical groups assess and treat mother experiencing postpartum hemorrhage.		
Senior students Complex medical/surgical nursing course	One complex patient case each semester. First is ED patient with acute MI, ECG changes, and low cardiac output who codes, requires ventilation, and admission to ICU. Second case is complex trauma victim requiring volume resuscitation who codes.	Application of complex cardiac and pulmonary assessment skills, other technical skills, and knowledge taught in class. Students need to use evidence-based practice guidelines and critical thinking skills. Application of primary and secondary survey assessment used in trauma and acute resuscitation methods.	Low-frequency, high-acuity events can be reviewed/assessed and practiced. Student might not witness these events in clinical rotation. In clinical setting frequently students relegated to observer during these situations. In simulation lab they are full participants. Stress management and team participation rehearsed.

TABLE 9.3 *(continued)*

Course and program level	Simulation session	Major objectives	Evaluation/ comments
Nurse practitioners (NP) Family NP, acute care NP, and nurse midwives	Use simulation lab in physical assessment course. Each clinical course uses lab at least once a semester to review/ identify high-frequency events and low-frequency/ high acuity events, and to review/practice pathophysiology, pharmacology, and some technical skills.	Practice and apply skills. Identification of abnormal findings, confidence building, and communication skills (need to articulate findings to peers and document).	Clinical practicum sites have commented on our students' preparation in regard to physical assessment and confidence. We attribute this partially to use of simulation prior to clinical rotation.
Nurse anesthesia program	Simulation lab used weekly during program.	Review, practice, and demonstration of skills for administration of anesthesia. Preparation for clinical rotations.	Major component of program. All aspects of anesthesia can be simulated and practiced.

ICU, intensive care unit; ECG, electrocardiogram; GU, Georgetown University; DKA, diabetic ketoacidosis; ICP, increased intracranial pressure; ED, emergency department; MI, myocardial infarction.

teaching objectives. The GUS Jr. was purchased from Medical Education Technologies Inc. (2003) at a cost of $204,000. We have received local and national television coverage of our simulation program.

Fundraising is easier with some successes behind us. The new center is inviting to potential industry donors because they want to be

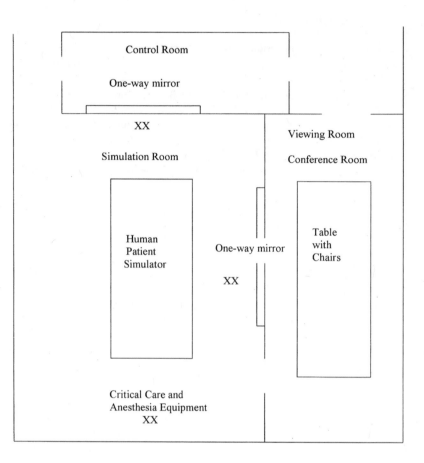

FIGURE 9.2   Diagram of Georgetown University School of Nursing and
Health Studies O'Neill Family Foundation Simulation Center.

XX = ceiling-mounted cameras for control-room visibility, recording (DVD
or VHS), and closed circuit TV/Web cast.

affiliated with a beautiful and successful center. The medical school has
now partnered with us, and all third-year medical students use the
simulation lab twice during their anesthesia clinical rotation for a fee.
The nursing division at the medical center has now incorporated simula-

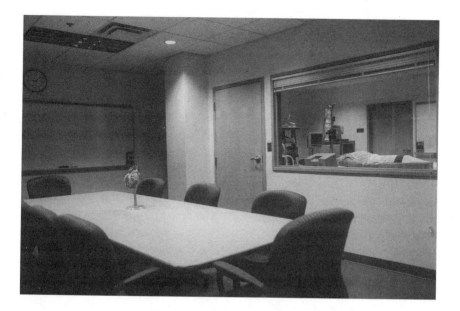

FIGURE 9.3A   Simulation laboratory, Georgetown University.

tion into their critical care course, and all new nurses hired for critical care have sessions in our lab. The new simulator and space also have presented opportunities for continuing nursing education, which has proven to be a source of revenue and potential graduate students.

Considerations in Purchasing a Simulator

The decision to purchase a second simulator was not made lightly. We investigated the various simulators available on the market. The lowest level are the stagnate (CPR-type) mannequins. The second level are the interactive simulators used primarily for advanced cardiac life support (ACLS) or mock code training. These simulators have some physiological simulation models, with electrocardiogram, pulses, and inspiratory and expiratory movement, and have the advantage of being portable; they range in price between $30,000–40,000. At the highest level are the fully automated, high-fidelity models costing more than five times

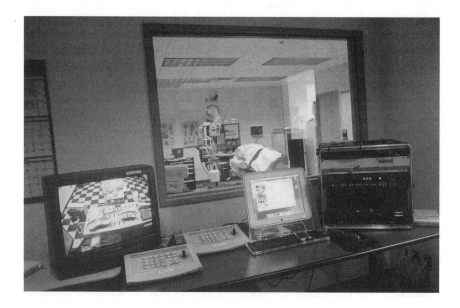

FIGURE 9.3B   Simulation laboratory, Georgetown University.

as much. Those simulators have many more applications; they have a gas analyzer, a drug recognition and response unit, and multiple preconfigured patients and scenarios. We opted to purchase a state-of-the-art simulator, the high-fidelity model, to have two fully functioning simulation labs.

Another motivation for purchasing a second simulator was that the first manufacturer had discontinued production of patient simulators, and we realized that repair of our first simulator might not be an option. Since simulation has been integrated throughout our curriculum, being without a simulator for any period of time would now be unacceptable.

Integrating Simulation into Teaching

Encouraging faculty to use simulation continues to be a challenge. Change is always difficult. Simulation does, and always will, take more time and energy than most traditional teaching methods. Integration of

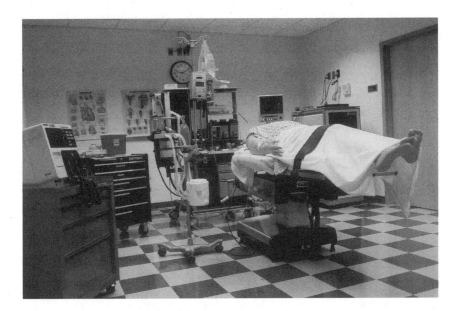

FIGURE 9.3C   Simulation laboratory, Georgetown University.

simulation requires a redesign of technical and clinical education as well as evaluation strategies. It also requires a change in instructional methods for students, but our experience has been that they adapt more easily than the faculty. Overall, the benefits of increased learning, retention, and confidence outweigh the difficulties of change, expense, and time.

The advice I would give someone starting a simulation program is to acquire adequate space and a high-level simulator, and offer training and strong support to the faculty. If you are able to do that, "faculty will come" and more important, "students will learn."

SUMMARY

There is little research to support the advantages of simulation as a teaching strategy in nursing education. Anecdotally simulation centers report good outcomes and positive evaluations from both faculty and students. Research is needed comparing simulation with traditional educational methods. Many claims have been made about increased confidence, increased knowledge retention, improved critical thinking skills, control over skill instruction, and the ability to decrease clinical instructional hours. These claims need to be supported and validated by at least some comparative research, and preferably by randomized studies. Our professional practice must be evidence based and so should our teaching methods.

REFERENCES

Alspach, J. (1995). *The educational process in nursing staff development*. St. Louis: C. V. Mosby.

Bandman, E., & Bandman, B. (1995). *Critical thinking in nursing* (2nd ed.). Norwalk, CT: Appleton & Lange.

Benner, P. (2000). *From novice to expert: Excellence and power in clinical nursing practice*. San Francisco: Addison-Wesley.

Benner, P., Hooper-Kyriakidis, P., & Stannard, D. (1999). *Clinical wisdom and interventions in critical care*. Philadelphia: W. B. Saunders.

Daly, W. (1998). Critical thinking as an outcome of nursing education. What is it? Why is it important to nursing practice? *Journal of Advanced Nursing, 28*, 323–331.

Daly, W. (2001). The development of an alternative method in the assessment of critical thinking as an outcome of nursing education. *Journal of Advanced Nursing, 36*, 120–130.

Done, M., & Parr, M. (2002). Teaching basic life support skills using self-directed learning, a self-instructional video, access to practice manikins and learning pairs. *Resuscitation, 52*, 287–291.

Eaves, R., & Flagg, A. (2001). The U.S. Air Force pilot simulated medical unit: A teaching strategy with multiple applications. *Journal of Nursing Education, 40*, 110–115.

Friedrich, M. (2002). Practice makes perfect: Risk-free medical training with patient simulators. *Journal of the American Medical Association, 288*, 2808–1812.

Gaba, D. (1992). Improving anesthesiologist's performance by simulating reality. *Anesthesiology, 76*, 491–494.

Gaba, D. (2002). Two examples of how to evaluate the impact of new approaches to teaching. *Anesthesiology, 96*, 1–2.

Gordon, J. A., Wilkerson, W., Shaffer, D. W., & Armstrong, E. G. (2001). Practicing medicine without risk: Students' and educators' responses to high-fidelity patient simulation. *Academic Medicine, 75*, 469–472.

Issenberg, S., McGaghie, W., Hart, I., Mayer, J., Felner, J., Petrusa, E., et al. (1999). Simulation technology for health care professional skills training and assessment. *Journal of the American Medical Association, 282*, 861–866.

Jeffries, P., Rew, S., & Cramer, J. (2002). A comparison of student-centered versus traditional methods of teaching basic nursing skills in a learning laboratory. *Nursing Education Perspective, 23*(1), 14–19.

Medical Education Technologies, Inc. (2003). Home page. Retrieved March 2, 2003, from http://www.meti.com/home.html

Miracle, D. (1999). Teaching psychomotor nursing skills in simulated learning labs: A critical review of the literature. In K. Stevens & V. Cassidy, *Evidence-based teaching* (pp. 71–103). New York: National League for Nursing.

Morgan, P., Cleave-Hogg, D., McIlroy, J., & Devitt, J. (2002). A comparison of experiential and visual learning of undergraduate medical students. *Anesthesiology, 96*, 2–25.

Morton, P. (1996). Creating a laboratory that simulates the critical care environment. *Critical Care Nurse, 16*(6), 76– 81.

Morton, P. (1997). Using a critical care simulation laboratory to teach students. *Critical Care Nurse, 17*(6), 66–69.

Naik V., Matsumoto, E., Houston, P., et al. (2001). Fiberoptic orotracheal intubation on anesthetized patients: Do manipulation skills learned on a simple model transfer into the operating room. *Anesthesiology, 95*, 343–348.

Rauen, C. (2001). Using simulation to teach critical thinking skills: You can't just throw the book at them. *Critical Care Nursing Clinics of North America, 13*, 93–103.

Rogers, P., Jacob, H., Rashwan, A., & Pinsky, M. (2001). Quantifying learning in medical students during a critical care medicine elective: A comparison of three evaluation instruments. *Critical Care Medicine, 29*, 1268–1273.

Rowles, C., & Brigham, C. (1998). Strategies to promote critical thinking. In D. M. Billings & J. A. Halstead (Eds.), *Teaching in nursing: A guide for faculty* (pp. 247–275). Philadelphia: W. B. Saunders.

Traver, S. (1999). Anesthesia simulators: Concepts and application. *American Journal of Anesthesiology, 26*, 393–396.

Wik, L., Myklebust, H., Auestad, B., & Steen, P. (2002). Retention of basic life support skills 6 months after training with an automated voice advisory manikin system without instructor involvement. *Resuscitation, 52*, 273–279.

Chapter 10

Using the Human Patient Simulator™ in Nursing Education

Wendy M. Nehring and Felissa R. Lashley

Nursing education is an evolving system. Today's nursing students expect novel and technological approaches to teaching. Creativity, inquisitiveness, and interactional learning are requirements for nursing education in the 21st century. Leading nursing organizations and health care groups are calling for increased professional nursing competence and public accountability (American Nurses Association, 2000; Kohn, Corrigan, Donaldson, and the Committee on Quality of Health Care in America, 1999), and it is mandatory that nursing faculty at every level instill these values, knowledge, and skills in their students prior to graduation. Such nursing competence includes an understanding of pathophysiology, pharmacology, disease conditions, and health promotion in the context of the nursing process. Students also need to develop competence in critical thinking, performance of skills, and psychosocial understanding of the patient and family members in the context of their health care status and interaction with the health system.

Knowledge, critical thinking, performance of skills, and working with the patient and health care team can each be measured objectively in an interactional environment with the use of the Human Patient Simulator™ (HPS). Allowing the nursing student to view the "total picture" can assist in preparation for professional nursing practice.

The opportunity to remodel our psychomotor laboratory with state-of-the-art equipment allowed us to purchase the adult and pediatric HPSs from Medical Education Technologies, Inc., (METI) for our school of nursing.

In this chapter, the use of the HPS in nursing education is explored. This teaching methodology has been used largely in the practice of medicine, specifically anesthesiology. Its use in nursing education is fairly recent. A model for practice using the HPS, called critical incident nursing management, is described in the chapter.

BACKGROUND

The ability to simulate reality for nursing students has been present since the early 20th century with the advent of Mrs. Chase, a life-size mannequin that was used for teaching fundamental nursing skills (Herrmann, 1981). Mrs. Chase, along with an infant model, was used for many decades. These life-size mannequins have evolved over the years to the realistic, jointed, and anatomically correct models that are available today for all age ranges including infants and geriatric patients of various ethnic backgrounds. Along with the changes in mannequins, various models were developed that represented parts of the body, for example, an arm for intravenous needle insertion and a pelvis for catheter and enema insertion.

The simulated patient also has been used successfully in nursing education. In this case, nursing faculty or hired actors address nursing students as if they actually had the disease condition. Students are often able to question the "patient" to obtain information, intervene, and evaluate their actions and the patient's health status. These simulated patient situations also have been implemented in video or computer-assisted instruction (CAI) formats. The evolution of simulation in nursing education has been tremendous with current options being realistic and interactive. Testing is often a part of this format. Future formats will involve virtual reality.

Of greater technological significance was the development of Sim One at the University of Southern California in 1967. Sim One was a simulated, computerized patient that "breathed," had carotid, apical, and temporal pulses, was able to be ventilated, and responded to the administration of medications (Abrahamson, 1997; Denson & Abrahamson, 1969). A precursor to today's HPS, this computerized mannequin was used by medical students and residents for the practice of anesthesia induction. In 1974, a number of physicians and engineers at the University of Miami School of Medicine devised a partial body mannequin that included software for 50 cardiovascular disease states and allowed the student to assess general appearance, arterial and venous pulses, heart sounds, and chest wall movements. This cardiovascular mannequin was called the Harvey model (Gordon, 1974; Jones, Hunt, Carlson, & Seamon, 1997) and was used by many schools of nursing.

Currently, there are two major manufacturers of a patient simulator: METI, that makes the HPS, and Laerdal™ that produces a less expensive and less sophisticated model called SimMan™. Approximately 30 schools of nursing have purchased an HPS and approximately 51 schools of nursing have the SimMan™ (D. Beaty, personal communication, May 6, 2002). METI produces both an adult and a pediatric model. These are pictured in Figures 10.1 and 10.2.

The HPSs are composed of a life-size mannequin and a computer system. The instructor has the option of leading the session with the computer keyboard on the console or with a handheld model that accompanies the system. The adult mannequin is preprogrammed with physiological parameters for a 12- to 100-year-old adult. The mannequin itself, as well as the default programming, is based on a healthy, 27-year-old adult. The pediatric model is preprogrammed for a healthy 6-year-old child, but has the ability to be programmed for a 2- to 11-year-old child.

The software is flexible so that preset scenarios can be run for different disease conditions or new ones can be added to fit the learning objectives of the course. For example, many scenarios are already in place for teaching the ACLS course. A number of medications also are preprogrammed and are monitored by a drug recognition system that uses syringes filled with normal saline and labeled with a bar code that the computer recognizes. The limitation of this drug recognition system is the lack of medications used by nurses in critical care and emergency room situations in the preconfigured drug library. Instead, the drug library is currently composed of medications used in anesthesia.

Research to date using HPSs has largely been medically based, but the outcomes can be applied to nursing education and used to advance future research. The basic research questions have focused on whether the HPSs can be used to objectively evaluate performance.

The literature on the use of HPSs in nursing education remains small but has grown in the past few years (Fletcher, 1998; Monti, Wren, Haas, & Lupien, 1998; Nehring, Ellis, & Lashley, 2001; Nehring, Lashley, & Ellis, 2002; O'Donnell, Fletcher, Dixon, & Palmer, 1998).

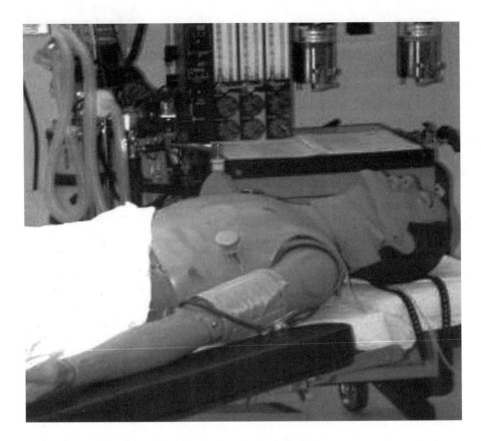

FIGURE 10.1   Adult Human Patient Simulator™.

Several of these articles are written by nurse anesthetists and detail how the HPS is used in the nurse anesthesia program and in an undergraduate critical care elective course (Fletcher, 1998; Monti, Wren, Haas, & Lupien, 1998; O'Donnell, Fletcher, Dixon, & Palmer, 1998). Nehring and her colleagues detail critical incident nursing management, the advantages and disadvantages of the HPS in nursing education, the use of the HPS in education and research, and the administrative costs involved in owning this technology (Nehring, Ellis, & Lashley, 2001; Nehring, Lashley, & Ellis, 2002). In the next section, we will describe the HPS program in our school of nursing and how it has been developed.

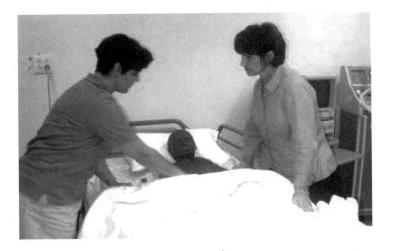

FIGURE 10.2   Pediatric Human Patient Simulator™.

HUMAN PATIENT SIMULATOR PROGRAM AT SOUTHERN ILLINOIS UNIVERSITY EDWARDSVILLE

In February 2000, the School of Nursing at Southern Illinois University Edwardsville (SIUE) opened its newly remodeled, state-of-the-art psychomotor laboratory. Two classrooms were remodeled to include four hospital room bays, a labor and delivery room, two clinic rooms, an emergency room station, an intensive care room, an operating room, and a psychiatric mental health consultation room. A small computer lab, a nurse's station, and a microscope room were also included. New equipment included the two HPSs.

Two faculty coordinators were named to head the School of Nursing HPS Program, and the Dean selected an additional six faculty as members of an ad hoc HPS Committee. The faculty coordinators received funding from the Dean to attend two training sessions on the use of the HPSs provided by the manufacturer at its plant in Sarasota, Florida. The coordinators returned from these sessions and provided a workshop for interested faculty on the functioning of the simulators. METI also provided the School of Nursing with startup monies for two research studies involving use of the HPSs in the undergraduate advanced medical–surgical nursing course and the graduate nurse anesthesia program.

In reviewing the literature and discussing the use of the HPSs in our nursing programs, the coordinators and committee members determined that the resulting education provided to the nursing students would be based on a model of nursing practice to be called critical incident nursing management (Nehring, Ellis, & Lashley, 2001; Nehring, Lashley, & Ellis, 2002). Development of this model is ongoing; the model to date is presented in Figure 10.3. This model is adapted from anesthesia crisis resource management (Gaba, Fish, & Howard, 1994) and the nursing process.

ANESTHESIA CRISIS RESOURCE MANAGEMENT

The need to assure that anesthesiology students were able to carry out their responsibilities in a systematic manner resulted in the development of anesthesia crisis resource management (ACRM) by Gaba and his colleagues at Stanford University (Gaba, 1992; Gaba, Fish, & Howard, 1994). This model was adapted from Cockpit Resource Management (Helmreich, 1987) used to check pilot performance after public outcry. Gaba (1992) outlined the chain of factors resulting in an adverse outcome in the operating room. Both human and mechanical factors could play a role in this outcome. He carefully spelled out how various predisposing factors, such as patient health status, equipment malfunction, and/or surgeon or anesthesiologist fatigue, could cause a critical incident. Gaba (1992) emphasized the need for skills in "dynamic decision making" to counteract critical incidents, thereby reducing untoward consequences (p. 125).

Gaba (1992) delineated the following steps in this process:

1. Observation
2. Data verification
3. Problem recognition
4. Procedural responses
5. Abstract reasoning
6. Coordination of activities via supervisory control and resource management
7. Action implementation
8. Reevaluation (pp. 135–138)

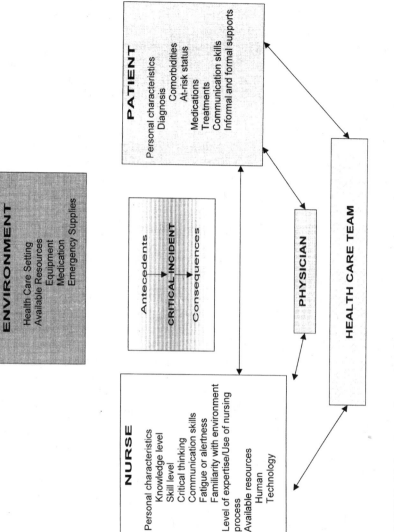

FIGURE 10.3 Critical Incident Nursing Management (CINM).

This process is similar to the nursing process with different terminology. Gaba and his colleagues (1994) also identified a number of critical incidents that could occur in the process of administering anesthesia. These critical incidents were categorized as cardiovascular, pulmonary, metabolic, neurologic, and equipment (Howard, Gaba, Fish, Yang, & Sarnquist, 1992).

Later, these colleagues discussed how these incidents could be simple or critical and classified them as human error, equipment failure, fixation errors, or unknown cause. A fixation error was defined as when a person focused too much on one aspect of what they were doing and neglected or was unaware of other events occurring (DeAnda & Gaba, 1990).

Fletcher (1998), a nurse anesthetist, described how she and faculty at the University of Pittsburgh adapted ACRM for the education of nurse anesthetists, entitled ERR WATCH. This acronym stands for environment, resources, reevaluation, workload, attention, teamwork, communication, and help (asking for assistance). Similar to Gaba and colleagues, Fletcher emphasized workload, teamwork, communication, and help in managing a crisis. She also stressed the importance of the environment, personal resources, reevaluation, and attention. For the process of surgery to go well, teamwork and communication must be present. The nurse anesthetist must know the environment, such as where the equipment is found, where additional supplies are found, and where the emergency equipment is located. The workload of any of the team members, in addition to fatigue or illness (resources), can adversely affect an outcome as can the lack of help, if needed. Finally, the nurse anesthetist must constantly re-evaluate the patient's status and be attentive to changes. All of these factors also apply to a nurse practicing in other clinical settings.

CRITICAL INCIDENT NURSING MANAGEMENT

The School of Nursing faculty involved in the HPS program examined how Gaba's successful model could be adapted for the education of nursing students outside of the operating room. The result of this discussion was the development of a model of nursing practice entitled *critical incident nursing management* (CINM). The HPS would be used to instruct the students about the nursing management of critical incidents through the development of scenarios based on an identified critical incident. The assumptions underlying the CINM are that:

1. Nurses are an integral part of the health care team.
2. Nursing care involves the use of the nursing process.
3. Nursing care involves knowledge, skill, critical thinking, care, and technological expertise.
4. In many environments, nurses provide 24-hour coverage.

To that end, the nurse is constantly influenced by his or her environment, the patient, the patient's physician, and other members of the health care team as depicted in Figure 10.3.

Nurse

The nurse performs his or her responsibilities as an individual with varying personal characteristics, level of expertise, and available resources. Personal characteristics include knowledge level, skill level, ability to think critically, communication skills, level of fatigue or alertness, and familiarity with the environment. These characteristics result in an individualized level of expertise and ability to use the nursing process including the important evaluation phase. Lastly, nurses have different resources available to them based on their expertise and familiarity with the environment. These resources involve human resources, technology, and equipment.

Environment

The environment is defined by the health care setting. This can be the hospital, another health care setting, the home, or the community. Within the environment, a number of available resources may exist such as equipment (e.g., blood pressure cuff), medications, emergency supplies, and technology (e.g., crash cart). Some environments, such as the hospital, have more comprehensive resources available in the case of a critical incident or an emergency than others. Many places in the community may have little or no resources available.

Patient

The patient, in whatever environment, also comes with a set of personal characteristics. These include the patient's diagnosis and the presence of comorbidities and at-risk status, medications, current treatments, communication skills, and availability of informal and formal supports. Each of these factors can influence the outcome of a critical incident.

Patient's Physician and Health Care Team

Moreover, the patient's physician and other members of the health care team caring for the patient play a role in the outcome of that person's care. Their own personal characteristics, similar to the nurse's detailed earlier, can affect the teamwork, communication, and actions undertaken to address the critical incident.

Alterations in any of the factors for the nurse, environment, patient, physician, or other member of the health care team can create an antecedent for the initiation of a critical incident. Quick action must then be taken to counteract the critical incident and minimize its consequences.

CRITICAL INCIDENTS FOR NURSES

What are the critical incidents for nurses? Gaba, Fish, and Howard (1994) defined a critical incident as "an incident that can directly cause an adverse patient outcome" (p. 13). Although textbooks exist for each nursing specialty, a comprehensive list of critical incidents for nursing care has not been succinctly compiled in one text. We hope to undertake this task over the next few years. Some critical incidents have already been identified by METI and our faculty, but additional critical incidents should be developed into scenarios for the HPS.

It is important to develop a model, such as the CINM model, for the use of the HPS in the nursing curriculum, whether at the undergraduate or graduate level. The ability to handle critical incidents in any setting in which they occur assists nursing students to develop their competencies for clinical practice.

CURRENT USE OF HUMAN PATIENT SIMULATOR IN OUR NURSING PROGRAMS

The HPS is used in three semesters of the undergraduate program and throughout the nurse anesthetist specialization in the graduate program at SIUE. The adult HPS is used in the health assessment nursing course in the sophomore year, the maternal-newborn nursing course in the junior year, the advanced medical-surgical nursing course in the senior year, and the graduate nurse anesthesia specialization. The pediatric HPS is used in the undergraduate pediatric nursing course in the junior year and the graduate nurse anesthesia specialization. In the undergraduate program, the HPSs are used to teach certain disease or health conditions and the nursing care needed in each situation.

Scenarios that focus on critical incidents and set the stage for the use of CINM have been developed for each of these courses and the nurse anesthetist specialization. In the undergraduate maternal-newborn course, a scenario has been developed for pregnancy-induced hypertension. In the undergraduate pediatric course, a scenario has been developed for status asthmaticus and a second scenario for diabetes is underway. In the undergraduate advanced medical-surgical course, scenarios have been developed for advanced heart and respiratory assessment, chronic obstructive pulmonary disease, congestive heart failure, pulseless electrical activity, and gastrointestinal bleeding. The cerebrovascular accident (CVA) scenario is illustrated in Table 10.1. Students have an opportunity during these scenarios to participate in a mock code. In the graduate nurse anesthesia specialization, a majority of the didactic teaching is done using the HPSs prior to and throughout the clinical experience.

Each of the scenarios is developed using a common format. Students have reading assignments to complete prior to their session with the HPS. They receive the health and medication history, background information about the patient, and information about the patient's current health status prior to beginning the scenario. The steps to configuring the software of the HPS to run the scenario are then listed. Faculty have the option to start the scenario and let it run on a timed basis, or to teach and field questions while the scenario is manually run. In any case, the debriefing that occurs after the scenario is paramount to the learning process.

TABLE 10.1 Sample Scenario Using CINM with Adult HPS for Patient with Cerebrovascular Accident

Cerebrovascular accident (CVA): Practice and test out

Name, Age, and Gender: Oscar Adamant, 64-year-old male

History of Present Illness: Arrives in the ER per ambulance. Is unresponsive. Family states they went over to his home to take him out for breakfast and found him unresponsive on the floor. The family states they had just spoken to him on the phone 1 hour earlier, and he had been fine.

Past Medical History:
Allergies: Penicillin, hives
Family states he has a history of mild hypertension and Type II Diabetes
Current Medications: ASA 325 mg daily, Glucophage 500 mg p.o. BID
Physical Examination:
  Unresponsive adult male. Appears in good physical condition. No signs of injury.
  Weight/Height: 72 kg. 5'11"
  Vital signs as shown on the monitor.
  Lungs: Respirations are shallow. Lung fields are clear.
  Heart: NSR. No murmurs.

Laboratory, Radiology, and Other Relevant Studies: None available at this time.

Directions for designing the scenario using the software for the HPS follow.

TABLE 10.1 (continued)

Step	State	Event	Physiologic response
Step 1	Click on patient options		
Step 2	Click on patient profile		
Step 3	Click on Standard Man Awake		
Step 4	Click Start		
Step 5	Click on Scenario Options		
Step 6	Click on Change Directory		
Step 7	Click on Parent Directory		
Step 8	Click on Allied Health		
Step 9	Click on "StrokeRoseFrank"		
Step 10	Click on Select		
Step 11	Click on Overlay		
Step 12	Click on Control Scenario		

(continued)

TABLE 10.1 *(continued)*

Step	State	Event	Physiologic response
Step 13 Initial Assessment	Initial Assessment	Baro rep min 110.00 Baro rep max 150.00 Resp rate factor 0.5 Shunt fraction 0.4 O_2 consumption 1200.00 ml/h Right pupil blown HR factor: 1.0	HR 117 BP 153/92 PAP 30/20 SaO_2 falling rapidly PAP 24/20 CVP 11–13

NOTE: Allow student to perform initial assessment and intervention. Priority is ventilation with 100% O_2. Once student has identified this, go to Step 14.

Step 14 Ventilation	Bag patient and prepare for intubation	Resp rate factor: 1.0 Oxygen consumption: 100.00 Shunt fraction 0.10	HR 110–115 SpO_2 rises

Note: Once patient is stabilized, discuss possible reasons for coma. Students should consider Hypoglycemia (accucheck is 94). Assessment should be done and blown right pupil should be found.

TABLE 10.1 *(continued)*

Laboratory and diagnostic test results

ABG's: pH = 7.28, pCO$_2$ = 50, pO$_2$ = 210, HCO$_3$ = 28.

CT: No evidence of hemorrhage. Radiologist reads CT as probably CVA from thromboembolism. CT also shows some cerebral edema and a slight shift of the ventricles to the left.

At this time, in practice, assist student in identifying need for TPA and hyperventilation.

In test-out, student should identify need for TPA and hyperventilation (by increasing rate and/or tidal volume).

Step 15	Administer TPA	Administration of TPA	Pupils return to normal Left radial pulse deficit 90.00	HR 110–120 BP 150's/90 SpO$_2$ 97% Normal breath sounds

NOTE: Student should identify BP is still elevated and the need to address increased ICP

Step 16	Select Decadron and Mannitol	Patient diureses and opens eyes.	Baro recp min/max 80/120 Eyes Open Urine output 000.00 ml/hr Vol 50.00 ml

Developed by Rosanne Griggs and Frank Lyerla, Southern Illinois University Edwardsville, School of Nursing, Edwardsville, Illinois, August 2002. Published by permission of Rosanne Griggs and Frank Lyerla.

Research on Effectiveness of Human Patient Simulator in Undergraduate Program

Research has been conducted in each of the undergraduate courses using the HPSs. To date, this research has been conducted as a one-group, pre- and posttest design. In the 2001–2002 academic year, the pediatric asthma scenario and the pregnancy-induced hypertension scenario were tested with two semesters of students in the undergraduate courses. Students took a pretest prior to instruction in the disease or health condition, and the first posttest at the completion of the HPS instruction. A second posttest was given approximately one month after completion of the HPS instruction. For the asthma scenario, students in each semester ($n = 34$ and $n = 50$) had significantly improved scores on the first posttest ($Z = -4.969$, $p < .001$; $Z = -4.401$, $p < .001$). In the Fall 2001 semester, students did not retain this knowledge from the first to the second posttest although there was still a significant difference between the pretest and posttest 2 scores ($Z = -3.245$, $p < .001$). The Spring 2002 semester students, however, retained their knowledge between the posttests ($Z = -0.579$, $p = .562$) as well as showed significant differences between the pretest and posttest 2 scores ($Z = -3.874$, $p < .001$). The findings were similar for the pregnancy-induced hypertension scenario except in this scenario the students showed less retention of knowledge.

Faculty in the undergraduate advanced medical-surgical course evaluated students' learning at pretest and posttest in the Spring and Fall semesters of 2001 ($n = 46$ for each group). Wilcoxin signed ranks test for each semester indicated significant differences between the pretest and posttest (Spring 2001: $Z = -5.280$, $p < .001$; Fall 2001: $Z = -5.199$, $p < .001$).

We continue to plan a program of research for the use of the HPSs in both the undergraduate and graduate nursing programs. Plans also are underway for development of scenarios in each of the nursing specialty areas.

Advisory Board for Human Patient Simulator Program

An advisory board was formed for the HPS Program. Currently, there are three outside members including a computer science professor, physician, and pharmacist. These professionals will assist the faculty in determining the face validity of the scenarios, provide suggestions for future scenarios, and participate in the further development of CINM.

IMPLICATIONS FOR NURSING EDUCATION

Research by nursing faculty must take place across schools and courses to establish the validity and reliability of the scenarios. Due to the cost of the HPS and the SimMan™, many schools of nursing will not be able to acquire this technology without financial assistance. If future research reveals that use of the HPS aids in significantly increasing competence in practice, then it might be logical that nursing simulation centers be developed geographically across the country.

We have discussed only the application of the HPS in preservice education, but its use in continuing education is also apparent. A few community colleges have already placed their HPS in a mobile van so they can deliver education to the community, for example, providing drug education to area high schools.

The opportunities for teaching nursing content and skills are endless with the use of the HPS. Scenarios can be integrated throughout the curriculum and used for process evaluation. For example, toward the end of the undergraduate and graduate program, students can be given a choice of two to three scenarios and asked to work through them. Faculty can obtain a timed record of the health status changes in the scenario and the student's actions to determine if the student responded in time to reverse a critical incident. Students can complete these scenarios while faculty observe or videotape their performance for later evaluation. This method allows for uniform and objective assessment of critical behaviors expected of students as they progress through the curriculum and information for curriculum revision. Scenarios with the HPS also provide a way of evaluating competence in that nursing specialty.

SUMMARY

Human patient simulators are an important adjunct to nursing education. They provide faculty with state-of-the-art technology for interactive learning of nursing knowledge and skills, such as critical thinking, communication, and teamwork. Their use provides faculty with a means to teach nursing students critical incident nursing management and the public with an objective measure of competence. Nurse anesthetists are debating the use of the HPS as a required measure of performance competence to complement the current measure of a paper-and-pencil test for certification (W. Ellis, personal communication, January 26, 2000). Whether or not CINM using the HPS is successfully implemented in the future as a model for measuring nursing performance competence, assuring the public that nurses provide competent care will remain an essential mandate.

REFERENCES

Abrahamson, S. (1997). Sim One—A patient simulator ahead of its time. *Caduceus, 13*(2), 29–41.

American Nurses Association (2000). *Working paper on continuing professional competence: Nursing's agenda for the 21st century.* Washington, DC: Author.

DeAnda, A., & Gaba, D. M. (1990). Unplanned incidents during comprehensive anesthesia simulation. *Anesthesia Analgesia, 71,* 77–82.

Denson, J. S., & Abrahamson, S. (1969). A computer-controlled patient simulator. *Journal of the American Medical Association, 208,* 504–508.

Fletcher, J. L. (1998). ERR WATCH: Anesthesia crisis resource management from the nurse anesthetist's perspective. *Journal of the American Association of Nurse Anesthetists, 66,* 595–602.

Gaba, D. M. (1992). Dynamic decision-making in anesthesiology: Cognitive models and training approaches. In D. A. Evans & V. L. Patel (Eds.), *Advanced models of cognition for medical training and practice* (pp. 123–147). New York: Springer-Verlag.

Gaba, D. M., Fish, K. J., & Howard, S. K. (1994). *Crisis management in anesthesiology.* New York: Churchill Livingstone.

Gordon, M. S. (1974). Cardiology patient simulator. Development of an animated manikin to teach cardiovascular disease. *American Journal of Cardiology, 34,* 350–355.

Helmreich, R. L. (1987). Theory underlying CRM training: Psychological issues in flight crew performance and crew coordination. In H. W. Orlady & H. C. Foushee (Eds.), *Cockpit resource management training: Proceedings of the NASA/MAC Workshop.* Moffett Field, CA: NASA-Ames Research Center.

Herrmann, E. K. (1981). Mrs. Chase: A noble and enduring figure. *American Journal of Nursing, 81,* 1836.

Howard, S. K., Gaba, D. M., Fish, K. J., Yang, G., & Sarnquist, F. H. (1992). Anesthesia crisis resource management training: Teaching anesthesiologists to handle critical incidents. *Aviation, Space, and Environmental Medicine, 63,* 763–770.

Jones, J. S., Hunt, S. J., Carlson, S. A., & Seamon, J. P. (1997). Assessing bedside cardiologic examination skills using "Harvey," a cardiology patient simulator. *Academic Emergency Medicine, 4,* 980–985.

Kohn, L., Corrigan, J., Donaldson, M., and the Committee on Quality of Health Care in America. (1999). *To err is human: Building a safer health system.* Washington, DC: National Academy Press.

Monti, E. J., Wren, K., Haas, R., & Lupien, A. E. (1998). The use of an anesthesia simulator in graduate and undergraduate education. *CRNA: The Clinical Forum for Nurse Anesthetists, 9,* 59–66.

Nehring, W. M., Ellis, W. E., & Lashley, F. R. (2001). Human patient simulators in nursing education: An overview. *Simulation & Gaming, 32,* 194–204.

Nehring, W. M., Lashley, F. R., & Ellis, W. E. (2002). Critical incident nursing management: Using human patient simulators. *Nursing Care Perspectives, 23,* 128–132.

O'Donnell, J., Fletcher, J., Dixon, B., & Palmer, L. (1998). Planning and implementing an anesthesia crisis resource management course for student nurse anesthetists. *CRNA: The Clinical Forum for Nurse Anesthetists, 9,* 50–58.

Part IV

Innovative Strategies
for Teaching in Nursing

Chapter 11

Critical Thinking: What's New and How to Foster Thinking Among Nursing Students

Carol A. Sedlak and Margaret O. Doheny

In teaching beginning students for over 20 years, we have found that the beginning clinical year provides the foundation for developing students' critical thinking skills. The paradigm shift in education from a training mode to an educative mode enables students to become active versus passive learners.

Over the last decade there has been a wealth of literature on the topic of critical thinking, but there remains a greater need to continue research on this concept, specifically in describing how beginning nursing students make clinical decisions. We believe that critical thinking is a major component of the nursing curriculum and that the development of critical thinking should start with beginning nursing students. Students at this level provide faculty with an ideal opportunity to foster the development of critical thinking skills. The purpose of this chapter is to provide a discussion of active teaching/learning strategies for helping students develop critical thinking in both the classroom and the clinical setting.

DEFINITIONS OF CRITICAL THINKING

Definitions of critical thinking have been presented over the past several years. Ennis (1985), a longstanding authority on critical thinking, defines critical thinking as reflective and reasonable thinking that concentrates on making decisions about one's beliefs and actions. Brookfield (1987, 1995) identifies thinking critically as involving logical reasoning or scrutinizing arguments for assertions unsupported by empirical evidence. Critical thinking has been described as being informed by reflection (Mezirow, 1990). In nursing education, Gaberson and Oermann (1999) defined critical thinking as the thought processes in problem solving and decision making.

Critical thinking in Sedlak's 1995 research refers to a reasoning process in which the nursing student reflects on the ideas, actions, and decisions of him- or herself and others related to clinical experiences. Reflection in clinical is the recall of clinical experiences that lead toward critical thinking to gain insight into one's learning, decisions, critical thinking abilities, and professional development (Sedlak, 1995). Reflection used by both students and educators serves as a tool for continuous personal and professional development, and for the promotion of ongoing critical thinking (Brookfield, 1995).

TEACHING CRITICAL THINKING IN CLINICAL SETTINGS

Critical thinking is often thought of as a "course" being taught in the classroom setting, but it is much more comprehensive. Critical thinking is not a series of discrete, technical skills, but includes broader issues of values and consequences (Paul, 1993). Since critical thinking as a concept is complex and is an ongoing process, there is no unique way to develop critical thinking skills in nursing students. However, the clinical setting provides a rich environment for developing critical thinking skills and should be optimized by faculty.

Historically, clinical instruction has been considered a vital component of the nursing curriculum and of nursing students' professional education. A large portion of the nursing curriculum focuses on nursing students' time spent in the clinical area, and clinical practice is the domain where students apply classroom theory. Too often, faculty who teach beginning students are stereotyped as faculty who teach only psychomotor skills such as bedmaking, taking blood pressure, and giving injections. Beginning students are often viewed as students who do not know how to solve problems and are assumed to be unable to make decisions because of their lack of experience and vulnerability to provide "perfect" nursing care. The purposes of clinical teaching are to enable learners to integrate the knowledge and skills associated with caring for patients, to give them the opportunity to internalize the role of the nurse as care giver, and to ensure that they, as developing professionals, demonstrate the ability to provide safe and competent care. These are the needed skills and knowledge for using critical thinking in clinical practice.

DEVELOPMENT OF CRITICAL THINKING

Two major factors that all nursing students have in common, regardless of age, include changes experienced in adult development whether moving into adulthood or making developmental transitions, and developing from a lay person to a professional nurse. Nursing students not only need to develop basic competencies for implementing safe patient care, but also need to be reflective about their practice as they are faced with the health care challenges of today. Nursing students must develop an awareness of their own perceptions of their clinical practice, and the ability to reflect consciously on their own learning is a vital component of developing awareness of one's own critical thinking skills. Opportunities need to be provided for nursing students to reflect on their experiences and individual learning to maximize the potential of their experiences and to promote self-direction throughout their nursing education.

Through active learning, students move from being passive participants who receive information, to actively engaging in reflection and critical thinking about their own learning. Critical thinking is nurtured through insightful teaching strategies. It is essential to foster beginning students' critical thinking early in their nursing program through the use of a variety of teaching strategies that promote active learning. This chapter provides a discussion of five active teaching/learning strategies that can serve as effective interventions for helping students develop critical thinking in both the classroom and the clinical setting. These include: (1) Socratic questioning, (2) journal writing, (3) developing service learning activities, (4) conducting peer reviews, and (5) dressing up as nursing diagnoses to learn the nursing process.

SOCRATIC QUESTIONING

Nurses must be able to take a broad knowledge base and apply it to individual patient situations. Often there are multiple approaches to solving a problem. One strategy that is useful for fostering critical thinking is the Socratic method of questioning. This is where questions (not answers) are used to arouse curiosity, draw out ideas, and at the same time, serve as a logical, incremental, step-wise guide that enables students to figure out a complex topic or issue using their own thinking and insights.

Using this method with beginning students can be beneficial. Often faculty believe that students need to have "basic" information before they can use their critical thinking skills. But when courses are designed to help students to ask and answer questions about the subject, students often show an ability and a willingness to think critically. Class and clinical experiences organized around open-ended questions foster an intellectual curiosity about the subject from the first day of class and/ or clinical practice.

Educators are familiar with Bloom and colleagues' taxonomy (1956) when it comes to writing objectives, but the same hierarchy can be used to develop questions. It is easy to ask knowledge questions where the teacher taps into the student's memory (recall of facts). However, moving the types of questions to higher-order questions that require the student to go beyond only facts and to make inferences and discover concepts requires application (applying facts to solve a problem), synthesis, and evaluation (solving a problem with creative thinking based on knowledge and facts). This type of questioning requires using facts rather than only recalling them.

Strategy Development and Implementation

For example, in a clinical postconference on osteoporosis, the content planned by faculty may center on diagnosing osteoporosis or identifying those at risk for osteoporosis and selecting appropriate interventions. Using questioning at the knowledge level, the teacher may ask: "When a person has a test for bone density, what are the WHO parameters?" A student who has prepared would know that a bone density score (DXA) of -1.0 SD to -2.5 SD below the norm indicates low bone mass (osteopenia), and a score of more than -2.5 SD below the norm is considered a diagnosis of osteoporosis.

A question at the application level for the scenario of a 56-year-old woman who has a bone density value of -2.6 may be: "What assessments should you consider?" Students would draw on their knowledge of risk factors for osteoporosis and identify possible factors. A question illustrating the evaluative level may address a 72-year-old Caucasian woman admitted to the hospital for a fractured hip. "You are planning her posthospital care. What should you consider in terms of her rehabilitation from the hip fracture?" Students would evaluate the situation by considering what factors may have contributed to the hip fracture such as bone density, risk factors, and/or a home environment conducive to falls.

Questions that require "if–then" relationships take time to formulate. The key word to higher-level questions is "why." This provides a framework where the student figures out an answer and does not only repeat facts. The teacher can have others build on the content by asking follow-up questions, which should help the student think about the topic. For example, "If the woman we discussed earlier has a bone density of −2.5, what would you need to do?" Students would draw on their basic knowledge of osteoporosis and question risk factors and risk for future fracture.

Conclusions

The actual use of questioning is not a new concept to educators. It is a technique that has been used throughout the history of education, but how this technique is used to foster critical thinking has not been frequently examined. For the teacher, asking questions that require reflection necessitates student time to think and being comfortable with silence. There are no right and wrong answers; it is an exploring and thinking process. Students new to this format of learning and who want the "right" answers can find the Socratic method frustrating. Faculty can help them not to panic and to develop skills they will need in the working world. Students will need to answer questions to solve problems using logic. Teachers must be nonjudgmental, realize that they do not know all the answers, and show respect for students' thoughts and opinions. In addition, teachers often need to help students engage in problem solving to identify solutions.

Shy students need to build up their confidence. Sometimes courses on the Internet are more beneficial for the shy student who is reluctant to offer comments in a traditional face-to-face class but is willing to share thoughts using a different format. Classes developed from a Socratic format are really conversations, and students are active listeners. The Socratic format can be difficult for some teachers who like to be in control of the class and provide information but do little to encourage reflection. Teachers need to let go and let students explore the issues. This will give them the needed tools to solve problems in their future jobs.

JOURNAL WRITING

Encouraging students to communicate using both the written and spoken word helps them to think critically and reflectively. Writing reflectively helps students to know themselves and facilitates introspection. Students need opportunities to step back and ask themselves, "Why did I do/feel/think that?" (Holly, 1997). Reflection on experiences promotes new thoughts and development of multiple perspectives (Holly, 1989). Journal writing provides an opportunity for reflection so students can tap into their own critical thinking skills. Through reflective writing, meaning comes from exploring and expanding experiences. Beginning nursing students' sharing of reflections about clinical practice helps nurse educators learn about students' critical thinking skills.

The literature is sparse in the area of describing critical thinking from the student's perspective. Sedlak (1995), using qualitative methodology, described critical thinking of beginning baccalaureate nursing students during the first clinical nursing course. This study focused on obtaining a description of students' reflections on their critical thinking documented in their own words through writing and through discussion. From this study, several advantages of journal writing were identified, including helping students engage in reflection about their thinking and clinical decision making, discover themselves, and increase their self-confidence.

Journal writing is particularly helpful to beginning nursing students because it documents their reflections about their first clinical experiences. Journaling provides an opportunity for students to "think aloud" through writing. It is important for educators to recognize that journal writing does not have a right or wrong answer. The most effective journals explore what students think about, ask questions, and look for relationships that are significant to the student. Journal writing is an opportunity to help students develop skill in introspection, reflection, and self-conversation.

The opportunity to engage in dialogue with the clinical teacher through reflection may spark new insights in the student. The process may assist both the student and teacher to gain more insight into the thinking of beginning nursing students during the first clinical experience. Journaling provides an opportunity for students to talk to an experienced educator who will "listen" to their journal writing.

Strategy Development and Implementation

We have found that using a structured format for journal writing with beginning students is beneficial. Too often, unstructured journaling becomes a free for all without focus. Students can keep a weekly written account of their reflections about their clinical experiences that they perceive as important and that require making some type of decision (Sedlak, 1992, 1995, 1997). There is no limit on the length of the weekly entry that students write but should be at least one page. Nonjudgmental written feedback can be given to acknowledge the entries and ask students to further reflect on specific points in the journal entry.

Written guidelines for journal writing should ask students to:

- Include a description of the situation(s) involving decision making
- Address how they went about making the decision and their thoughts before, during or after making the decision
- Record feelings generated
- Include questions raised and alternatives considered
- List resources needed for carrying out the decision
- Evaluate outcomes of the decision

Tables 11.1 and 11.2 provide more detail about journal writing.

Use of a journal stem can be given periodically to help students focus their journal writing on a particular topic or an issue in relation to the week's clinical experience. Examples of journal stems are listed in Table 11.3.

Journal Writing and Ethical Decision-Making Opportunities

The richness of journal writing provides many examples of students' ethical decision-making dilemmas in everyday clinical practice. Faculty

TABLE 11.1   Directions for Weekly Journal Writing

Write about a situation(s) that you experienced in clinical practice that you felt was important and that required you to make some type of decision. Examples could be situations involving skills (e.g., psychomotor), moral/ethical issues, and communication. Include each of the following as you describe the decision-making situation(s):

- What was your most challenging clinical decision(s) today?

    - Set the scene of the situation. Include client age, diagnosis, gender, location of the situation(s), who was present, etc.
    - Describe the situation(s) and the decision(s) vividly to provide context of the situation.

- How did you go about making the decision(s) in the situations(s) that you identified?

    - Tell what you were thinking about before, during, and after making the decision(s)? Include your feelings, any questions you thought of, etc.
    - What alternatives did you consider?

- What made the decision-making situation(s) challenging?
- What did you decide to do and why?
- How much time did you have to make the decision? Was it enough time?
- What resources did you use to make the decision? Were any resources unavailable?
- How would you rate your decision(s)—were they a success? If so, in what way? If not, describe what happened.
- In reflecting, would you have done anything differently? If so, tell me more about it.
- What did you learn about yourself and your own learning as a result of your thinking and decision making?

Develop Weekly Goals

- Each week think about two to three goals you would like to accomplish in the next week's clinical experience.
- Write out these goals.
- Try to make your goals as specific as possible.

can use these as examples in discussions, for Socratic questioning, and for role play in clinical conferences to enhance students' critical thinking and ethical decision making. Ethical dilemmas often develop for students because of their limited clinical experience, uncertainty of their skills,

TABLE 11.2   Tips for Students' Clinical Journal Writing

- Set aside at least 10–15 minutes after each clinical day to relax and reflect on your clinical experiences, and to write in your journal.
- Do your journal writing in a setting that has few distractions. Journal entries are best written in a quiet reflective setting.
- Write continuously for at least 10–15 minutes in your journal.
- Use blue or black ink. Pencil is difficult to read. You may use the computer to write your journal.
- There is no specific length for each journal entry. This is up to you but be sure to include specific details and examples to convey a clear picture of the clinical experience (as though I were there with you).
- Grammar/spelling will not be corrected but try to be accurate.
- Feedback will be given on your weekly journal entries.

TABLE 11.3   Examples of Journal Stems

- What is your greatest concern as you begin clinical? What are you most excited about as you begin clinical? What are you most scared about?
- The best/worst part about today's clinical in taking care for my first assigned patient was . . .
- My experiences with nurses while in clinical have been . . . My experiences with physicians while in clinical have been . . .
- Tell me how you feel about giving your first injection to a patient. How are you mentally preparing yourself to give the injection?
- Tell me your feelings about becoming a nurse. Now that several weeks of clinical practice have gone by, how do you feel about being a nurse? At this time are you comfortable with nursing as your career choice? Do you see yourself as a nurse?
- Think back about the decisions you had to make in clinical practice since the beginning of the semester. What have been the most difficult decisions you had to make over the semester (give an example)? What have been the easiest decisions you had to make (give an example)?
- Have you changed in how you go about making decisions in the clinical setting? What has not changed in regard to your clinical decision making?
- Tell me how you feel about the clinical written assignments. Are they useful? Not useful?
- If you were asked to write a handbook on *Tips and Pointers for Beginning Nursing Students in Surviving the First Clinical Nursing Course*, what would you include based on your experiences this semester?

lack of confidence, feelings of vulnerability, and being overwhelmed with the role of nurse (Ludwick & Sedlak, 1998).

In examining students' journals, Ludwick and Sedlak (1998) found many examples of ethical dilemmas involving beginning students and patients, staff, faculty, and peers. Patient interactions as a source of dilemmas for beginning students often reveal the pressure on students to do things correctly. Students' thoughts are filled with worry and include "What if I say something wrong?" "What if the patient does not like me?" "What if I hurt someone?" and "What if the patient asks me something, and I don't know the answer?" The pressure to be perfect may potentially lead to students hiding a mistake and potentially falsifying information (Ludwick & Sedlak, 1998).

Ethical dilemmas involving health care staff often originate from students' perceptions of health care professionals being godlike authority figures who never make mistakes. Dilemmas may develop from situations in which students identify nurses, physicians, or ancillary staff performing skills incorrectly, giving misinformation, downplaying students' assessment data, or providing inadequate care (Ludwick & Sedlak, 1998).

Ethical dilemmas involving faculty may develop when students perceive faculty performing procedures incorrectly, when students may be asked to do things they feel frightened of or unprepared for, and when faculty are perceived as not supporting students' rights and not standing up to health care staff (Ludwick & Sedlak, 1998).

A common ethical situation involving peers in the clinical setting includes having something accidentally occur, such as a student yanking a drainage tube when pulling down a side rail causing patient discomfort, and then being told by a peer involved in the care not to tell the instructor. Other dilemmas may include relying on peers for calculating medication dosages and observing peers stealing supplies (Ludwick & Sedlak, 1998).

The following is an excerpt of a story from a student's journal writing depicting critical thinking in an ethical dilemma involving staff (Sedlak, 1995):

> A couple of things concerned me with this patient, one being that when I gave her a bath, her bed was soaked with urine. My first thought was, Oh my gosh, I ripped her foley out. But with further inspection I found that her foley was in place. My second thought was that it might be leaking. I did not know how to check for this, so I told my nurse. She

assessed my patient and told me that her foley was not leaking. She said . . . she became incontinent, and they put it back in . . . and she thinks that on insertion of the foley, some urine escaped, and the sheets were not changed. I was appalled because she acted as if this was OK . . . the patient was not just sitting in a drop of urine, she was sitting in a lot of it. I did not tell the instructor; I was so shocked that could even happen. I felt bad for her [the patient]. She was elderly but because she's confused doesn't mean she has to lay in urine all day. They could have easily changed that bed and that really upset me.

The student reasoned through this dilemma and as she tried to gain perspective of the cause for her patient's wet bed; her caring for the patient's welfare was obvious. She continued to write about another dilemma with the same patient.

The second thing that bothered me was that I found her coccyx area was reddened. I told my nurse, and she said she would have a look at it. . . . I went back to my patient's chart . . . under the integumentary system . . . my nurse had charted . . . that my patient's skin . . . was intact and showed no signs of redness . . . could you please tell me why she did this? I sometimes feel as if the nurses think that we have absolutely no idea what we are doing—it is so frustrating. I've been thinking about that all week, and I regret that I did not approach her about that . . . how can she put this in the notes? I am ashamed . . . I did nothing because of . . . intimidation . . . I don't know why I didn't do anything, and I felt really bad because I felt . . . let down. I sometimes feel that we are helping the nurses, and we are competent in some respect. We're not RNs, but we see things too. She made me feel like I'm here to do nothing but scut work, and she's the RN who makes the decisions.

While in clinical practice, the student proceeded to tell a classmate about the dilemma, and the classmate suggested possible rationales for the contradictory documentation of the patient's skin condition. The classmate recommended that she inform the instructor, but she was unable to immediately locate the instructor. As a patient advocate, the student demonstrated courage by reporting her assessments to the nurse but was unable to take one step further and question the nurse.

Students' views of nurses as authority figures prevent them from speaking up, particularly because they perceive themselves as being only "student nurses" who are guests in the health care agency. Because nursing emphasizes the human element and nursing students deal with human lives, educators play a key role in developing beginning students as critical thinkers and as ethical nurses (Ludwick & Sedlak, 1998). Students' reflections and critical thinking in journaling provide both the faculty and students with an opportunity to develop multiple perspectives on the ethics of nursing practice.

Conclusions

From a broader perspective, the use of a journal should not be looked at as an isolated activity for one course but can be used over time as a means to show students their personal growth, professional development, and critical thinking development.

SERVICE LEARNING ACTIVITY

As an educational strategy, service learning combines community service with academic learning objectives. These experiences can enhance communication skills, strengthen critical thinking abilities, develop civic responsibility, and foster a sense of caring for others. Service learning experiences develop critical thinking skills by gaining insight and knowledge about a situation. In many clinical courses students become actively involved in organized service experiences that meet community needs and in turn sharpen their critical thinking skills (Sedlak, Doheny, Panthofer, & Anaya, 2003). Callister and Hobbins-Garbett (2000) reported one benefit of service learning projects of nursing students as developing higher-level critical thinking skills.

Strategy Development and Implementation

The following are suggested guidelines for students to structure service learning experiences, which should be mutually developed with the faculty and approved before final contracting with an agency. Further information about service learning, its current status in nursing education, and how to plan and implement an international service learning experience is found in chapter 3.

- Perform library and Internet searches. Students who perform searches can find information on service learning experiences and potential clinical agencies.

- Based on personal learning objectives, identify and contact a community agency that will meet learning needs. Faculty often have previously developed partnerships with several agencies and may be able to help students find a match between their learning needs and the agency needs. The United Way is one agency that provides reference materials that can be used as a valuable resource for students to obtain information about the services provided by various agencies.
- Develop a written contract for specified hours of service. Once a community agency is found, a contract should be developed by the student identifying his/her learning objectives, the needs/ goals of the agency, and hours of service to be provided.
- Write a reflective journal. The journal serves as a self-evaluation of students' experiences, describes decisions they make, and outcomes of these decisions.
- Present a poster display at the end of the experience. A poster display highlights the experience in terms of students' objectives and implications for nursing practice as well as celebrates their experience with other students, faculty, and staff (Sedlak et al., 2003).

Conclusions

There are several implications for nursing education. Many students enter nursing programs familiar with service learning from high-school experiences, and faculty can build on these experiences. Faculty need to be aware, though, that not every course is appropriate for service learning. However, in some clinical courses the academic learning objectives are a good fit with service learning and development of critical thinking skills.

PEER REVIEW ACTIVITY

One teaching strategy for developing critical thinking skills in beginning students is peer review through student-led clinical rounds. In clinical experiences, beginning nursing students can learn communication and assessment skills and develop skills in critical thinking, priority setting, and reporting and documenting nursing care. A major component of critical thinking is to view a situation from multiple perspectives and dialogue with others to develop these perspectives (Chaffee, 1991). Peer-led nursing rounds promote assessing situations from multiple perspectives through active student learning and personal reflection, and encourage collaboration among peers. For beginning students, using peer review activities enables them to use their critical thinking skills to identify what they know and areas that they need to know more about (Sedlak & Doheny, 1998).

Beginning students may have difficulty communicating and posing questions to each other about the rationale they used for a particular aspect of their nursing care. While one-on-one faculty-student interactions to teach critical thinking are important, they do not cultivate a cooperative, collaborative relationship among students. Collaboration involves the sharing of ideas and plans about care of patients with other health care providers; students need to learn how to develop these collaborative relationships with other providers.

Peer review is an informal manner of developing collaborative dialogue as students present patient cases to each other and summarize the nursing care given with rationales. Peer review enables students to develop collaborative relationships, validate their nursing care activities with each other, and pose questions about the care given. In a nonthreatening setting, peer review through student-led nursing rounds is a strategy for developing collaboration and critical thinking skills (Sedlak & Doheny, 1998).

Strategy Development and Implementation

Clinical rounds help students reflect and think critically about their own nursing care as well as consider the care provided by their peers. Rounds provide multiple opportunities for critical thinking as students present their individual patients. The format can help students identify patient care problems or issues for further study, evaluate data from patient care, plan for future patient needs, and enhance professional growth. The following are suggested guidelines to structure the clinical experience for peer review.

At the end of each clinical day, in groups of three to four, students can participate in clinical/walking rounds. To promote active learning, walking rounds are encouraged rather than the traditional classroom style post-conference format. Students can present their patient's infor-

TABLE 11.4   Peer Review Walking Rounds Protocol

The following protocol can be used by students during clinical rounds with peers. When possible the student may introduce the patient to the other students.

- Present important physical and psychosocial assessment findings in a 2- to 3-minute report.
- Discuss pertinent nursing diagnoses, nursing interventions,and outcomes.
- Introduce the patient to the peer group (when possible).
- After meeting the patient and leaving the room, provide time from peers for questions about the patient.
- Review written documentation with peers for completeness and correctness.

mation while the other students listen, ask questions, and share reflections about data presented and the care delivered. Students are encouraged to acknowledge positive aspects of the nursing care from their peers and identify areas needing further clarification. Prior to beginning this strategy in the clinical area, the use of role play with clinical case studies is suggested to develop communication skills, which may be helpful for dealing with the awkwardness that students normally feel when communicating in front of patients or with peers present (Sedlak & Doheny, 1998). Table 11.4 has a suggested format for peer review clinical rounds.

Conclusions

Peer review through student-led clinical rounds can help students develop critical thinking and become actively involved in the learning process. This experience is an opportunity for professional learning and growth. Peer review rounds can facilitate team interaction, enhance self-direction in a supportive environment, and be used in clinical settings to develop critical thinking, promote active learning, and encourage collaboration (Sedlak & Doheny, 1998).

DRESSING UP NURSING DIAGNOSES TO LEARN THE NURSING PROCESS

Nursing faculty are presented with a challenge in teaching beginning students who have not yet begun clinical practice the foundational components of the nursing process with a focus on assessment and developing nursing diagnoses. A difficult aspect of teaching the nursing process is how to develop the cognitive skill that nurses use to attach meaning to the assessment data collected, process the data, cluster cues, make inferences, and identify specific nursing diagnoses (Sedlak & Ludwick, 1996). Critical thinking provides the basis for promoting the cognitive development and communication skills needed for using the nursing process.

A fun and creative teaching strategy called *Dressing Up Nursing Diagnoses* developed by Sedlak and Ludwick (1996) can help beginning students develop and identify nursing diagnoses based on data analysis using a risk-free party atmosphere. *Dressing Up Nursing Diagnoses* is a teaching strategy for the laboratory setting developed to help stimulate beginning students' critical thinking skills through formulating nursing diagnoses.

Using a group party-like setting, students come to the lab dressed up to portray a particular nursing diagnosis. Students demonstrate their creativity and critical thinking skills through their party garb attire and ability to use verbal and nonverbal communication to present the assessment data for their nursing diagnosis. Through group dialogue, classmates discuss the assessment data and try to identify their peers' diagnoses.

Strategy Development and Implementation

Steps for this teaching strategy begin with sending invitations for a "Nursing Diagnosis Party" to all students 2 weeks before the party (Sedlak & Ludwick, 1996). Prior to the party faculty help students prepare by giving verbal instruction to review their class notes and textbooks on the nursing process and nursing diagnoses. Directions for costumes should be specific and simple. Students select a nursing diagnosis and portray the supporting data using verbal and/or nonverbal communication. Professionalism is to be used in students' costumes and representation of their diagnoses. Faculty also can dress up as nursing diagnoses. Prizes are offered for students with the most original diagnoses as judged by their classmates. To promote a comfortable party-like atmosphere, students and faculty may provide food and beverages.

During the nursing diagnosis party, all students portray and/or act out their diagnosis to their classmates through the use of verbal and nonverbal communication. A lively dialogue results as students use their nursing diagnosis book to discuss and guess their classmates' diagnoses (Sedlak & Ludwick, 1996).

Critical thinking skills are demonstrated by students in a variety of ways during the *Dressing Up Nursing Diagnoses* teaching-learning strategy (Sedlak & Ludwick, 1996). Students' creative costumes depicting a large array of nursing diagnoses demonstrate their critical thinking and creativity. Students' in-depth dialogue about the costumes serves as another opportunity for expressing critical thinking and encourages lively debate among peers. For example, one student's costume portrayed the nursing diagnosis of "powerlessness." In this scenario, the student was wrapped in a 10-foot orange extension cord with a light bulb protruding from his mouth. Another nursing diagnosis that a student portrayed was "ineffective airway clearance" depicted by wearing a baseball cap that had a model airplane attached. The plane was split in two with the portions protruding on each side of her hat. Test your critical thinking abilities and see students' creativity firsthand as you try to guess the depicted nursing diagnoses in Figure 11.1.

As students dialogue about each other's costumes, they actively engage in data analysis and verbalize their thinking by raising questions and presenting their rationales to determine the nursing diagnoses (Sedlak & Ludwick, 1996). As faculty encourage students to develop an exhaustive list of data interpretations, a lively discussion occurs as students identify major and defining characteristics. Students share a variety of perspectives as they discuss how data can be interpreted differently depending on points of view and how data can represent more than just one nursing diagnosis. With the dialogue, students soon realize the importance of not only being able to identify all nursing diagnoses that their peers portray, but also the challenge of prioritization when determining pertinent nursing diagnoses for individuals (Sedlak & Ludwick, 1996).

Conclusions

The *Dressing Up Nursing Diagnoses* is an effective teaching-learning strategy that stimulates students' reflection and critical thinking. The success of the experience is attributed to the cooperative interaction among students and faculty in a social risk-free environment where

Directions: Test your skills. Identify the nursing diagnoses.

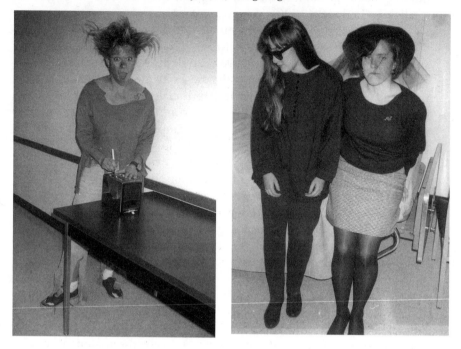

Answers: A = Injury related to improper use of electrical appliance (toaster).

B = Grieving related to loss of relationship.

FIGURE 11.1   Examples of students' nursing diagnoses.

multiple viewpoints can be shared without fear of being incorrect (Sedlak & Ludwick, 1996). Critical thinking is enhanced as students think aloud to determine nursing diagnoses. Opportunities for Socratic questioning and active discussion are cultivated as faculty reflect and mirror students' ideas and actions back to the class. Students share a spirit of inquiry as they learn to question classmates and to answer questions in a nondefensive manner. Students develop accountability for their critical thinking as they convey their perspectives in a fun and comfortable learning atmosphere.

General Points for Critical Thinking Teaching Strategies

The following are general points to consider when developing critical thinking teaching strategies:

- Use your creativity to make it fun
- Be organized with specific directions
- Do a dry run to plan use of time
- Involve students in planning the strategies
- Identify multiple ideas to stimulate critical thinking
- Select class topics that foster critical thinking
- Use active learning and adult learning principles to engage the students in the experience.

SUMMARY

This chapter provided an overview of critical thinking, its importance, and a variety of creative teaching strategies for stimulating critical thinking in nursing students. The teaching strategies outlined specific, useful tips and pointers to assist nurse educators in making the most of these active learning strategies. The time and effort required for fun and creative teaching strategies that facilitate students' critical thinking and active learning are well worth the effort and provide multiple rewards and benefits.

REFERENCES

Bloom, B. J., Englehart, M. S., Furst, E. J., Hill, W. H., & Krathwohl, D. R. (1956). *Taxonomy of educational objectives: The classification of educational goals, Handbook 1: Cognitive domain.* New York: David McKay.

Brookfield, S. (1987). *Developing critical thinkers: Challenging adults to explore alternative ways of thinking and acting.* San Francisco: Jossey-Bass.

Brookfield, S. (1995). *Becoming a critically reflective teacher.* San Francisco: Jossey-Bass.

Callister, L. C., & Hobbins-Garbett, D. (2000). "Enter to learn, go forth to serve": Service learning in nursing education. *Journal of Professional Nursing, 16,* 177–183.

Chaffee, J. (1991). *Thinking critically* (3rd. ed.). Boston, MA: Houghton Mifflin.

Ennis, R. H. (1985). A logical basis for measuring critical thinking skills. *Educational Leadership, 43,* 44–48.

Gaberson, K. A., & Oermann, M. H. (1999). *Clinical teaching strategies in nursing education.* New York: Springer Publishing.

Holly, M. L. (1989). Reflective writing and the spirit of inquiry. *Cambridge Journal of Education, 19,* 71–80.

Holly, M. L. (1997). *Keeping a professional journal* (2nd ed.). Geelong Victoria, Australia: Deakin University Press.

Ludwick, R., & Sedlak, C. A. (1998). Ethical issues and critical thinking: Students' stories. *Nursing Connections, 11*(3), 12–18.

Mezirow, J. (1990). *Fostering critical reflection in adulthood: A guide to transformative and emancipatory learning.* San Francisco: Jossey-Bass.

Paul, R. W. (1993). *Critical thinking: What every person needs to know to survive in a rapidly changing world.* Rohnert Park, CA: Center for Critical Thinking.

Sedlak, C. (1992). Use of clinical logs by beginning nursing students and faculty to identify learning needs. *Journal of Nursing Education, 31,* 24–28.

Sedlak, C. (1995). Critical thinking in beginning baccalaureate nursing students during the first clinical nursing course. *Dissertation Abstracts International, 56*(6), 3130B.

Sedlak, C. (1997). Critical thinking of beginning baccalaureate nursing students during the first clinical nursing course. *Journal of Nursing Education, 36,* 11–18.

Sedlak, C., & Doheny, P. (1998). Peer review through clinical rounds: A collaborative critical thinking strategy. *Nurse Educator, 23*(5), 42–45.

Sedlak, C. A., Doheny, M., Panthofer, N., & Anaya, E. (2003). Critical thinking in students' service learning experiences. *College Teaching, 51*(3), 99–103.

Sedlak, C. A., & Ludwick, R. (1996). Dressing up nursing diagnoses: A critical-thinking strategy. *Nurse Educator, 21*(4), 19–22.

Chapter 12

From Traditional Care Plans to Innovative Concept Maps

Donna D. Ignatavicius

Postsecondary education in the United States has traditionally followed the centuries-old English model of teaching. In this model, the educator presents information to the students, who then try to learn the material and successfully complete the course (O'Banion, 1997). What often happens, however, is that the student memorizes the content to pass the tests and then forgets the information beyond course completion.

Nursing students, however, must build on previously acquired knowledge as they progress through their programs. They must learn, apply, and integrate new knowledge into their practice to become safe, beginning practitioners. However, many educators focus more on teaching than facilitating learning. Learning facilitation requires the use of innovative learning tools and strategies, rather than the same written assignments that have been used for over 30 years. Concept mapping, presented in this chapter, is an exciting learning device that can be used in the classroom, skills laboratory, and clinical setting.

FOCUS ON LEARNING

How Students Learn

Novak and Gowin (1984), respected authorities on learning, outlined several steps to describe how a student learns. First, the learner breaks new knowledge into small parts or sub-concepts. Then, these "bits" of information are arranged and reordered until they make sense to the learner. Finally, the learner makes connections between and among the subconcepts to fully grasp the new knowledge.

Due to the enormous amount of knowledge that nursing students must learn in a relatively short time frame, the last step of establishing connections, or relationships, among subconcepts may not always occur. Consequently, students may be able to recall pieces of information but not be able to link those pieces together in a meaningful way. In other words, students often cannot grasp "the big picture."

How Nursing Educators Traditionally Teach

For many years, nursing instructors believed that they must "cover" a certain amount of content in each course of their program. The most efficient way to include large amounts of information in the classroom is thought to be through lecture and discussion, i.e., using a teaching paradigm. In this approach, pieces of information are provided, but there is little or no opportunity for learners to form relationships or connections between and among those pieces. Students may choose to miss class because the presented content is in their books. They often come unprepared for class because they know that the instructor will tell them what they need to know.

A similar process occurs in the skills laboratory. The instructor demonstrates the skill, or the student watches a videotape or demonstration on a CD, and the student then performs the memorized steps of the skill in a return demonstration. During this experience, the student may not understand how skill performance connects with total client care.

While the clinical setting offers many opportunities for application of knowledge to grasp "the big picture," most nursing programs continue to require columnar nursing care plans. These tools have been used for many years as "evidence" that learners can apply the nursing process in the care of their clients. As shown in Table 12.1, though, the disadvantages of traditional care plans far outweigh their benefits.

Students rapidly learn that they can copy care plans from the myriad of care plan and nursing diagnosis books currently available. They often do not relate what they have copied to the clients for whom they are

TABLE 12.1   Benefits and Pitfalls of Traditional Care Plans

Benefits	Pitfalls
• Assists in understanding the nursing process • Steps of the nursing process are well-organized in columns	• Usually taken largely from care plan books • May not be individualized to the assigned client • Time-consuming for students to complete • Time-consuming for faculty to grade • Often redundant from one care plan to another • Referred to by some students as "busy work" • May not foster critical thinking

caring. Care plans require a lot of time to complete, and they are not the valuable learning tools that some educators think they are. Most important, traditional care plans do not foster critical thinking.

RELATIONSHIP OF CRITICAL THINKING TO LEARNING

Although there is no single accepted definition of critical thinking in nursing, a major goal of nursing education is to develop critical thinking by emphasizing process, inquiry, and reasoning (Duchscher, 2003). In an attempt to develop a consensus definition, Scheffer and Rubenfeld (2000) conducted a Delphi study that resulted in the identification of a set of habits and cognitive skills that characterize an expert critical thinker. More recently, Alfaro-LeFevre (2003) identified a set of critical thinking indicators that reflect the cognitive, affective, and knowledge behaviors of this complex construct.

A number of these critical thinking habits or behaviors have appeared consistently in the literature. For example, being creative, proactive, and insightful are commonly cited by authors and researchers as affective behaviors needed for critical thinking. Examples of frequently cited cognitive critical thinking skills include interpretation, analysis, and inference. In view of these skills and behaviors needed for critical thinking, faculty must rethink how they facilitate learning and what strategies they use to enhance both learning and critical thinking.

CONCEPT MAPS AS A LEARNING TOOL

Over the past few years, a number of articles have been published on the use of concept maps in nursing education, and regional and national conferences have included sessions on concept mapping. However, the use of concept maps as an innovative learning tool is not new to general education.

Concept maps are a type of graphic organizer. Simply stated, graphic organizers are tools that visually display pieces of information using one of several organizational schemes. They can be used in work, business, or educational settings. One of the most familiar graphic organizers is a health care system's organizational chart, which presents the hierarchical structure of the business by employee position. Other common uses of graphic organizers include algorithms, decision-making trees, and flow charts. Most of these forms, however, are somewhat linear in that the information begins at the top of the page and is read vertically.

Description of Concept Maps

Despite the type of map used, generally speaking, a concept map is a visual learning tool or schematic device that represents and organizes pieces of information, ideas, or concepts, and delineates relationships among these pieces where they exist (Novak & Gowin, 1984). Concept maps may be used in the classroom, skills laboratory, and clinical setting by both students and faculty.

In addition to showing relationships, one of the major advantages of concept maps is to help students assimilate knowledge (Ausubel, Novak, & Hanesian, 1986). New knowledge that the student acquires is integrated into previously learned knowledge. The diagramming that takes place in concept maps helps to identify known and new relationships or propositions.

Use of Concept Maps in the Classroom

In the first clinical nursing course of generic programs, students learn about basic human needs such as oxygenation, nutrition, and mobility.

Within each major need are various sub-concepts that are discussed and, therefore, lend themselves to concept mapping. The instructor can present a completed concept map to organize information related to the primary concept. Or, the instructor can develop the map while presenting the content to the class.

For educators who believe they are not artistic enough to diagram the map, they can download a program from *www.inspiration.com* (Inspiration Software, Inc., 2003) to develop the map. This program allows the user to select various schemes, colors, and shapes in completing the map. A tutorial also is included as part of the program.

The freehand-drawn example shown in Figure 12.1 illustrates the subconcepts related to immobility. Students who are not visual learners may find that the map is confusing and displays too much information at one time. If the instructor discovers that most students do not learn best using visual methods, each subconcept can be presented one at a time, and then put together as a summary.

An alternative to the preconstructed instructor map is to have students, either individually or in groups, develop concept maps centered on the topic being discussed. Groups of students can be given a piece of butcher paper and markers to begin sketching their maps. Learners begin this critical thinking activity by first identifying the subconcepts that relate to the major concept. Then, the learners arrange and reorder the subconcepts and use symbols, such as circles, rectangles, and squares, to represent each piece. Finally, where appropriate, the nature of the connections between and among the subconcepts are written on the lines and arrows. This process reflects Novak and Gowin's (1984) description of how people learn.

Other clinical course content that can be easily presented using concept maps includes disease complications, pathophysiological concepts, and pharmacological content. These learning tools are not limited to use in undergraduate education. Content in many master's level courses easily lends itself to concept mapping as well. As visual learning aids, these tools are particularly helpful in breaking down complex material for the student to improve comprehension.

Use of Concept Maps in the Skills Laboratory

One of the frustrations for students in the skills laboratory is determining how each skill relates to total client care. Teaching skills in isolation without helping students understand the bigger picture does not foster

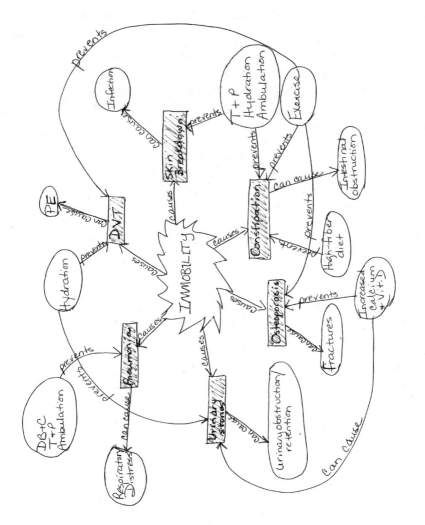

FIGURE 12.1 Sample concept map on immobility.

critical thinking. Teaching students only one way to perform a procedure also does not foster critical thinking.

Once learners master the steps of a given procedure, they need to be asking themselves and be asked by the teacher "what if" and "what else" questions. For example, how does one start an IV line? The procedure varies depending on factors such as client age, purpose of the therapy, availability of usable veins, and so forth. The assessments and documentation that relate to the skills must be learned as well. Clinical simulations with critical thinking activities, for example, case studies, are an ideal method to meet these learning outcomes. The client situation can be manipulated to help students better prepare for clinical practice (Gaberson & Oermann, 1999).

In addition to answering questions and adapting the skill for various situations, students can construct concept maps centered around the skill or case study. This activity can be implemented using groups and butcher paper, as described earlier.

Use of Concept Maps in the Clinical Practicum

Concept maps in the clinical setting can replace traditional care plans. Schuster (2002) defined this form of mapping as concept map care plans. Other commonly used terms for these learning tools include clinical correlation maps, clinical concept maps, mind-mapped care plans, and clinical maps.

Why to Use Concept Maps in Clinical Courses

Clinical correlation maps (CCMs), the term I prefer, allow students to visualize the entire plan of care for a client. Interrelationships between and among medical diagnoses, nursing diagnoses/collaborative problems, assessment data, and interventions are clearly evident. Students enhance their critical thinking skills by analyzing and interpreting client data, determining priorities for care, and organizing aspects of care (Schuster, 2002). Table 12.2 summarizes the benefits of CCMs for the student.

When to Introduce Clinical Correlation Maps

The degree of success in using maps of any type is having "buy-in" from all educators within a nursing program. If only a few faculty decide

TABLE 12.2   Benefits of Clinical Correlation Maps for Nursing Students

- Provide a different way to organize a client's plan of care
- Show relationships between steps of the nursing process
- Link theory to practice
- Improve critical thinking skills
- Summarize a unique, individualized plan of care
- Help to determine priorities for care
- Promote assimilation of knowledge

to try mapping and others do not, the students may become confused and question the value of the learning tool. Therefore, it is important for instructors to learn about mapping and try it with their students in a variety of ways. Using maps in the clinical setting is perhaps one of the easiest applications.

Prior to or during the first clinical semester, generic nursing programs typically introduce students to the steps in the nursing process. To facilitate learning about this problem-solving approach, students develop traditional columnar care plans based on their collected assessment data for assigned clients. Once students understand how to use the nursing process, they then should begin diagramming CCMs in the first semester. Otherwise, if the instructor waits until late in the program to introduce them, students usually find that it is difficult to switch from a linear approach, in the traditional care plan, to the CCM that is more "helical." To facilitate moving from traditional plans to concept mapping, using maps in the classroom and skills laboratory helps students become more familiar with them.

How to Use Clinical Correlation Maps

Clinical correlation maps can be used in a number of ways in the clinical setting. The instructor should try various approaches to determine which works best with his or her students. Several approaches are described here.

For students who have a pre-assignment activity, CCMs can be prepared based on the data collected. Each student develops a CCM and brings it to the clinical practicum for review by the instructor, instead of a traditional nursing care plan. To help students make the transition from the columnar care plan to a CCM, sections of the traditional plan can be cut and pasted into the diagrammatic CCM. Students are encouraged to use shapes and colors to distinguish the steps of the nursing process. Or, they might use the *www.inspiration.com* Web site to prepare their maps.

A second way to familiarize the students with mapping is to have them create their CCMs in groups during clinical conference. This is often the best way to begin the students' experience with clinical mapping, particularly if the idea is introduced late in the program when students are used to developing traditional columnar care plans.

Ideally, students select clients who have problems that they have discussed in the classroom. For example, if the theory component of their course has been focused on problems of oxygenation and perfusion, such as those seen in clients with cardiac problems, then the student constructs a clinical correlation map for a client with this type of problem in the clinical setting. The setting may be the hospital, home, nursing home, or other environment.

After client selection, students work in groups using butcher paper and colored markers to create their maps. Some learners prefer to write the pieces of information for the map on "post-it" notes so they can move them around on the paper to look for the best fit. The instructor facilitates the entire process, providing assistance if students become bogged down or overwhelmed by the project.

Once students are familiar with the purpose and developmental process in diagramming a map, they can then be held responsible for creating their own individual maps to submit to the instructor for feedback. While the maps can be graded, most educators do not evaluate them with a letter grade because of their complexity and individuality. However, the instructor assesses for:

- Inclusion of steps of the nursing process
- Links between and among steps of the nursing process
- Relationships between and among pieces of information
- Creativity
- Weekly progression

The clinical correlation map is graded as a pass or fail. For those who insist on a letter grade, an article by Daley, Shaw, Balistrieri, Glasenapp, and Piacentine (1999) suggests a method for doing so.

Reactions by students to the change to CCMs vary. Once they become comfortable with how to construct the maps, they usually prefer them to traditional care plans. The benefits of mapping for students include the following:

- Helps to put the "pieces of the puzzle" together
- Helps to identify connections in aspects of client care
- Assists in linking theory to clinical experience
- Provides a good picture of the client and clinical situation
- Serves as an effective learning tool
- Allows for more creativity than the traditional care plan
- Encourages critical thinking more than with traditional care plans.

Students who are not visual learners generally have more difficulty with developing maps. They complain that the maps take too long to create, perhaps as much as 10 to 12 hours for one map when constructed without assistance. In these situations, the teacher can pair those students with others who are more visual and creative.

How to Construct a Clinical Correlation Map

A number of articles have been written about how to design a concept map including those used in the clinical practicum. Authors vary in their discussions of how to put a map together. Students should be given general guidelines for map development so as to avoid stifling their creativity. The following guidelines are suggested:

- Use a large piece of paper for the map rather than the standard paper size, or tape two regular size pieces together.
- Place the main reason for admission or the client's primary medical diagnosis in the center of the paper. Feel free to draw a shape to represent the problem; e.g., a heart for congestive heart failure, a kidney for kidney problems, and so forth.
- Develop a key that outlines what each shape or color indicates. For example, all assessment data might be within yellow rectangles; all interventions might be within blue circles.
- Place assessment data (including pertinent client history data), nursing diagnoses/collaborative problems, and interventions (both prescribed and independent) on the map.
- Draw lines/arrows to show which pieces connect or are related. For instance, the defining characteristics (signs and symptoms) should connect with the relevant nursing diagnosis.

- When not obvious, write the relationship on the line. For example, does one piece of information generate another?
- Write the expected outcomes for each nursing diagnosis/collaborative problem on the bottom of the page, if there is room, or on a separate piece of paper. The evaluation of each outcome can be written next to the outcome after care is provided.

Students find these guidelines helpful particularly when provided with an example. However, they might chose to copy the format of the example rather than use their own creative style for the map.

FACULTY CONCERNS ABOUT MAPPING

The use of concept mapping is a change for many educators. Some instructors have used it for a long time, but most have not tried it, despite the number of articles, conference sessions, and books on the topic. Many fear that they are not visual or artistic enough to use mapping.

Some educators are concerned about the difficulty of grading the CCMs. If the student's clinical experiences are graded, they feel that they need a grade for the written work as well. Educators also are concerned that students may not put forth sufficient effort if the maps are not going to be graded. Unfortunately, faculty have set up an "everything gets graded" mentality for students. Concept maps of any type are learning tools and that should be the focus of nursing education.

For most educators who have tried mapping with their students, they are pleased with the results. Students find connections that they did not see before doing mapping. They can relate theory to clinical care better than prior to mapping. And, faculty have a tool that they can peruse quickly to determine if students understand the care required by their clients.

FUTURE OF CONCEPT MAPPING

Concept mapping has been used for more than 20 years in other fields and in general education. It has recently been introduced for application in nursing education and will undoubtedly continue to gain popularity as a learning tool for students. A few core textbooks now include concept maps to help students understand the complexity of care for common medical diagnoses (Ignatavicius & Workman, 2002).

Concept maps are versatile. In the classroom, instructors can present prepared concept maps or have students develop them. In the skills laboratory, maps can be used to show how skills relate to total client care. In the clinical setting, concept maps can replace traditional care plans. For any application, these tools help students develop critical thinking, a major goal of any nursing program.

REFERENCES

Alfaro-LeFevre, R. (2003). *Critical thinking in nursing* (3rd ed.). Philadelphia: W. B. Saunders.

Ausubel, D. P., Novak, J. D., & Hanesian, H. (1986). *Educational psychology: A cognitive view* (2nd ed.). New York: Werbel & Peck.

Daley, B. J. (1999). Concept maps: A strategy to teach and evaluate critical thinking. *Journal of Nursing Education, 38,* 42–47.

Duchscher, J. E. B. (2003). Critical thinking: Perceptions of newly graduated female baccalaureate nurses. *Journal of Nursing Education, 42,* 14–27.

Gaberson, K. B., & Oermann, M. H. (1999). *Clinical teaching strategies in nursing education.* New York: Springer Publishing.

Ignatavicius, D. D., & Workman, M. L. (2002). *Medical-surgical nursing: A critical thinking approach to collaborative care.* Philadelphia: W. B. Saunders.

Inspiration Software, Inc. (2003). Home page. Retrieved February 25, 2003, from www.inspiration.com

Novak, J., & Gowin, D. B. (1984). *Learning how to learn.* New York: Cambridge University Press.

O'Banion, T. (1997). *A learning college for the 21st century.* Phoenix: Oryx Press.

Scheffer, B. K., & Rubenfeld, M. G. (2000). A consensus statement on critical thinking in nursing. *Journal of Nursing Education, 39,* 352–359.

Schuster, P. M. (2002). *Concept mapping: A critical thinking approach to care planning.* Philadelphia: F. A. Davis.

Chapter 13

Peace and Power as a Critical, Feminist Framework for Nursing Education

Adeline R. Falk-Rafael, Mary Ann Anderson, Peggy L. Chinn,
and Alicebelle Rubotzky

Ten years ago, three of us, all nursing educators, entered the doctoral program at the University of Colorado. In much of our course work, we experienced firsthand the use of Chinn's *Peace and Power* process in the classroom (Chinn, 2001). Without fully understanding the critical, feminist pedagogy that underpinned this process, our conversations during the first term were one of amazement at the respect with which we were treated. In our naïveté, we speculated that perhaps our experience was related to the uniqueness of the school and its faculty, or to doctoral education itself!

While each of those factors may well have contributed to our feeling empowered as students, we began to see, as we continued in the program, differences in those classes in which the principles of *Peace and Power* were used consistently. Each of us independently began to incorporate this approach in our own classroom and clinical teaching and found that our students had similar experiences:

> I explain the *Peace and Power* process the first day of class. I also explain to the students how power in this class will be used for the purposes of enabling, not dominating. In one class, after I had completed my explanation, a male student raised his hand and said to me and the class, "Does that mean you will value what I say and do?" His nonverbal behavior connoted absolute surprise that a faculty person would think that way.

217

When we realized a few years ago that we had each incorporated *Peace and Power* into our teaching, we decided to investigate whether research would support the effectiveness of such a pedagogy in empowering our students. The focus of this chapter is to describe our collective experiences in using the principles of *Peace and Power* in the classroom, give examples of how those principles translated into actual teaching practices, and report some of the students' reactions to what is, for most of them, a new experience.

BACKGROUND

Peace and Power is grounded in feminist and critical pedagogies that share an emancipatory purpose. To provide a context for the discussion that follows, highlights of the literature related to critical and feminist pedagogies and a synopsis of the *Peace and Power* process are provided.

Critical, Feminist Pedagogies

Critical pedagogy grew out of a critique of traditional pedagogy with respect to its use as a tool to reproduce societal power structures through both its methods and the content it privileged. Perhaps the most influential force in shaping critical pedagogy has been the work of the Brazilian educator, Paulo Freire. Building on Dewey's philosophy of democratic education, and influenced by liberation theology (Kenway & Modra, 1992), Marxism, and critical theorists (Lather, 1991), Freire characterized traditional education as "banking," whereby teachers deposit information and students receive, store, and retrieve the deposits (Freire, 1973). The analogy is frequently used to characterize traditional teaching methods that focus primarily on mastery of content in isolation of the student-teacher relationship and the process of education (Brunson & Vogt, 1996).

Many of the tenets of critical education are consistent with feminist theories and incorporated into feminist pedagogy. Some are related to process, such as the rejection of teacher as information-giver and an emphasis on dialogue as critical for learning. The notion of teacher as expert and student as passive learner is replaced by an acknowledgment that each is a teacher-learner or learner-teacher (Freire, 1973). Implicit in this approach are values shared with feminist theories, for example, the importance of relationship in the process of teaching for critical consciousness and the reduction of power imbalances between teachers and students. Feminist pedagogy shares with critical pedagogy the goals of individual empowerment and social transformation. However, in addition to raising consciousness of social and economic structures that serve capitalism, consciousness of forces that serve patriarchy also are raised (Lather, 1991; Lewis, 1992; Weiler, 1988). Feminist pedagogy also moves beyond critical social theory's reliance on rationality as an exclusive source of knowledge and embraces multiple ways of knowing (Ironside, 2001).

Not excluded from those forces is education itself. The masculinist focus of traditional and critical education privileges both rationality, as the preferred (and perhaps exclusive) way of knowing, and content, as deemed important from the male perspective (hooks, 1994; Kenway & Modra, 1992; Martin, 1981). As a result, Martin (1981) asserted, "the intellectual disciplines into which a person must be initiated to become an educated person *exclude* women and their works, *construct* the female into the male image of her, and *deny* the truly feminine qualities she does possess" (italics in original, p. 101). Feminist pedagogy extends beyond critical education to value various ways of knowing (Maher & Tetreault, 1994) and includes content that makes visible both women's contributions and what is relevant to their experiences.

The critique of traditional pedagogy extended to other disciplines, and in nursing in the 1980s, took the form of a "curriculum revolution" (Allen, 1990; Bevis & Watson, 1989; Chinn, 1989; Hedin, 1989a, 1989b; Lindeman, 1989; Pitts, 1985). As in other disciplines, nursing leaders challenged both curricular content and methods. A shift from the disease orientation that dominated nursing education to an emphasis on caring in the human health experience was advocated (Watson, 1989). Methods that would reduce power inequities between teachers and students, increase students' awareness of societal inequities, and develop critical thinking skills were promoted (Chinn, 1989). The premise behind the changes proposed in the curriculum revolution was that they would empower students to transform oppressive social realities in their personal and professional work lives.

Empowerment

The origins of empowerment are often credited to Freire (1973), who believed that human beings are capable of critically reflecting on their world and transforming it. He postulated that the process of increased awareness and concomitant action (praxis) freed people from oppressive realities. Although Freire's initial work emerged out of class oppression, it has since been used widely to facilitate the empowerment of women (Chinn, 2001; hooks, 1994), nurses (Hedin, 1986; Roberts, 1983), and nursing students (Hedin, 1989a; Watson, 1989).

The importance of the concept of "empowerment" in nursing is evident in the numerous concept analyses within nursing literature (Ellis-Stoll & Popkess-Vawter, 1998; Gibson, 1991; Rodwell, 1998). Several attributes of empowerment have emerged through concept analyses of the term's use in nursing and health care literature (Rafael, 1995). First, those being empowered must actively participate in their own empowerment, in a relationship in which power is equalized as much as possible. Second, empowerment is an enabling process that enhances personal control. Finally, empowerment involves helping to raise others' awareness of social, economic, or political realities, and increasing their ability to act on those realities in order to transform them (Gibson, 1991).

Peace and Power

Peace and Power focuses on the process by which groups interact. Although structures, such as course objectives, time frames, and evaluation criteria may be a fact of academic lives, within a *Peace and Power* approach, they are used as tools to accomplish goals, rather than ends in themselves (Chinn, 1989). PEACE is an acronym for Praxis, Empowerment, Awareness, Cooperation (previously consensus), and Evolvement (Chinn, 2001). Praxis refers to simultaneous reflection and transformative action that, along with Awareness of one's self in a political and historical context, leads to Empowerment or the increased power to enact one's will without infringing on others' ability to do so. Within the spirit of enabling each other, groups take into account all perspectives and base decisions on common values (co-operation/consensus), one of which is a conscious commitment to growth and transformation (Evolvement).

Principles of Unity

Chinn is clear that the PEACE process involves more than intent; it results in actions consistent with the PEACE principles (Chinn, 2001).

Those actions require each group member to accept responsibility for the group's process and progress. In order to do so, it is critical that groups develop principles of unity—statements that reflect their values and beliefs and guide their decision making. Principles of unity may be developed by asking questions such as who are we, what is our purpose, what values and beliefs do we share, what do we expect of every member, and so on.

PEACE Powers

Actions consistent with the *Peace and Power* process are fueled by PEACE powers, alternative forms of power that contrast sharply with traditional conceptualizations of power as dominance and control. Power over others often leads to damaging group dynamics such as avoidance of confrontation or making compromises to maintain friendship, remaining silent at meetings but complaining afterwards, indulging destructive behavior in others, and disengaging from group discussion that does not directly affect oneself. PEACE powers are enabling forms of power that serve to bring out the power within each of us and foster growth in group members. Conflict, rather than being a negative and divisive force, can be an opportunity for transforming the situation.

Several of the PEACE powers relate particularly well to teaching-learning environments and were central to our teaching:

1. The power of diversity to ensure every student's voice was heard
2. The power of responsibility, which translated into the teacher's responsibility to demystify the processes involved in evaluation and grading
3. The power of sharing to create a community of learners in which teachers and students shared their talents, skills, and abilities to enhance the learning of all

Check-In and Closing

To facilitate integration of the *Peace and Power* process, Chinn (2001) suggested several practical tools. Two that are essential to the success of the process are check-in and closing. Check-in is a time at the beginning of the class to hear from each class member. Although in large classes the method of checking-in may vary, as will be described, the intent of check-in remains to provide an opportunity for each group/ class member to call his or her name into the group to indicate presence in mind, body, and spirit and readiness to attend to the group. Check-in is a time in which members may briefly indicate circumstances that may distract them or are likely to influence their participation in the group (such as not having prepared for class), identify any agenda items that need to be discussed (housekeeping items or issues related to the readings), and/or indicate expectations and hopes for the meeting. Although check-in is critical for group process, being succinct so that the group's business can be attended to also is critical.

At the end of each class, members of the class again succinctly share thoughts and feelings about the meeting. This is effectively accomplished through a three-part statement that includes: (1) an appreciation to someone or for something that happened during the class, (2) a critical reflection that highlights insights into the group process or content discussed, and (3) an affirmation that expresses commitment toward continued learning and personal growth

Convenor

Additional strategies for facilitating effective class processes include identifying a convener, using a rotating chair, and using techniques such as circling to move the discussion forward. The convener is a group leader who takes responsibility for both focusing on the group process and giving the meeting some structure, that is, coming to the meeting with an agenda, creating opportunity for check-in, and providing leadership in facilitating attention to the mutually agreed on agenda. In a classroom, the teacher often is the convener, but if students use the process for small group work, ideally they will take turns convening meetings in an agreed on fashion.

A convener is responsible for:

- Letting the group know when agreed upon time-limits are approaching
- Integrating requests for changes in the agenda, tasks, or processes
- Helping the group be aware of alternative possibilities that have not emerged in the discussion

- Providing leadership in developing consensus when the opportunity arises
- Shifting the discussion to allow the agreed on time for closing

SOPHIA

Often a SOPHIA is used to introduce a topic for discussion in a class. SOPHIA is an acronym that stands for Speak Out, Play Havoc, and Imagine Alternatives. It is often prepared by the convenor as a short (10–20 minute) provocative critique of a topic to begin discussion. The SOPHIA can be used as a graded learning evidence in which students or groups of students, depending on the size of the class, prepare and lead the class with a SOPHIA.

Active Participation of Learners

The *Peace and Power* process requires active participation of group/class members. It includes actively listening to others and being willing to express one's own viewpoint on an issue. Not to do so deprives the group of the benefit of each member's perspective. Practical implications of using *Peace and Power* are that students and teachers need to be present and prepared for class. Both engage as teacher-learners in a situation in which the unique expertise of each participant is valued. Self-discipline is needed to remain focused, and information shared needs to be kept confidential to create and maintain a safe environment. This process requires that students and teachers share the responsibility for learning in an equitable way.

PUTTING *PEACE AND POWER* INTO PRACTICE

Three of us used the *Peace and Power* process in diverse geographical and cultural settings located in the southwestern and northeastern United States, and in eastern Canada. Although all of us were teaching in baccalaureate nursing programs, one program was exclusively for post-RN students, one exclusively for basic nursing students, and the other integrated post-RN and basic students. Two of us taught primarily fourth-year leadership courses, whereas the third supervised students in a clinical experience. Even within the leadership courses, the wide variance in class size, which ranged from 12 to 95 students, necessitated modifications to the operationalization of some of the *Peace and Power* principles. Because the nature of clinical teaching is quite different from the classroom, adoption of *Peace and Power* in a clinical teaching environment is addressed separately.

Getting Ready

Putting *Peace and Power* into practice requires both intent and action. Advance preparation may be needed to prepare oneself and the learning environment.

Preparing Self

The authors, like many nurse educators, began nursing at a time when masculinist, military, and medical perspectives dominated nursing and society. Submission and compliance were expected and reinforced. Many of us learned to stand when physicians entered the nursing station and follow their orders unquestioningly. Embracing an emancipatory pedagogy that includes a critique of the gendered power imbalances in society requires teachers to increase their awareness of oppressive realities and develop the confidence, skill, and willingness to take actions to transform them. In short, it requires empowered teachers.

The story of one of the authors is typical of many nurses' experiences:

> I was raised in rural America and was taught to be absolutely obedient. I worked hard, was not a problem to my parents, and did not learn to think beyond being a "good girl" who was rewarded for her obedience. I went from my family home to a convent school of nursing for women where compliance and obedience were reinforced. Our lives were regimented and monitored. For example, study hall was Monday through Thursday from 7:30–9:00 PM. A nun presided in the library, where most students studied, to enforce a "no nonsense policy." If a student chose to study in her room, the door had to be ajar, and she was required to study sitting at her desk, not lying on her bed. One of the nuns "made rounds" with her clipboard every 30 minutes to make sure all students were where they were supposed to be. Being socialized personally and

professionally to be deferent and compliant has made my paradigm shift extremely challenging; I have worked very hard to become an empowered woman.

In addition to the shift in one's own thinking that may be necessary, using a pedagogical approach that invites students to participate and take responsibility for their own learning, ironically, often requires more careful preparation and a broader knowledge base on the part of the teacher than traditional pedagogical approaches such as lectures. This paradox is related to the fact that, although students are experts in their own lived experience of education, nurse educators are expected to have both practice and pedagogical expertise. In addition, they have an understanding of the whole curriculum that is critical in ensuring that course content and assignments contribute to the overall program outcomes.

It is important, therefore, that invitations to students to participate in directing the focus of course content and discussions include limits and guidelines that might apply. Nurse educators must balance students' learning needs with their own responsibility for upholding institutional academic standards, professional practice and ethical standards, and societal expectations for safe and competent practitioners. However, being willing to share setting the direction and scope of classroom discussion with students within those parameters requires flexibility, a broad knowledge base, the courage to take risks, and the self-confidence to share power.

Preparing the Environment

The physical environment, course syllabus, and organizational context may all impact the success of the *Peace and Power* process. Because faculty members may have varying degrees of control over these factors, we have shared below some of the adaptations we made in trying to stay true to the principles.

Physical Environment

Planning to use *Peace and Power* in the classroom begins well before the start of the term. First, class size and physical space issues and seating arrangements must be addressed. While it is not always possible to influence these factors, it is worth the effort to try. Smaller classes that can be seated in a circle or U-shape are ideal in fostering trusting relationships between faculty and students, and among students themselves. Although many classrooms are set up in the traditional lecture style with rows of tables and chairs facing the front of the room, with a little effort, they can be rearranged. Even if they need to be placed back in a traditional configuration at the conclusion of class, the activity is a good one for students, as it requires them to work as a team.

One author could not control the size of the class and generally taught the leadership course to a class of 75–95 in a tiered auditorium with fixed seating. She adapted the principles of *Peace and Power* by asking students to form small learning groups of 8–10 students. Even with fixed seating, student groups were creative in attending to check-in, closing, and their learning activities. The noise of 9 or 10 groups in simultaneous discussion can be somewhat overwhelming and may be able to be reduced by other innovative approaches, such as arranging for small break-out rooms for the group work or scheduling group activity immediately before or after a class break so that some student groups may actually move to a cafeteria or common room if there is one nearby.

The importance of the physical environment cannot be overstated. One of us recalled that after class on the first day, a student excitedly reported that it was "wonderful" to be in class where she could see faces instead of the backs of heads! Another, who usually taught the large classes, was amazed at the difference in her class one year when she taught the same course in a summer term to 12 post-RN students. Not only was it possible for her to develop relationships with each of the students, they were able to develop relationships with each other because of size and seating arrangements. Students spoke about feeling responsible to each other to come to class prepared. The class also appeared to make a difference in students' work lives. A clinical nurse specialist who worked on the same unit as two of the students approached the faculty member as the term was ending and spoke of the dramatic changes she had observed in the students' becoming actively involved in the unit's governance.

Course Syllabus

The second aspect of preparing the environment relates to creating a flexible framework for learning, the course syllabus. Prepared before the course begins, the syllabus offers a tentative outline of course content and learning activities. Using the principle of demystification, requirements for completion of learning activities are provided in as much detail as possible and criteria that will be used for grading made explicit in the syllabus. For added flexibility, it may be possible to give students a choice of two or more assignments or perhaps to choose the percentage of grade, within a range that has been calculated to work, that two or more assignments will be worth.

Some courses, such as undergraduate core courses, may have less flexibility in terms of changing content than, for example, elective courses or those at a graduate level. Students are invited to review the proposed structure of the course and identify related areas for consideration. Our experience at the undergraduate level is that it is rare for students to suggest changes either in content or in learning activities at the beginning of the course. However, opportunities continue throughout the term as students are invited to make suggestions during check-in at each class. Suggested changes to learning activities, in particular, often occur midway through the course, as students balance numerous assignments in multiple courses.

In one example, students raised the issue during check-in that the amount of writing required in the course was excessive and together with assignments from other courses was overwhelming. The teacher invited the class to choose several classmates to represent them in a meeting with other faculty members who taught courses that term. Although the teacher initially believed that the required learning activities were reasonable, when she heard the workload that students faced in other courses, she negotiated a mutually agreeable solution that was subsequently proposed to and accepted by the entire class.

Organizational Context

The above example serves as a useful reminder that courses do not exist in a vacuum and that events in the school or community may interfere with and, at the same time, create opportunities for learning. If students feel safe and empowered to raise such issues, great skill is required on the part of the teacher not only in setting limits for appropriate behavior but also in modeling and guiding effective resolution of the problem.

The following example illustrates such a situation:

> As I was setting up for class, I noticed that the students seemed upset with the yellow piece of paper most had in their hands. I added it to the

agenda for discussion after check-in. The paper announced a half-day event, sponsored by the school, which all students were required to attend or complete a make-up assignment. The memo was exactly the opposite of the empowering environment I try to create. I turned the time over to the students for discussion. They immediately began venting angry feelings and, of course, wanted me to agree with them and validate their anger. I called time out and refocused their energies on addressing the issue. As they did so, their focus changed from their feelings of being overpowered to identifying the issues—work and family commitments made attendance difficult, and compulsory extracurricular activities seemed unjust. They wrote their concerns as a group and examined them to see that they were honest, objective, professional, and respectful of others. I helped them to identify the appropriate person to approach. As a result, the students were not required to attend but agreed to make every effort to do so because it was the professional thing to do. It was a win-win negotiation!

Resolving problems like these in a mutually acceptable way both teaches students effective problem-solving skills and gives them the experience and self-confidence to address future problems in their work or personal lives in similar ways. The process promotes respect and creativity, attributes that are sorely needed in the workplace.

USING THE *PEACE AND POWER* PROCESS IN THE CLASSROOM

As every educator knows, calling the students to order at the beginning of class or return from break can present a major challenge. Often energetic students have a great deal to say to each other and getting their attention can be difficult. Creativity and dialogue with the students can result in a mutually agreed on strategy to call students to order for the start of class. For some educators, raising hands as a signal to stop talking may be effective. Some students actually asked one of the authors to raise her voice enough to bring the class to order. Another found the unusual and pleasing sound of a rain stick was effective for this purpose.

Check-In

Once class has been called together, the initial activity is to check-in. The power of naming is central to check-in. Each group member, including the teacher, calls her/his name out to the class and briefly indicates readiness to participate, expectations for the class, and any housekeeping or content issues to be added to the agenda. If extenuating circumstances are likely to interfere with group members' ability to be fully attentive, they are invited to succinctly share the reasons, for example, being up all night with a sick child. This allows the class members to support each other without criticism or blame. Furthermore, those who are well prepared can assist those less prepared to understand content. The overall objective is to develop a community of scholars who take responsibility in assisting each other to learn. Usually, this is a foreign experience for students, and patient reinforcement of the value of spending time this way each class is needed.

Check-in helps both students and faculty remember names of class members and increases students' willingness to branch out from their cadre of friends to work in groups with other students. Since many students are unfamiliar with this process, it may take a few weeks before they feel comfortable and appreciate its benefits, as illustrated by the following:

> Once I had a group of students in which several members simply did not seem to value the check-in process. One student in particular complained about it strongly and often. Finally, I asked the class what we should do about the concerns of their classmates. I made it clear that everything said in the class would be valued, including complaints. The students who were unhappy with the check-in process deserved their due consideration. The group decided that they would continue with the current process for three more weeks and then would reevaluate it. By the end of the three weeks, even the strongest complainer agreed he wanted to continue with the check-in process. He didn't say why he changed his mind, but he eagerly participated. I often wondered if he simply needed to be heard and valued.

Addressing the Agenda

After check-in, it is important to address the agenda items that have been added. It helps to make a list of them on the blackboard or an overhead transparency so they are not forgotten. Being sensitive to the mood of the class is helpful, and if the teacher/convener senses stress or distraction, the teacher can add this to the agenda to provide an opportunity for discussion. Other items the faculty might add are "news" items such as assignment dates, reminders, and other business of the group. Students also use this time to clarify assignments and ask questions about points of concern that relate to the group.

Such discussion, no matter how clear the syllabus may seem, is an important aspect of demystifying the grading process and can provide an opportunity for teaching negotiating skills:

> I taught a research class online during a six-week summer session. The compressed schedule was further complicated because it took students the first week to get glitches in the technology worked out. At week 3 of 6, a full-day session was scheduled in which students were to present oral critiques of research articles. I used a modified approach online to the *Peace and Power* process, and then in the on-site class, students experienced other aspects of the process, such as meeting me and each other, hearing the rain stick, and discussing added agenda items. In this case, the salient concern of the students was "would they learn what they should" with the time constraints. Personally, I had some of the same concerns. I invited their suggestions and taught them the basics of win-win negotiation. In other words, the group could only change assignments if a positive outcome resulted for both students and faculty. It took considerable struggling, but they proposed a solution that I agreed was workable. It worked out so well that I am considering it for future classes!

Principles of Unity

During the first few weeks of a course, it is helpful for students to develop principles of unity. These are values and statements of purpose that students can use as guidelines for classroom behavior. Often these principles address issues that are fundamental to the *Peace and Power* process such as "helping ourselves and others achieve academic goals," "respecting differences," and "being open-minded and receptive" to others' suggestions. Principles such as these can be used to shift responsibility for class behavior from the teacher to the students.

SOPHIA

Once the housekeeping items on the agenda have been completed, the teacher and students move to the topic of the day. A SOPHIA is a useful way of focusing student attention on the topic. Rather than summarizing the readings related to the topic, the SOPHIA encourages students to critically examine how the topic is presented in the readings, what assumptions underpin the readings, and what application the content may have for clinical practice. The SOPHIA concludes with "Imagine Alternatives," which fosters a provocative discussion about the topic.

Preparing and presenting a SOPHIA is an effective learning activity for students. It is important, however, for the teacher to model what is expected in a SOPHIA in the first weeks of the course. Often, students seem more comfortable in presenting content, rather than critically examining its relevance to practice.

Class Discussion

The quality of class discussion depends largely on the level of preparation of the students. Some students may lack confidence to speak out in a group, particularly if it is large. Strategies such as working in pairs or small groups on a focused task are effective to encourage student participation. Ideally, the students will take ownership of the process and dynamics within the classroom and develop principles of unity to guide their discussions. However, this may take some time and will require clear direction and consistent role modeling by the teacher.

The challenge for students is to accept that learning to interact effectively in groups is as important to nurses as the content. Once students have experienced some success with this process, they can begin to use it in other situations. Students have told us of using *Peace and Power* in group work, in clinical practice, in other courses, and in their personal lives. One group of students recalled beginning the process of appreciation, critical reflection, and affirmation on a trip to Florida!

Closing

Checking out, or closing, is the last activity of class. When people check out of class, they state (a) their name again, (b) an appreciative thought, generally directed toward someone or something learned that day in class, (c) a critical reflection or insight gained during the class, and (d) an affirmation. This often results in students valuing each other, a characteristic that may carry over into their professional lives. Occasionally, there are students who check out with tears because of experiences in the class that were meaningful to them. If students have negative responses to the class that day, these also are stated during the closing and are accepted by the teacher and peers. It is the students' time to be honest, knowing that whatever they say will be valued. Check out is a fitting conclusion to any class or group meeting because it allows the participants to summarize the significance of what happened during that class.

USING *PEACE AND POWER* IN THE CLINICAL SETTING

The clinical setting poses its own challenges to using *Peace and Power*; since the focus is on client care, it may be difficult to find time to teach the basics of the process. Preparing a handout for students on the *Peace and Power* process and making copies of the book available on the unit may be helpful. A general pattern is to check in at the preclinical conference and check out at the postclinical conference. It is challenging, however, to take the time to check out when students are tired and anxious to go home, but it is worth the effort.

Student presentations of SOPHIAs are valuable for clinical conferences. It is important, though, to allow students two to three weeks to become comfortable with the clinical course and setting before asking them to prepare and present a SOPHIA. Parameters regarding length and topic need to be established in advance either democratically or by the teacher. A 10-minute SOPHIA works well in post-clinical conference. As in the classroom, it is helpful for the clinical teacher to model the initial SOPHIA. Depending on the length of the clinical course and the number of students, it may be necessary for students to work in pairs.

The clinical setting provides an opportunity for faculty to role model the feminist pedagogical principles of empowerment and caring. This is done by maintaining a caring and supportive approach to interactions with patients, staff, and students in all patient care activities. This approach is exemplified in the following passage:

> Students by definition are not yet at the level of independent practice required at graduation. It is my role as a clinical teacher to ensure that they provide safe and competent care. To attend to the multiple aspects of patient care, students need to be well prepared to care for their patients. If not, or if they are not performing at the expected level, I believe it is caring on my part to confront the situation. In a straightforward manner, I ask students to review the material with me. Recently, I told one student I was concerned that she might be bluffing and not really have the

knowledge to support her clinical actions. I explained that was not acceptable in nursing work, and there was no negotiation. By the end of the semester, she was trustworthy during her clinical practice time. Using concepts of mutual respect, honesty, and directness in interactions is a powerful way to teach students about appropriate professional behavior.

Demystification of which learning evidences will contribute to a grade is as important in the clinical area as it is in the classroom. The nature of learning evidences, criteria by which they are to be graded, and the value assigned to each activity must be clear well in advance. A schedule of learning activities may initially be generated by the clinical teacher. The clinical group may negotiate modifications, such as topic, due date, or assigned value. Whatever the process, it is important to clarify expectations early in the clinical rotation to relieve students' anxiety and allow them to assume greater responsibility for their own learning.

The more experiences students have with effective negotiation and problem-solving approaches, the more likely they are to adopt them for other group work. Many everyday experiences can be turned into such teaching opportunities:

> Last semester, there was an extra clinical day. That meant, among other things, that one student could observe twice in the operating room. Every student wanted that experience. Rather than choose the student myself, I brought it to the group for resolution. Each student expressed reasons for wanting to have the second day in the operating room. I identified four ways the dilemma could be resolved: (1) draw straws, (2) give me the decision-making responsibility, (3) deny all students the extra observation, or (4) make the decision by consensus. The group chose consensus and effectively made the decision.

Peace and Power is useful in facilitating clinical learning. It provides a process for effective problem solving and an opportunity for every voice to be heard. The *Peace and Power* process also provides an opportunity for developing negotiation and consensus-building skills that are an asset in any work environment.

CONCLUSION

Our experiences with the *Peace and Power* process, first as students, then as teachers, have been rewarding. Although our enthusiasm stems from overwhelmingly positive responses from students, it would be misleading and less than helpful to suggest that the process is a panacea for all student concerns. In the same class, one student might report that the teacher was nonjudgmental and open, while another might feel and express the opposite.

We have shared our successes with using *Peace and Power* in diverse settings both to illustrate that there is no "right way" and to identify elements that are critical for success. We have attempted to show that even if we teach in circumstances that are less than ideal, substantial benefits may still be derived from using the *Peace and Power* process, in whatever ways are possible, to introduce students to a different way of being with one another.

REFERENCES

Allen, D. G. (1990). The curriculum revolution: Radical re-visioning of nursing education. *Journal of Nursing Education, 29*, 312–316.

Bevis, E. O., & Watson, J. (1989). *Toward a caring curriculum: A new pedagogy for nursing.* New York: National League for Nursing.

Brunson, D. A., & Vogt, J. F. (1996). Empowering our students and ourselves: A liberal democratic approach to the communication classroom. *Communication Education, 45*(1), 73–83.

Chinn, P. L. (1989). Feminist pedagogy in nursing education. In *Curriculum revolution: Reconceptualizing nursing education* (pp. 9–24). New York: National League for Nursing.

Chinn, P. L. (2001). *Peace and power: Building communities for the future* (5th ed.). New York: Jones and Bartlett.

Ellis-Stoll, C. C., & Popkess-Vawter, S. (1998). A concept analysis on the process of empowerment. *Advances in Nursing Science, 21*, 62–68.

Freire, P. (1973). *Pedagogy of the oppressed.* New York: Continuum.

Gibson, C. H. (1991). A concept analysis of empowerment. *Journal of Advanced Nursing, 16*, 354–361.

Hedin, B. A. (1986). A case study of oppressed group behavior in nurses. *Image: Journal of Nursing Scholarship, 18*, 53–57.

Hedin, B. A. (1989a). A feminist perspective on nursing education. *Nurse Educator, 14*(4), 8–13.

Hedin, B. A. (1989b). With eyes aglitter: Journey to the curriculum revolution. *Nurse Educator, 14*(4), 3–5.

hooks, b. (1994). *Teaching to transgress: Education as the practice of freedom.* New York: Routledge.

Ironside, P. M. (2001). Creating a research-base for nursing education: An interpretive review of conventional, critical, feminist, postmodern, and phenomenological pedagogies. *Advances in Nursing Science, 23*(3), 72–87.

Kenway, J., & Modra, H. (1992). Feminist pedagogy and emancipatory possibilities. In C. Luke & J. Gore (Eds.), *Feminisms and critical pedagogy* (pp. 138–166). New York: Routledge.

Lather, P. (1991). *Getting smart: Feminist research and pedagogy within the postmodern.* New York: Routledge.

Lewis, M. (1992). Interrupting patriarchy: Politics, resistance and transformation in the feminist classroom. In C. Luke & J. Gore (Eds.), *Feminisms and critical pedagogy* (pp. 167–191). New York: Routledge.

Lindeman, C. (1989). Curriculum revolution: Reconceptualizing clinical nursing education. *Nursing & Health Care, 10,* 23–28.

Maher, F. A., & Tetreault, M. K. T. (1994). *The feminist classroom.* New York: HarperCollins.

Martin, J. R. (1981). The ideal of the educated person. *Journal of Education, 31*(2), 97–109.

Pitts, T. P. (1985). The covert curriculum: What does nursing education really teach? *Nursing Outlook, 33,* 37–42.

Rafael, A. R. F. (1995). Advocacy and empowerment: Dichotomous or synchronous concepts? *Advances in Nursing Science, 18*(2), 25–32.

Roberts, S. J. (1983). Oppressed group behavior: Implications for nursing. *Advances in Nursing Science, 8*(7), 21–30.

Rodwell, C. (1998). Empowerment: An analysis of the concept of empowerment. In C. Hein (Ed.), *Contemporary Leadership Behavior* (5th ed., pp. 155–165). Philadelphia: Lippincott.

Watson, J. (1989). A new paradigm of curriculum development. In E. O. Bevis & J. Watson (Eds.), *Toward a caring curriculum: A new pedagogy for nursing* (pp. 37–50). New York: National League for Nursing.

Weiler, K. (1988). *Women teaching for change.* New York: Bergin & Garvey.

Chapter 14

Information Technology Applications in a Community-Based Curriculum

Cheryl P. McCahon and Sheila A. Niles

Over the past 10 years, the Cleveland State University Department of Nursing (CSU) and Visiting Nurse Association Healthcare Partners of Ohio (VNAHPO) developed its education/practice partnership, *Vision on 22nd Street*. This partnership has evolved into a community-based, education-service model that provides value to both institutions. The purpose of this chapter is to describe selected VNAHPO technology initiatives with subsequent application and integration into the CSU community-based nursing curriculum. The chapter framework includes descriptions of the three phases of technology development: phase one describes telehealth initiatives, phase two chronicles state-of-the-art, point-of-care technology integration, and phase three introduces some future initiatives. Curricular applications with each phase are described, and issues for implementation are discussed. Opportunities to incorporate technology initiatives within a curriculum, limitations to integration, and recommendations are provided to guide faculty considering any technology initiatives.

EVOLUTION OF INFORMATION TECHNOLOGY INTEGRATION IN NURSING CURRICULUM

The partnership between the CSU and VNAHPO, *Vision on 22nd Street*, was forged in response to mutual partner needs and the articulated strategies identified by the PEW Foundation (de Tornyay, 1992). Shared needs included meeting an urban mission by responding to the community's health care needs, implementation of a community-based curriculum, and developing a cadre of graduates prepared for community practice. The partnership demonstrated that models such as those recommended by PEW could provide a collaborative relationship between clinical education and service with outcomes that include state-of-the-art clinical nursing practice. In a community-based curriculum, these models provide opportunities for faculty practice, new and expanded avenues for community collaboration, and research initiatives (McCahon, Niles, George, & Stricklin, 1999; McCahon & Niles, 2000).

The *Vision on 22nd Street* model supports Maxwell's contention that vision adds value to everything (Maxwell, 1993). The partnership maximized the educational experiences of students in service delivery, fostered a collaborative spirit between two different organizational cultures, and created a bond of trust that affords the two institutions opportunities to explore nontraditional venues in research and clinical sites. The ongoing success of the partnership has been instrumental in attaining numerous collaborative grants that are grounded in the *Vision on 22nd Street* model. Currently, the ongoing management of the partnership and the challenges of sustainability are the responsibilities of co-coordinators from each organization (the CSU Undergraduate Nursing Program Director and the VNAHPO Director).

PARTNERS IN THE *VISION ON 22nd STREET* MODEL

Cleveland State University

Cleveland State University was created more than 35 years ago to provide affordable public higher education to residents of greater Cleveland. The Department of Nursing, housed in the College of Arts and Sciences, offers a baccalaureate nursing degree and a master's degree in nursing with a focus on the health of populations. The majority (85%) of graduates remain in the greater Cleveland area, providing a cadre of nurse leaders to meet the needs of Cleveland's health care community. The university has identified health care initiatives as a goal, responding to community needs in a city in which health care is the major industry. The community-based curriculum developed with the VNAHPO partners provides rich, diverse clinical experiences producing graduates prepared to practice in a variety of institutional and community environments that comprise the Cleveland health care community.

Visiting Nurse Association Healthcare Partners of Ohio

Founded in 1902, the 100-year-old Visiting Nurse Association of Cleveland (now the Visiting Nurse Association Healthcare Partners of Ohio) is the pioneer nonprofit community health care organization in Ohio. Experts in nursing, rehabilitation, and supportive care deliver the full cycle of life services to more than 10,000 families throughout northeast and mid-Ohio. Now in its second century of caring, one of its four priorities for VNAHPO service delivery is technology. Technology initiatives are providing the information framework to enhance the delivery of services, improving efficiency, economy, and access to care. In the early 1990s, the VNAHPO recognized the technology tidal wave in the home care arena. The agency sought and attained funding and committed human resources to design, integrate, educate, and deliver evolving technology systems to enhance care delivery in the home and community.

Concurrently, as information technology skyrocketed to the forefront within the service sector, national groups such as the PEW Foundation, the American Association of Colleges of Nursing (AACN), the National League for Nursing, and nursing leaders emphasized the need for nursing students to become proficient in using this technology. The AACN Essentials of Baccalaureate Education for Professional Practice (1998) identified information and health care technologies as one of seven key components of core knowledge necessary to incorporate in baccalaureate curricula. According to Travis and Brennan (1998), basic understanding of computers, or computer literacy, was not sufficient for nursing practice. Instead, nurse educators needed to introduce a full range of informatics into nursing education, viewing the integration of technology into the support of patient care as an appropriate focus of nursing. Brennan (1999) contended that of the many technologies demanding nursing's attention, computer and information technologies held the most promise for supporting nursing in its efforts to build knowledge and enhance the health of society and its citizens.

Over the past 10 years, the VNAHPO and selective service collaborators have discussed the designs, processes, outcomes, and evaluations of their journey toward using clinically based information systems for patient care (Elfrink, 2001; Hockenjos & Wharton, 2001; Stricklin, 2001; Stricklin, Niles, Struk, & Jones, 2000; Stricklin, Jones, & Niles, 2000; Stricklin, Lowe-Phelps, & McVey, 2001; Struk, 2001; Thoman, Struk, Spero, & Stricklin, 2001). This literature provides guidelines for faculty, students, and clinicians as they integrate the "lessons learned" for the development of relevant clinical applications for nursing education.

Today, the exploding technology revolution in home care, with implications for nursing education and service delivery, has led to state-of-the-art practice for clinicians, faculty, and students. Selective technology initiatives developed by VNAHPO, specifically Healthy Talk and point-of-care technology, have been integrated into CSU's nursing curriculum.

PHASE I: EARLY TECHNOLOGY: HOMETALK™ AND HEALTHY TALK

In the mid-1990s, costly telecommunication and telemedicine products offered home care providers disease management systems that supported patient care and education. HomeTalk™, a product developed by the VNAHPO, "is a disease specific monitoring system that uses an interactive voice response system to monitor patients' health status and educate patients about their chronic disease" (Stricklin, Jones, & Niles, 2000, p. 55). This system expanded skilled home visits and care management.

The HomeTalk™ system's initial success led to a health promotion, health risk appraisal application, called Healthy Talk, which is part of the VNAHPO's community *Healthy Town* program (Stricklin, Jones, & Niles, 2000). The *Healthy Town* program provides health promotion screening for seniors in community centers throughout the greater Cleveland area. As part of this program, Healthy Talk is a user-friendly technology system that allows seniors to call from any touch-tone phone to complete the health promotion screenings. The screenings identify senior health risk issues such as safety and injury prevention; alcohol, drug, and family abuse; and anxiety and depression, and refer and link seniors to existing community-based resources (Niles, Alemagno, & Stricklin, 1997).

Curricular Applications of Early Technology

Curricular applications for early VNAHPO technology initiatives were introduced to CSU students in classroom discussions under the curricular framework of health promotion. Both basic students and registered nurses in the baccalaureate (RN/BSN) program learned about these telehealth initiatives. The RN/BSN students were able to work with the *Healthy Town* program and staff in the community centers, providing individual and group education for health promotion to center elders. The selected *Healthy Town* centers provided meal programs, funded by the Older Americans Act, which served as a student entrée to assess elders and offer health promotion teaching sessions. For example, students developed medication teaching, depression, and falls prevention modules.

One faculty member, excited about the benefits of the *Healthy Town* program, worked for the VNA during the summer to assist with delivery of the technology screening system. During this phase, the delivery of the technology screening system was extended to include families with children 2–6 years of age, and the technology screening tool was translated into Spanish. As a result of these developments, students were afforded the opportunity to observe culture/language-specific health promotion screenings using the translated tool with the congregation of a Spanish speaking church. A few students chose to work with *Healthy Town* staff for their senior practicum, a culminating experience for the generic BSN student. Students assisted in the development of new senior centers, identified community resources for referrals and linkages, wrote and implemented a variety of teaching modules directed at health promotion, and provided staff with assistance in addressing individual health care needs. This experience greatly enhanced their knowledge about health promotion and community resources and allocation.

Curricular Issues/Implementation: Phase I

Curricular issues that challenged the integration of Phase I technology, HomeTalk and the Healthy Talk screening system, into the clinical curriculum included the time frames required for service delivery, which conflicted with times students were available; the time needed to orient students to the concepts of technology supported health promotion; the lack of stable clinical faculty to assist the students in program orientation; and assignment to specific *Healthy Town* clinical sites. One aspect not foreseen was the ongoing need to promote faculty "buy-in" to the opportunities of the program. This problem may have been related, in part, to the faculty's hesitancy to take on new clinical experiences when those already in place met course objectives. In addition, introducing new activities meant additional faculty time would be needed for planning. However, based on student evaluations, the experience with *Healthy Town* and its Healthy Talk screening technology was a valuable learning opportunity that should be made available to all students.

Three students who were involved in an independent project with the *Healthy Town* program provided an exhaustive literature review on medication issues with elders for the *Healthy Town* staff who were designing medication teaching modules. The students also presented lectures on safe medication administration for individuals at the various *Healthy Town* senior community centers. The students evaluated this experience as one of the most important clinical learning activities in their curriculum. Based on the evaluations by students and staff at the senior centers, the *Healthy Town* program and its technology became an integrated component of the classroom portion of the community courses in the basic nursing program and of both classroom and clinical experiences in the RN/BSN courses (McCahon & Niles, 2000).

PHASE II: STATE-OF-THE-ART TECHNOLOGY: POINT-OF-CARE TECHNOLOGY

In the late 1990s, the VNAHPO began to explore all of the elements required to replace pencil and paper documentation with automated, online, real-time patient information (Stricklin, 2001, p. 743). This automated POC technology is a computer input device used by clinicians to both enter and retrieve clinical data. To the clinician and student, this means electronic charts, clinicians inputting clinical data in patient homes, and accessing, retrieving, and communicating patient information in real time.

With the support of products from McKesson Information Solutions Horizon Homecare (2003), VNAHPO completed the design, education, and implementation of POC technology with 175 clinicians. The implementation of this technology required weeks of agency, individual, and group training, which included preparing teaching manuals for VNAHPO clinicians, and computer competencies.

Curricular Applications/Implementation: Phase II

Curricular applications necessary in Phase II initiatives became evident with the agency's decision to become involved in POC technology. Students making traditional skilled home visits with VNA nurses would observe both cutting-edge technology and experience the reaction of patients and staff to the paperless system. They would observe the trials and tribulations of home care nurses providing "hands on care" and laptop documentation of patient data in the home, and learn about what was necessary to make the system work. It became clear quickly that because of the complexities associated with the agency experience in preparing nurses to use POC technology, CSU nursing students would not be in their clinical rotation long enough to learn and then apply POC principles in an actual home care visit.

The partnership faculty believed that simulation of the POC system would be an acceptable alternative. That belief, coupled with the conviction that incorporating informatics across the CSU curriculum was imperative, led to a technology grant proposal to support the costs of integrating information technology concepts and experiential activities in the curriculum and developing a simulated POC lab for the nursing program. The grant was funded by a local foundation in part because it built on the successful outcomes of the *Vision on 22nd Street* model and the strength of the partner relationship.

Point-of-Care Technology Simulated Laboratory: Phase II

The POC lab was funded as a one-year project. However, the project director and those involved in implementing the POC lab found the process to be more complex than first thought. Since POC was new to the involved faculty, as well as to the students and nurses, the project director decided that the four faculty who were directing and implementing the project should complete the same orientation to the POC as the VNA staff. This orientation, extending for 1-week, 8 hours a day, during the summer, provided faculty with multiple insights about using POC technology and a preview of the issues that would later confront the RN/BSN students who would pilot the project.

With the assistance and support of the VNA technical staff, an orientation manual was developed for student and faculty use. The manual contained information about computer basics, terminology specific to POC, and information about the Outcome and Assessment Information Set (OASIS), the 17-page assessment tool used by home care nurses to assess, develop, implement, and evaluate a patient's plan of care.

The project director and VNAHPO specialists then developed the simulated POC laboratory, which was located in a classroom at VNAHPO headquarters. The simulated laboratory was wired for student use, and four case studies were written for students to use to input data into a laptop programmed for their use. The course syllabus was redesigned to integrate didactic information about POC technology and a simulated lab assignment.

Issues with Development of Simulated Laboratory

Significant hours of time, beyond the funding from the grant, went into development of the simulated laboratory with outcomes that were less than impressive. While students expressed many of the same concerns that were voiced by the VNA clinicians who went through agency orientation to POC, they had other issues with the simulated laboratory experience. The learning process to develop computer competencies was intense, and the OASIS form, with its multiple questions, screens, and new terminology, was tedious to learn how to use. The time required for learning how to use the laptop and OASIS tool left little opportunity for practice. In addition, students demonstrated a general lack of knowledge specific to home care nursing, how to set priorities, and what was expected within the context of a home visit.

One major difference between staff nurses and students was that while some within each group had limited computer skills, compromising their ability to even conceive of a paperless system, the staff nurses *had* to learn the system. In contrast, the students had taken a Computers and Health Care course so they had lost the fear frequently seen in one new to the basics of a computer and were able to experience the simulation as an educational exercise rather than having to learn how to use the system such as the staff nurses did. Other issues that interfered with a positive experience for students were the agency time frames provided for the simulation. Since the community course only met one day per week, and the lab was only available to students at that time, most students were unable to complete the simulation assignment within their allocated course/clinical time even when they worked in pairs.

Strategies for Resolving Issues

As educators prepare students to use technology in clinical practice, understanding the basic technology and skills in using it, as well as relevant clinical experiences with technology, must be addressed throughout the nursing curriculum. To date, several of the curricular concerns that existed during Phases I and II have been resolved. Prior to this project, RN/BSN students piloted a computer competency test available to incoming freshmen. Those students with little or no computer knowledge were encouraged to enroll in a university computer course to assure a level of confidence in using the technology. During implementation of the simulated lab experience, a nurse informatics consultant developed a computer competency test specifically for the nursing program, and today that test is part of the admission process. Students who are deficient must successfully complete a Computers in Health Care course. That course includes basic computer skills and introduces the students to the information technology applications across the curriculum. Additional initiatives are being planned to incorporate documentation protocols into the student's clinical practice experiences in order for technology to play an ongoing role in the student's professional development.

FUTURE TECHNOLOGY: PHASE III

The *Healthy Town* program, supported since 1994 by local philanthropic foundations and funding from the State of Ohio, has kept pace with new technology applications. The initial telephone IVR Healthy Talk screenings were replaced with interactive laptop video screening and education modules. Today, seniors at community centers sit at the laptops and enter their own data specific to their health needs. Based on these data, they receive automatic printed health risk appraisals, select education modules specific to their health promotion needs, and are referred and linked to existing community resources. Medication education and management software was recently developed and added to the *Healthy Town* program. In addition, *Healthy Town* Web pages were developed with hot links that provide senior center staff with easy access to health information and local health resources (VNAHPO, 2002).

CareWatch, a new telemedicine VNAHPO initiative, was implemented in the summer of 2002, following an extensive agency pilot program. *CareWatch* is a home monitoring device reminder to measure and record a patient's vital data. It looks like a clock radio and weighs less than 3 pounds. Early on, a few of the RN/BSN students working with VNAHPO clinical preceptors observed the *CareWatch* monitors being piloted in patient homes and were able to share perceptions of the experience with their peers. Now, all students working with a clinical preceptor have an opportunity to not only observe but also work with clients using the monitoring devices, as more are made available to clients through the agency. Telemedicine products are now emerging as an essential component of the delivery of skilled home care services.

The *Healthy Town* program has screened over 2500 seniors at 26 senior centers and provided students opportunities for "hands on" curricular technology applications within a community service agency. The program structure and evidence-based outcomes are consistent with multiple components of the CSU curriculum, and CSU is part of the plan for sustaining the program after the funding ends. Students deliver services, use technology applications, review aggregate population data, design Web downloadable education brochures for the *Healthy Town* Web pages, and conduct medication assessments and group health promotion lectures to seniors and community staff. They also participate in updating the annual review of community resources for centers and the Web pages. *Healthy Town* has provided students with a variety of multicultural clinical experiences. Most importantly, student evaluations consistently provide high ratings for the program and learning about population health.

CHALLENGES FOR INFORMATION TECHNOLOGY APPLICATIONS IN EDUCATION/PRACTICE PARTNERSHIPS

Throughout the development of the initiatives discussed in this chapter, time frames were a challenge for both organizations. University courses are developed on a 16-week cycle, whereas an agency such as VNAHPO delivers services seven days per week. The *Healthy Town* program was frequently introduced to new senior center sites in time frames to fit the center and the VNAHPO staff work schedules. Often these time frames did not fit the structure of academic schedules or specific clinical course offerings. For example, students needed to return to campus for a 2 p.m. class, not allowing enough time after lunch to complete the teaching for the *Healthy Town* program. As a result, students frequently could not observe or provide the level of support to programs such as *Healthy Town* that might be possible if time frames for program presentation did not conflict with their class schedules.

This time frame problem was complicated by a variety of personnel changes leading to faculty instability. "Buy-in" was needed by new faculty, none of whom had been part of the original *Vision* model planning and evolving partner collaborations. Community-based learning activities are often new to faculty and may be unsettling to faculty who were educated at a time when clinical nursing experiences took place mainly within the confines of the institution. In addition, many newly hired faculty were novices to the emerging technology applications in the service sector. Although faculty orientation to the overall CSU nursing program is provided, university expectations for faculty as well as individual faculty research agendas create competing priorities for faculty time.

The numerous challenges for VNAHPO clinicians in learning POC technology through use of a computer laboratory such as developing computer skills, learning the new home care assessment tools and changing documentation standards, and applying POC technology in the patient environment (Struk, 2001) were similar for the nursing students. In addition, for the RN/BSN students using the simulated POC laboratory, clinical course scheduling, computer access, and time to practice in the lab were major challenges for an already demanding classroom and clinical schedule. While these RN students had some experience in hospitals using elements of computers, they were being asked to apply the POC technology and OASIS assessment tools to simulate a home care visit, a new clinical environment that provided its own challenges.

While they were practicing with the simulated case studies in the lab, students also were assigned to a VNAHPO nurse preceptor. During the initial home care visits, students were expected to observe the preceptor's behavior, for example, how the preceptor communicated with the client, and what safety issues were confronted by the preceptor. Students also examined the use of the POC technology by the preceptor and how the technology was integrated in clinical care. For example, how does the nurse concentrate on communicating with the client while at the same time inputting data into the laptop? Although students were never expected to document on the client's actual record, they found that even the simulated case studies and an assignment to develop a plan of care using the OASIS assessment were stressful. However, the experience with the preceptor did heighten their awareness of the issues clinicians face when using POC technology during home care visits.

For both students and staff, orientation to POC technology was complicated by the need for multiple laptops and inability to provide sufficient laptops and laboratory space to accommodate large numbers of students at any one time. An additional factor that has continued to pose challenges are the Health Insurance Portability and Accountability Act standards, with implications not only for POC technology but also for the provision of new safeguards regarding all types of electronically transmitted information.

OPPORTUNITIES FOR INFORMATION TECHNOLOGY APPLICATIONS IN EDUCATION/PRACTICE PARTNERSHIPS

Innovative and diverse opportunities for information technology initiatives exist in both the education and service sectors. For example, with continued success in each technology program came the ability to develop new collaboratives, with partners from governmental agencies as well as philanthropic foundations. Funding opportunities became available for new programming. For example, funding for a medication education program was secondary to the ongoing success of the *Healthy Town* program. New collaboratives were initiated to enhance health promotion services for age-specific populations. Some monetary awards, such as a training grant to teach end-of-life care to practicing nurses and nursing students did not relate to the technology initiatives but resulted from the ongoing success of the education/practice partnership.

What were the opportunities for students and faculty? First, students were able to interact with clients across the health care continuum in settings other than the acute care environment. With each new initiative, students gained entrée to new clinical sites. Each initiative demonstrated to students the importance of technology in nursing education, not only from the perspective of learning about new hardware but also from the perspective of information management. Students also had opportunities for involvement in cutting edge practice initiatives. Faculty involved in the various programs gained opportunities for faculty practice as well as adapting the evolving technologies to nursing education.

The *Vision* partnership has continued to increase the visibility of both organizations and has been provided nontraditional multicultural clinical experiences for students and faculty and for community engagement. The success of the partnership initiatives has strengthened ties between the two organizations and provided the impetus needed for program sustainability.

LIMITATIONS OF INFORMATION TECHNOLOGY APPLICATIONS IN EDUCATION/PRACTICE PARTNERSHIPS

As information technology becomes an increasingly important consideration in both education and service sectors, it is important to reiterate:

- Technology is an information management tool. The tools are only as effective as the practitioners who understand their use.
- Technology can enhance classroom teaching and facilitate learning.
- Learning to manage information needs is necessary for nurses practicing in today's health care arena. Taking risks and being willing to change are no longer luxuries in nursing practice.
- Technological changes will continue at a rapid rate, and costly and frequent upgrades will be necessary.
- Technology at the POC in the home environment does not save time; it adds more time to nursing care.
- Curricular changes take time. Incorporating technology concepts in courses and planning clinical experiences for students involves ongoing discussions with faculty and exploration of innovative approaches that take time to plan.
- Educators need to "pick up the pace" and put informatics on a "fast track" to successfully integrate it within nursing programs.

RECOMMENDATIONS TO SCHOOLS OF NURSING

To effectively implement information technology initiatives in a school of nursing, faculty should:

- Explore partnering with a clinical agency and identify the advantages/constraints of a partnering situation.
- Realize that support by administrators and others who have the ability to effect change is essential for success and sustainability.
- Recognize that there needs to be fiscal, material and human contributions from each partner.
- Rethink faculty research agendas to include real-time clinical issues that will contribute to nursing's body of knowledge.
- Set realistic time frames for developing strategies for teaching students how to use technology.
- Accelerate the implementation of curricular changes in nursing education to respond to the nursing practice expectations of the present and future health care environment.

Faculty continue to express concern about constraints to students' clinical practice time, yet the information technology interface realistically requires more classroom and clinical hours to meet nursing care needs. Are there "sacred cows" that need to be abandoned in order to respond to our changing health care landscape?

SUMMARY

In summary, the role of information technology in client care will continue to be a priority in both the academic and service sectors. Education/practice partnerships such as *Vision on 22nd Street* can provide the framework, impetus, and collaboration necessary for successful technology initiatives. Outcomes of successful education/practice partnerships will benefit each organization and foster new initiatives, increase visibility, and contribute to quality patient care. Although educators contend that the burgeoning nursing curriculum cannot be extended, the reality is that students, and practicing nurses, today and in the future need to understand and apply information technology in an ever changing health care delivery system. Though significant issues must be considered when developing new initiatives, opportunities abound for those who persevere.

ACKNOWLEDGMENT

The *Healthy Town* Program received a 2003 Best Practice Award from the Health Promotion Institute, National Council on Aging.

REFERENCES

American Association of Colleges of Nursing. (1998). *The essentials of baccalaureate education for professional nursing practice.* Washington, DC: Author.

Brennan, P. (1999). Harnessing innovative technologies: What can you do with a shoe? *Nursing Outlook, 47,* 128–132.

de Tornyay, R. (1992). Reconsidering nursing education: The Report of the Pew Health Professions Commission. *Journal of Nursing Education, 21,* 296–301.

Elfrink, V. (2001). A look to the future: How emerging information technology will impact operations and practice. *Home Healthcare Nurse, 19*(12), 751–757.

Hockenjos, G., & Wharton, A. (2001). Point of care training: Strategies for success. *Home Healthcare Nurse, 19,* 766–773.

Maxwell, J. (1993). *Developing the leader within you.* Nashville, TN: Thomas Nelson Publishers.

McCahon, C., & Niles, S. (2000). The Vision on 22nd Street partnership: The experience of Cleveland State University. In P. Matteson (Ed.), *Teaching nurses in the neighborhood: Innovative responses* (pp. 188–203). New York: Springer Publishing Co.

McCahon, C., Niles, S. A., George, V. D., & Stricklin, M. L. (1999). Vision on 22nd Street: A model to restructure nursing education. *Nursing & Health Care Perspectives, 20,* 296–301.

McKesson Information Solutions (2003). McKesson HBOC-ITB. Horizon Homecare products. Retrieved March 3, 2003, from http://www.horizonhomecare.com/

Niles, S., Alemagno, S., & Stricklin, M. L. (1997). Healthy Talk: A telecommunications model for health promotion. *Caring, XVI*(7), 46–50.

Stricklin, M. L., Jones, S., & Niles, S. A. (2000). Home Talk™, Healthy Talk: Improving patients' health status with telephone technology. *Home Healthcare Nurse, 18,* 52–62.

Stricklin, M. L., Niles, S., Struk, C., & Jones, S. (2000). What nurses and nurse managers expect from point of care technology. *Home Healthcare Nurse, 18,* 515–523.

Stricklin, M. L. (2001). Technology for tomorrow's homecare. *Home Healthcare Nurse, 19,* 743.

Stricklin, M. L., Lowe-Phelps, K., & McVey, R. (2001). Home care patients' responses to point of care technology. *Home Healthcare Nurse, 19,* 774–778.

Struk, C. (2001). Critical steps for integrating information technology in home care: One agency's experience. *Home Healthcare Nurse, 19,* 758–765.

Thoman, J., Struk, C., Spero, M., & Stricklin, M. L. (2001). Reflections from a point of care pilot nurse group experience. *Home Healthcare Nurse, 19,* 779–784.

Travis, L., & Brennan, P. (1998). Information science for the future: An innovative nursing informatics curriculum. *Journal of Nursing Education, 37,* 162–167.

Visiting Nurse Association Healthcare Partners of Ohio. (2002). *Sample Comprehensive Health Profile.* Retrieved March 3, 2003, from http://www.vnahealthytown.org/html/services/HealthyTown/healthplan/content.htm

SELECTED BIBLIOGRAPHY

Axford, R. L., & Carter, B. E. (1996). Impact of clinical information systems on nursing practice: Nurse's perspectives. *Computers in Nursing, 14,* 156–163.

Carty, B., & Rosenfeld, P. (1998). From computer technology to information technology: Findings from a national study of nursing education. *Computers in Nursing, 16,* 259–265.

Elfrink, V., Davis, L. S., Fitzwater, E., Castleman, J., Burley, J., Gorney-Moreno, M. J., et al. (2000). A comparison of teaching strategies for information technology into clinical nursing education. *Nurse Educator, 25,* 136–144.

Elfrink, V., & Martin, K. (1996). Education for community nursing practice: Point of care technology. *Healthcare Information Management, 10*(2), 81–89.

Lewis, D., & Pesut, D. (2001). Emergence of consumer health informatics. *Nursing Outlook, 49,* 7.

National Advisory Council on Nurse Education and Practice. (1997, December). *A national informatics agenda for nursing education and practice* (pp. 1–32). Report to the Secretary of the Department of Health and Human Services Health Resources and Services Administration. Washington, DC: U.S. Government Printing Office.

National League for Nursing. (1993). *Vision for nursing education.* New York: Author.

Nightingale Tracker Field Test Nurse Team. (1999). Designing an information technology application for use in community focused nursing education. *Computers in Nursing, 17,* 73–81.

Nightingale Tracker Field Test Nurse Team. (2000). A comparison of teaching strategies for integrating information technology into clinical nursing education. *Nurse Educator, 25,* 136–144.

O'Grady-Porter, T. (2001). Profound change: 21st century nursing. *Nursing Outlook, 49,* 182–186.

Russo, H. (2001). Window of opportunity for home health nurses: Telehealth technologies. *Online Journal of Issues in Nursing, 6*(3), topic 16. Available at: http://www.nursingworld.org/ojin/topic16/tpc16_4.htm

Siktberg, L., & Dillard, N. (1999). Technology in the nursing classroom. *Nursing & Health Care Perspectives, 20,* 128–133.

Stanley, J., Kiehl, E., Matteson, P., McCahon, C., & Schmid, E. (2002). Moving forward with community based nursing education. Washington, DC: AACN.

U.S. Department of Health and Human Services. (1991). *Healthy People 2000: National Health Promotion and Disease Prevention Objectives.* Washington, DC: Author.

U.S. Department of Health and Human Services. (2000). *Healthy People 2010.* Washington, DC: Author.

Verhey, M. (1999). Information literacy in an undergraduate nursing curriculum: Development, implementation, and evaluation. *Journal of Nursing Education, 38,* 252–259.

Part V

Development of Students, Nurses, and Teachers

Chapter 15

Student Academic Dishonesty

Marianne R. Jeffreys and Lori Stier

A s we begin the 21st century, there is growing concern that nursing student academic dishonesty is widespread. Despite this, little has been done to change the culture of nursing education and equip academic administrators and faculty to deal effectively with this increasing problem. The shortage of nursing professionals, the increasing complexities of health care, and a more academically diverse and less prepared student population currently offer additional new challenges for nursing education. Nurse educators are in a key position to promote academic integrity, discourage academic dishonesty, and uphold professional values through the use of well-planned "PROACTIVE" communication with students about student academic dishonesty (SAD), and through definitive action when cheating or other dishonest behavior is discovered.

Through the use of case exemplars from a variety of academic and clinical settings, this chapter illustrates how nurse educators can proactively promote student academic integrity through the use of effective communication. Future implications and resources for nurse educators conclude the chapter.

AN OVERVIEW OF STUDENT ACADEMIC DISHONESTY

Prior to 1980, little was written on the topic of SAD in nursing. Over the past twenty years, however, a growing body of literature has addressed dishonesty as a valid nursing concern (Bailey, 1990, 2001; Bradshaw &

Lowenstein, 1990; Brown, 2002; Daniel, Adams, & Smith, 1994; Gaberson, 1997; Hilbert, 1985, 1987, 1988; Jeffreys & Stier, 1991, 1995, 1998; Osinski, 2003; Prescott, 1989; Roberts, 1999). Early nursing research examined the causes of SAD and the possible effects it could have on future professional development.

During the past decade an explosion in information technology and Internet use has tangled the problem of academic dishonesty. Students first began using computers for purposes of fact finding and information gathering, but have come to depend on it as a primary source of information. Some report that at the present time, "the probable impact of Internet access on student plagiarism is mostly a matter of conjecture and has not yet been studied sufficiently or systematically" (Scanlon & Neumann, 2002, p. 374). Other sources cite increasing evidence of plagiarism via undocumented use of materials from the Internet, purchase of papers from online paper mills, and use of plagiarism-detection software by college faculty (Young, 2001).

"PROACTIVE" COMMUNICATION

To prepare highly qualified nursing professionals who are ready to meet the ethical dilemmas and health care demands of the future, faculty cannot ignore SAD. Nurse educators must take action through a "PROACTIVE" communication strategy to preventing academic dishonesty (Figure 15.1). "PROACTIVE" communication focuses on: Policy, Responsibility, Ongoing action, Accountability, Commitment, Trust, Initiative, Values, and Expectations.

Policy: It is critical that college policies be clearly stated, publicized, and understood by students and faculty alike. Students must perceive that policies are fair and consistently applied (Berger, 2001). Penalties for cheating need to be clearly defined and communicated in school policy to promote agreement regarding expectations in coursework.

Responsibility: It is the faculty's responsibility to clearly delineate dishonest behaviors and to communicate these to students through written policies and open discussions.

Ongoing: Academic integrity needs to be continually reinforced with students throughout the semester. Faculty must take advantage of every opportunity to reinforce school policies and make students aware of the seriousness of dishonest behaviors and their consequences.

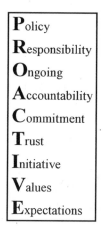

Policy

Responsibility

Ongoing

Accountability

Commitment

Trust

Initiative

Values

Expectations

FIGURE 15.1   Proactive communication.

Accountability: School administrators and educators are ultimately accountable for academic integrity. Leadership commitment to academic integrity can best be expressed as part of the organizational mission, vision, and values. Academic administrators can support faculty to both develop and enforce school policies.

Commitment: Faculty can demonstrate their commitment to academic integrity by weaving open discussions about the importance of honesty and integrity into their coursework. When students see an established policy in addition to a commitment on the part of faculty and administrators, it serves to reinforce school values and expectations.

Trust: Trust and respect form the basis for effective teaching, learning, and evaluation (Gaberson, 1997).

Initiative: Faculty must take the initiative to incorporate and enforce school policies in both the clinical and classroom setting.

Values: It is the mutual responsibility of administrators, students, and faculty to understand and uphold academic integrity as an institutional value (May & Loyd, 1993).

Expectations: Expectations are clearly set by school policy and reinforced by the faculty's commitment to student academic integrity. The National Student Nurses Association (NSNA) adopted a two-part Code of Ethics consisting of a Code of Professional Conduct (1999) and Code for Academic and Clinical Conduct (2001). The Code of

Ethics along with the NSNA Bill of Rights and Responsibilities for Students of Nursing (1991) provide guidelines that set the tone for professional development.

STUDENT ACADEMIC DISHONESTY MODEL

Jeffreys and Stier (1995) first developed a conceptual model illustrating the complexities and issues of SAD in nursing. Five assumptions underlie this model:

1. Student academic dishonesty is a widespread problem affecting all disciplines including nursing.
2. Student academic dishonesty can be damaging to future professional development.
3. Student academic dishonesty may adversely affect client care.
4. Academic integrity, professionalism, and quality health care are important values to the nursing profession and society.
5. Proactive communication is the key strategy for preventing and confronting dishonest behavior.

The SAD model that is proposed in this chapter builds on the previous prototype and further illustrates the paths that undergraduate nursing students and nurse educators may encounter during the course of a degree program (Figure 15.2).

PREDISPOSING FACTORS

Nursing students are influenced by a multitude of psychological, ethical, legal, social, and environmental factors that may predispose them to dishonest behaviors (Table 15.1). Many of these factors develop over time and long before a student gains admission to a program of academic study. Similarly, nurse educators can be affected by factors that may cause them to ignore student dishonesty (Table 15.2). When students behave dishonestly and educators fail to recognize or confront these behaviors, the nursing profession ultimately suffers. "The nursing student who cheats during academic exercises and who manages to obtain passing grades, graduate, pass state boards, and become licensed may not be capable of practicing competently" (Jeffreys & Stier, 1991, p. 1).

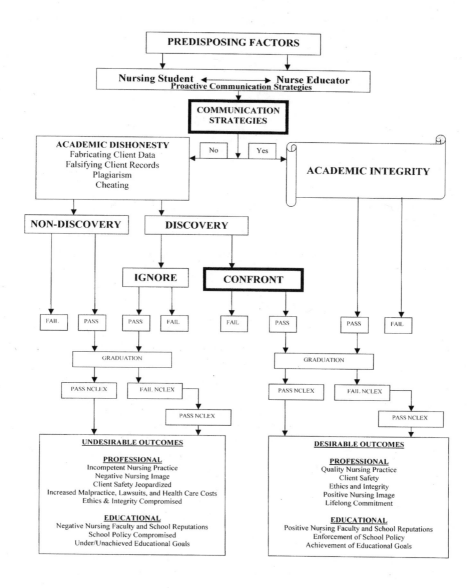

FIGURE 15.2   Jeffreys and Stier student academic dishonesty model.

TABLE 15.1   Factors Predisposing Nursing Students to Dishonest Behavior

Category	Factors
Psychological	Stress
	Pressure for high grades
	Family expectations
	Test anxiety
	Borderline or failing grades
	Personality
	Need for approval
Ethical (Level of Moral Development)	Difficulty differentiating right from wrong
	"Success at all costs" as a prevailing value
	Personal gains valued despite social effects
Legal	Organizational policy on SAD poorly defined
	Dishonest behaviors undefined or ambiguous
	Penalties undefined or ambiguous
Social	Peer pressure
	Competitiveness
	Group misconduct and cheating
	Peer perception that "everyone cheats"
Environmental	Crowded testing conditions
	Sale of exams and exam answers
	Availability of papers
	Prevalence of Internet "cheat" sites
	Use and re-use of exams
	Inconsistent policy implementation

ACADEMIC INTEGRITY

The relationship between the student and the nurse educator is fostered through proactive communication and can result in academic integrity, passing grades, graduation, successful NCLEX completion, and ultimately desirable professional and educational outcomes. While a small percentage of students may fail despite positive, proactive communication and honest student behaviors, the student who repeats the course and subsequently passes the required coursework and examinations honestly will be better prepared for professional life and future academic endeavors.

TABLE 15.2   Factors Predisposing Nurse Educators to Ignore Student Academic Dishonesty

Category	Factors
Psychological	Stress 　　Faculty workload 　　Incompetent leadership 　　Role ambiguities 　　Emphasis on research and publications Personality 　　Need to avoid conflicts 　　Need to nurture and protect others
Ethical (Level of Moral Development	Difficulty separating from "caring" role "Feels responsible" for others' actions "Selfishness" valued over universal obligations
Legal	Organizational policy on SAD poorly defined Policy classifies SAD as academic evaluation Method for due process procedures unclear
Social	Actions by other faculty that: 　　minimize dishonest behaviors 　　excuse dishonest behaviors 　　avoid confrontation
Environmental	Institutional philosophy and policies that: 　　discourage reports of SAD 　　encourage dismissing SAD charges Lack of organizational support for faculty by: 　　chairperson 　　administrators 　　hearing committee and review board

ACADEMIC DISHONESTY

Academic dishonesty can occur in spite of proactive communication with students. Educators must be prepared to identify "at risk" students and guide them to appropriate behaviors through ongoing communication during the semester.

Dishonest academic behavior may include cheating, plagiarism, fabricating data, or falsifying records. Student academic dishonesty has been defined as "forms of cheating and plagiarism which result in students giving or receiving unauthorized assistance in an academic exercise (all forms of work submitted for credit or hours) or receiving credit for work which is not their own" (Kibler, Nuss, Paterson, & Pavela, 1988, p. 1). Cheating involves getting something by dishonesty, deception, or violating rules (Merriam-Webster, 2003). Graham, Monday, O'Brien, and Steffan (1994) listed 17 behaviors that could be thought of as cheating. Among them were allowing someone to copy homework, copying someone else's term paper, and taking a test for someone else.

Plagiarism is another form of academic dishonesty that has been defined as "failure to distinguish the student's own words and ideas from those of a source the student has consulted" (Harris, 2001, p. 132). It may include taking someone else's words, laboratory data, computer program, photograph, table, or graph, and claiming it as one's own (Harris, 2001).

Dishonesty is particularly serious in clinical settings because of the risk potential for patients (Daniel, Adams, & Smith, 1994). Student academic dishonesty in clinical nursing practice might include falsification and fabrication of data. Examples of unethical behaviors include falsifying nursing care plans and progress notes, failing to report medication errors, and documentation of treatments not performed (Hilbert, 1987; Prescott, 1989).

Nondiscovery: Failing to Discover Academic Dishonesty

When dishonest behavior is not discovered by the nurse educator, the student may pass all course work, graduate and pass the NCLEX (Figure 15.2). The obvious concern is that dishonesty in school will transfer to dishonest or incompetent professional practice, jeopardizing patient safety and increasing malpractice claims (Bailey, 2001; Gaberson, 1997; Hilbert, 1985; Jeffreys & Stier, 1995). Alternatively, the student who cheats may fail a course, repeat the course, continue to cheat, and subsequently pass all required course materials and examinations. Without being confronted about their dishonest behavior, students will not recognize its seriousness and may continue undesirable behaviors in the future. It is critical therefore that nurse educators know and understand the definitions of SAD, become familiar with school policy related to SAD, and initiate ways to discover and detect dishonesty in the classroom and clinical setting.

Discovery: Ignoring Academic Dishonesty

Academic dishonesty that is discovered but ignored by the nurse educator is a serious situation. Graham, Monday, O'Brien, and Steffan (1994) reported that although the percentage of faculty who caught a student cheating was high (78.7%), only 9% penalized the student by failing the assignment, deducting points, or failing the course. This type of behavior sends the wrong message to students—a message that says it is acceptable to cheat.

Factors that predispose faculty to ignore SAD include excessive workload, a need to avoid conflict, feeling responsible for other people's actions, and organizational policies that are poorly defined (see Table 15.2). Dishonest behavior that has been discovered but ignored may lead to passing grades, graduation, and passing the NCLEX, but poor professional outcomes. In this situation, the nurse educator who ignores SAD has missed an opportunity to intervene and to correct undesirable behaviors that can follow the students throughout their education and professional life (see Figure 15.2).

Discovery: Confronting Academic Dishonesty

Confronting students with a clear explanation of their dishonest behavior and its consequences after it is discovered carries the most promise for influencing future professional and academic growth and for preventing undesirable outcomes. Students learn that dishonest behaviors are not tolerated and that these behaviors have consequences. Even though the student may still fail, there is greater opportunity to effect a change in behavior when the student is confronted. The desired outcome of the model is to promote academic integrity with students honestly achieving passing grades, graduating, and passing the NCLEX licensing exam (see Figure 15.2).

COMMUNICATION

Communication strategies have the power to change the course of action (decisions and behaviors) and outcomes in the educational path toward professional development. Figure 15.3 presents six key components of communication: timing, setting, goals, objectivity, modes, and content. In the sections that follow, each component is described in terms of preventing and confronting student academic dishonesty.

1.   Timing

Timing is critical to opening or closing further communication and for emphasizing the importance of academic and professional integrity.

Prevention

Ideally, the best "time" to begin to discuss academic dishonesty with students is during the first class session or orientation. Planning to discuss professional integrity within class content topics and then linking it to positive strategies for promoting academic integrity and excellence will further reinforce the need for preventing academic dishonesty. Because prevention needs to be ongoing throughout the educational process, future reminders to students may be planned during critical times, such as before an examination, before distributing a new written paper assignment, or before a new clinical rotation. Reminders to keep

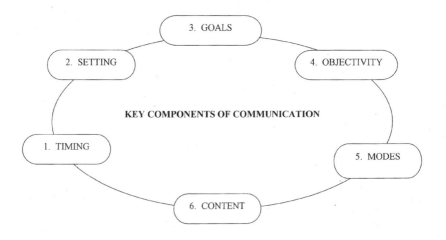

FIGURE 15.3   Key components of communication.

test papers covered may be necessary during an exam. Praising students for academic integrity throughout the semester and educational process will promote positive behaviors.

Confrontation

Timing of communication is often dependent on when the incident is discovered. If the nurse educator is present during the critical incident (i.e., dishonest behavior), the communication should be direct and brief with a request to schedule a follow-up discussion at a later date and time. If the nurse educator discovers the incident later, a formal meeting should be scheduled at the earliest time possible, yet allowing for the nurse educator to be adequately prepared with necessary documents, information, and materials.

2. Setting

Setting refers to the place where communication takes place.

Prevention

The setting for a discussion about SAD should be conducive to open communication and interaction between student(s) and nurse educator. Typically the initial setting is a classroom with a group of students. During student independent study or internship, the setting may be a private office.

Confrontation

The setting should be conducive to private communication and interaction between student(s) and nurse educator whether on or off campus. "Privacy promotes open channels of communication and enhances confidentiality" (Jeffreys & Stier, 1995, p. 301). In a classroom exam setting, communication should be as brief and quiet as possible to avoid distracting other students. Depending on the circumstances, confrontation may require immediate action in the classroom; at other times, waiting until the exam ends may be the preferred choice. During a scheduled meeting, an office setting is ideal to assure privacy.

Preferably a third neutral party such as the department chairperson, dean, or another faculty member should be included. A documented

third-party witness is important if grievance proceedings are later initiated (Jeffreys & Stier, 1995). The nurse educator should carefully review
the school policy concerning setting, participants, and/or other procedures before meeting with the student.

3.   Goals

Goals of communication should incorporate the academic institution's
goals for education with those of the nursing profession.

Prevention

Clearly identifying goals as student expected outcomes in a course
outline emphasize the importance of academic integrity and clarify any
ambiguities. For example, the outline may list the students' expected
outcomes as follows:

At the completion of this class discussion, the student will be able to:

1. Identify desirable educational and professional outcomes
2. Define academic dishonesty
3. Discuss examples of academic dishonesty in nursing
4. Identify undesirable educational and professional outcomes
5. Discuss the potential impact of undesirable educational and professional outcomes on students, the academic institution, the nursing
   profession, the health care system, and society
6. Identify strategies for promoting academic and professional integrity
7. Describe institutional policy on academic dishonesty, including penalties, procedures, and due process
8. Develop skills for lifelong commitment to professional growth, development, and integrity.

Confrontation

In all cases of suspected SAD, the *first goal* is to confirm and carefully
review all available information before confronting the student. The
second goal is to stop SAD through quiet confrontation to prevent the
student from copying or continuing these types of behaviors when
actively engaged in an educational, testing, or clinical activity. The *third
goal* then would be to identify penalties, procedures, and policies as
they pertained to the student's situation. The primary objective is to

follow institutional policy and handle the incident as either an academic evaluation or as a disciplinary procedure requiring referral to a review board.

4.   Objectivity

Objectivity refers to neutrality, candor, and fairness when communicating with students.

Prevention

Educators need to remain impartial and open when discussing dishonesty with students. A partnership that emphasizes nurse educators and students working together to promote professional integrity, client safety, and personal growth is the best approach. Asking students objectively to be coparticipants in the process of promoting professional integrity is important.

Confrontation

Dishonest behavior is often influenced by multiple factors unrelated to the faculty or school. Educators, therefore, need to remain objective, avoid personal emotions, and channel feelings of anger when discussing dishonesty with students. Arguments and reprimands may alienate the student and pose barriers to further communication.

5.   Modes

Modes refer to the oral, written, or other channels of communication used by the nurse educator and students.

Prevention

Integrating several modes of communication may allow the student to develop a deeper awareness and understanding of integrity, dishonesty, and professional behavior. The nurse educator may give an oral explanation of the written school policy on academic dishonesty during the first day of class. This combined with a review of the student handbook, the course outline, the college catalog, the ANA (2001) Code of Ethics, and/or the NSNA Code of Ethics may emphasize legal, professional, and ethical standards and values, and serve as a prevention strategy. Students should sign a written statement attesting review and comprehension of definitions, policies, and responsibilities concerning academic dishonesty. The signed statement is then placed in the student's file for future reference. This validates that communication has taken place between the student and nurse educator in a written mode of communication.

Open class discussion is another mode of communication that encourages students to explore and clarify their own values (Jeffreys & Stier, 1995). Nurse educators can encourage students to openly accept responsibility for mistakes, solve problems, and avoid errors in the real clinical setting through experiences in the nursing skills laboratory and simulated case studies in the classroom (Gaberson, 1997; Hoyer, Booth, Spelman, & Richardson, 1991). A video about professional ethics, legal responsibilities, and/or client safety, followed by in-class written reflection about the video and group discussion, serves as additional mode of communication that can be explored.

Confrontation

During a prescheduled meeting, both oral and written communication modes should be strategically used when confronting the student. The nurse educator, student, and neutral third party should sign an official record of the conference meeting. Written documentation should include factual details and avoid subjective statements. When the nurse educator is present while the dishonest behavior is occurring, verbal and nonverbal communication is typically used. For example, direct eye contact and an outstretched hand requesting "cheat notes" to be handed over during an exam may be all that is needed for initial confrontation.

6.   Content

Essential content must include the use of consistent and specific terminology, policies, and penalties concerning dishonest behavior.

Prevention

The student handbook and the college catalog serve as the guidelines in addressing legal issues related to academic dishonesty and disciplinary consequences. The ANA Code of Ethics also serves as a guideline in addressing professional integrity, behavior, and misconduct (Jeffreys &

Stier, 1995). Empirical evidence reveals that honor codes are correlated with lower levels of SAD among college students; therefore, a policy that includes honor codes may be beneficial (McCabe, Trevino, & Butterfield, 2002).

The classification of SAD as either disciplinary misconduct or academic evaluation is a central issue. When classified as disciplinary misconduct, the responsibility for judgment and penalties are shifted away from the educator to a pre-established hearing committee. In disciplinary misconduct cases, public institutions are required to ensure due process. The Fourteenth Amendment stipulates due process procedures when state action may deprive a person of constitutional rights. When SAD is classified as an academic evaluation, subjective and inconsistent penalties are more prevalent unless guided by a detailed procedural policy for course instructors. Because due process is not routinely considered in this subjective method of handling SAD, the academic institution and course instructor should be aware of the possibility of legal proceedings. The accused student may choose to challenge the judgments and penalties in court (Jeffreys & Stier, 1991; Osinski, 2003).

The "content" also should include measures aimed at affective learning, that is, the development of values, attitudes, and beliefs consistent with professional nursing. Sufficient detail of essential content is a necessary precursor in preventing dishonest behaviors. Subsequent supplementary information may be provided at appropriate intervals for reinforcement of previously learned content and for further professional growth and development. For example, if a new policy is approved, it must be conveyed immediately to students.

Furthermore, as students encounter real clinical situations, fictitious case studies, and/or other professional ethical dilemmas, the content can be reinforced and expanded. The SAD model may be reviewed with students to help them recognize the overarching factors predisposing dishonest behaviors, trace the various path options and their potential consequences, and discover the importance of open, ongoing communication with the nurse educator to achieve common professional and educational goals. Expected behaviors and unacceptable behaviors should be clearly identified.

Confrontation

The institution's policies, procedures, and penalties should guide the content of all communication between educator and student. Consistent use of terminology, avoidance of personal feelings, and objective factual comments or questions should underlie all communication. Depending on the circumstances, the content may need to be brief; at other times the content can be more detailed. For example, discovery of a dishonest behavior in the clinical setting may require detailed discussion to be followed up later since actions to maintain client safety will outweigh all other interventions.

To determine if dishonest behavior occurred, the nurse educator may schedule a meeting with the student. During the meeting, the nurse educator should introduce questions or comments that range from vague to specific in an effort to evoke a student confession, determine students' knowledge about the written paper, establish areas of inconsistencies in student's dialogue, or clarify areas of ambiguities. During scheduled meetings to confront confirmed cases of dishonest behavior, the content should include specific details in relation to school policy, professional ethics, and local, state, and federal laws. In addition, the actual and potential adverse consequences to clients, families, communities, peers, nurses, and others should be outlined.

The following three case exemplars demonstrate how the various communication strategies outlined above may be adapted for various nursing educational areas: classroom examination, written paper, and clinical (hospital) setting. In addition, three different school policies will be presented. The exemplars are intended to stimulate ideas for nurse educators interested in developing situation-specific interventions.

CASE EXEMPLARS: COMMUNICATION STRATEGY IN ACTION

Problem: Cheating on a Classroom Examination

Prevention

Professor Johnson is strongly committed to promoting academic integrity. In addition to the various communication strategies that have been recommended for the first class session with reinforcement throughout the course (listed above), Professor Johnson implemented specific interventions to promote academic integrity and prevent cheating on an examination. First, she assessed factors predisposing cheating on exams. She then prepared new exams organized in A and B formats with scrambled question sequencing. The school policy concerning student academic integrity was printed on the examination booklet cover. Before the beginning of the exam, students were asked to place all notes, books, beepers, and cellular phones in the front of the classroom.

Next, students were randomly seated in well-spaced rows to avoid premeditated "seating for cheating" and avoid overcrowded classroom conditions. Students were then instructed to write their name on the exam booklet and optical scanning sheet after receiving them. These instructions also were written on the chalkboard as a reminder. At the beginning of the exam, Professor Johnson reminded students that they were expected to: (1) remain in the classroom and in their seats until handing in their exam, (2) keep their eyes on their own exam and answer sheet, (3) keep their exam and answer sheet appropriately positioned on their desk, (4) refrain from talking and asking questions, (5) do their own work, and (6) refrain from assisting others during the exam.

Professor Johnson distributed the exam booklets, assuring that each student had only one exam booklet. Next, she walked up and down the aisles, verifying that each student had written his or her name on the exam booklet and answer sheet. As an active exam proctor, Professor Johnson walked up and down the aisles periodically, watching for any cheating behaviors.

Discovery and Initial Confrontation

Professor Johnson observed that Shirley is reading a small piece of paper hidden under her exam booklet. Professor Johnson can either ignore or confront the suspected cheating incident. Remembering the essential elements of the "PROACTIVE" communication, she mentally reviews college *policy* and realizes that it is her *responsibility* to uphold the policy of the academic institution and communicate this to the student. Additionally she knows that her responsibility is *ongoing*. She mentally reviews the potential undesirable outcomes that can be caused by not confronting the incident. Ignoring it could lead to further undesirable educational and professional outcomes. It also could create the perception that cheating is acceptable and easy, leading to greater prevalence of cheating by Shirley and others. She recognizes her *accountability* to students, the educational institution, nursing profession, and society to uphold ethical standards and assure minimum educational requirements by all students. With strong *commitment* to professional and educational integrity, Professor Johnson knows that others *trust* her to actively promote integrity. Professional and educational integrity as well as client safety issues require her to take *initiative* to maintain professional *values* and *expectations*. Subsequently, Professor Johnson decides to confront the suspected cheating incident.

Timing in the classroom must be immediate. Professor Johnson decides to immediately confront Shirley as quietly as possible so as not to disrupt other students and to secure the "cheat sheet," exam booklet, and answer sheet. She asks Shirley to exit the classroom quietly and see her after the exam is over. The *goals* are to uphold policy and stop cheating behaviors. Although Professor Johnson initially feels angry, she consciously prepares herself to maintain *objectivity*. The *modes* of communication include verbal and nonverbal gestures to avoid distracting other students. The intended *content* of the message is to remove the "extra" paper, verify and acknowledge that cheating behavior is not tolerated, remove the test and cheat sheet, and then ask Shirley to see her after the exam is over.

After the exam, Shirley returns to the empty classroom. Referring to the written school policy concerning academic integrity printed on the examination booklet, Professor Johnson informs Shirley that she will be contacted to set up an appointment to discuss the situation according to the established procedural protocol.

Planned Confrontation Meeting

The "PROACTIVE" acronym reminds Professor Johnson that *policy* is the essential component that will guide her subsequent actions. First, the university's policy classifies cheating as requiring an academic evaluation. Second, the policy specifies that the faculty member must impose a zero grade for cheating during the exam. Third, the school of nursing requires a three-way meeting with the student, faculty member, and dean.

The *timing* of the meeting should be as soon as possible following the incident, yet Professor Johnson also realizes that she must adequately prepare for the meeting. Professor Johnson schedules the meeting for one week later. First, she prepares detailed written documentation of the incident consistent with university policy. Next, she meets with the dean to discuss the incident prior to the scheduled meeting with the student.

The *setting* of the student meeting is in the dean's office, with only Shirley, Professor Johnson, and the dean present. The primary *goals* of communication are to uphold school policy and maintain professional ethics and values while assisting Shirley to develop higher levels of moral reasoning consistent with professional nursing values. Despite Shirley's verbal anger and crying, Professor Johnson and the dean maintain *objectivity* by demonstrating calm, nonjudgmental, and factual demeanors. Oral and written *modes* of communication are used for the essential *content* needed for the meeting. Professor Johnson refers to the school policy, the ANA Code of Ethics, and the NSNA Code of Ethics. Shirley's signed academic integrity statement also is addressed.

Professor Johnson provides a copy of the written documentation of the incident and a copy of the confiscated cheat sheet. The content clearly identifies the student's behavior and the subsequent penalties and procedures for cheating. Shirley is informed that she will receive a grade of zero for her exam and that documentation of the incident and current meeting will be placed in her student file, per college protocol. Shirley is angry about this penalty, declaring that she was accused of cheating before and received the opportunity to retake the exam. Both the dean and professor reinforce the current university and nursing school policy and the need to change behaviors.

Shirley reluctantly agrees to meet with a college counselor to discuss her feelings and explore acceptable strategies for academic achievement and promote moral development. Finally, all participants sign an attendance sheet, acknowledging the date, time, and nature of the meeting. Written documentation of the meeting is an asset, particularly when later referral to a grievance committee is a possibility.

Problem: Plagiarism on a Written Paper

Prevention

In addition to standard prevention strategies, Professor Green implemented specific interventions to promote academic integrity and prevent plagiarism on a written paper assignment. She:

1. Assessed for predisposing factors related to SAD
2. Recognized and removed circumstances that make plagiarism easy, such as continued use of the same written assignment from semester to semester, broad assignments with no specific topic, unspecified paper components, a single out-of-class

written assignment, unclear expectations concerning documentation procedures, and ambiguous format expectations.

3. Developed new, updated, and creative written paper assignments requiring individual responses such as personal reflection
4. Defined plagiarism and accountability for written work (verbally and in written format) at the beginning of the assignment
5. Randomly assigned different paper topics or allowed students to select from different topics to avoid copying
6. Expected students to submit outlines, drafts, annotated references, printouts of computerized literature searches, and current references (when possible) at designated intervals throughout the semester
7. Reviewed students' submitted materials and provided constructive comments to guide the development of the written assignment
8. Expected students to periodically discuss their topic and their progress in completing various components of the written paper assignment with unannounced update reports throughout the semester
9. Expected students to incorporate written and verbal constructive comments in subsequent drafts and the final written paper
10. Required students to submit two copies of their final paper accompanied by a signed statement attesting to academic integrity and originality of written work. One paper was filed in the nursing department, and one paper was returned to the student.

Ongoing evaluation of the student's writing ability allows instructors to evaluate the student's process of writing, growth in mastery of the topic, strengths, and weaknesses. Early identification of student difficulties permits nurse educators to develop group and/or individual teaching strategies to enhance academic achievement. Consequently, ongoing evaluation serves a dual purpose of enhancing learning outcomes while also promoting academic integrity.

Discovery and Confrontation

Professor Green reads a final written paper submitted by Joe, an academically weak student. Previous outline submissions lacked appropriate details; the final paper did not include updated references or areas for further development as suggested by Professor Green. When reading the grammatically correct and technically detailed paper on "Psychosocial Support for the Client with Aplastic Anemia," Professor Green notes that the technical details and empirical terminology are well beyond what a third semester associate degree nursing student without previous college experience would be able to grasp. Additionally, the paper does not focus on the registered nurse role or on psychosocial support, as was required according to the paper format guidelines.

Professor Green suspects plagiarism. At this point, she has three options: (1) to ignore the possible plagiarism incident and award a passing grade; (2) to ignore the possible plagiarism incident, deduct points, and award points for sections of the paper that met the paper format guidelines; or (3) to confront the suspected plagiarism incident. Reflecting on the essential elements of the "PROACTIVE" acronym, she refers to the college *policy*; the policy classifies plagiarism as academic misconduct. She realizes that it is the instructor's *responsibility* to take active and *ongoing* measures to prevent plagiarism as well as to confront it. She also recognizes her *accountability* to students, the educational institution, the nursing profession, and society to uphold ethical standards and assure minimum educational requirements by all students. With strong *commitment* to professional and educational integrity, Professor Green knows that others *trust* her to take *initiative* and confront plagiarism in an effort to uphold educational, professional, and societal *values* and *expectations*.

Professor Green decides to confront the suspected incident and uses plagiarism-detection software to confirm that Joe obtained large portions of his paper directly from two major sources: a health care consumer Internet site and an online term paper mill. In Joe's case, three findings raised initial suspicions. First, his paper reflected a quality inconsistent with his usual level of work. Second, the content of his paper was not entirely consistent with the course assignment. Third, references and citations in the text were outdated and unavailable at the college library. Any one of these findings is sufficient enough to question originality of work.

Professor Green asks Joe to meet with her next week to discuss his paper (*timing*). Next, she prepares detailed written documentation of the incident consistent within university policy and compiles pertinent evidence. Then she meets with the nursing chairperson to discuss the incident, review materials, and plan the discussion prior to the scheduled meeting with the student. Initially, the chairperson is reluctant to pursue the issue as academic misconduct, urging Professor Green to simply "fail the student." The chairperson cites overburdening the college review board and a negative reflection on the nursing program as rationale. Professor Green refers back to the college policy that clearly classifies plagiarism as academic misconduct and further delineates mandated faculty and administrator action in plagiarism cases. The chairperson then agrees to follow the college protocol.

The *setting* of the student meeting is in the chairperson's office, with only Joe, Professor Green, and the chairperson present. The primary *goal* of the communication is to uphold school policy and maintain professional ethics and values. An underlying *goal* is to assist Joe in developing higher levels of moral reasoning consistent with professional nursing values. Professor Green and the chairperson maintain *objectivity* by remaining calm and attempting to give Joe the opportunity to openly confess plagiarism without being accused.

Oral *modes* of communication are used initially. First, Professor Green asks Joe if he had any idea why the meeting about his paper had been scheduled. Joe quickly states that he spent so much time researching and writing the paper that he has no idea. Furthermore, he says it is unfair that he has to meet with the instructor and chairperson when other students have not been asked to do so. Joe becomes angry when he is unable to discuss sections of his paper or explain how he obtained technical information listed in his paper. Now, both oral and written *modes* of communication are used for the essential *content* needed for the meeting. Professor Green refers to the school policy, ANA Code of Ethics, and NSNA Code of Ethics.

Next, Professor Green provides a copy of the written paper assignment and the signed statement attesting to academic integrity and originality of written work. Despite Joe's verbal anger, repeated denials, accusations of unfair treatment, and threats to sue, Professor Green and the chairperson remain calm and nonjudgmental. When Professor Green displays the Internet printout that correlates verbatim with Joe's paper, Joe becomes silent. He is informed that he will be referred to the college review board and that documentation of the incident and current meeting will be placed in his student file, per college protocol. Joe is distressed over this penalty and states that a written paper is not as important as passing a test or taking care of a patient. Both the chairperson and professor reinforce that fact that school policy is uniformly applied in all cases of SAD.

All participants sign an attendance sheet, acknowledging the date, time, and nature of the meeting. The content clearly identifies the student's dishonest behavior and the subsequent penalties and procedures as mandated by school policy.

Problem: Falsifying Records and Fabricating Information in the Clinical Setting

Prevention

Professor Long's SAD prevention tactics included the various communication strategies recommended for the first class session (preconference) with specific applications to the clinical setting. The National Student Nurses Association (NSNA) two-part Code of Ethics consisting of a Code of Professional Conduct (1999) and Code for Academic and Clinical Professional Conduct (2001) were reviewed and discussed. The ANA Code of Ethics (2001) along with the NSNA Student Bill of Rights and Responsibilities (1991) for students of nursing were additional references discussed to provide guidelines for professional development.

As an additional precaution, Professor Long met separately with individual students and their preceptors and reviewed policies and expectations concerning student academic integrity and professional integrity. All students signed a form attesting to comprehension of the school's policy and penalties. Students also signed a statement attesting to comprehension of the hospital policies concerning patient rights and professional accountability. Hospital and school policies also require students to carry malpractice insurance, further emphasizing individual student accountability.

Following orientation by her preceptor, Leslie is assigned to care for Mrs. Davis, a seventy-year-old woman who had surgery for a fractured hip several days before. During the shift, Mrs. Davis begins to complain of dull, persistent pain in her right hip. Leslie makes a mental note to check the medication administration record to find out if Mrs. Davis is due for pain medication, but becomes distracted by another patient call bell and assists the patient in the next room. Hurrying to finish her assignment and complete her documentation in time for post-conference, Leslie falsely signs that she has administered a dose of pain medication and reports that she has done so to her preceptor.

While in post-conference, Leslie reports that the pain medication alleviated her patient's pain within thirty minutes after administration. Meanwhile, the preceptor finds Mrs. Davis in severe pain, stating that she had not received any pain medication since last night. The patient medication dispensing system indicates that there is an extra dose of medication that was documented but not given. The preceptor then interrupts Professor Long from post-conference.

Dishonesty in the clinical setting poses a new set of challenges for nurse educators. The impact of falsifying or fabricating data can have serious and devastating patient outcomes. *Timing* and urgency in confronting the student must be emphasized. In an acute care setting such as this, Professor Long realizes that internal hospital policy such as filing an incident report and follow-up investigation with quality management will occur. The incident is discussed privately in the nurse manager's office *setting*, including the nurse manager, preceptor, student, and faculty member. The primary *goal* of the communication is to provide an *objective* and factual account of the incident. The priority is to promote quality patient care and safety. A secondary *goal* is to foster the moral and ethical development of the student.

Without making any accusations, Professor Long succinctly presents the data *objectively*. Oral *modes* of communication are used initially followed later by written documentation of the incident. Leslie is given the opportunity to admit that Mrs. Davis was not medicated yet she remains silent. Next, Professor Long asks Leslie directly if Mrs. Davis had complained of pain and if she had been medicated. Reluctantly, Leslie admits that she meant to administer pain medication but became distracted. In her rush to complete her assignment, she falsely documented and verbally reported that she gave the medication.

Once this is clarified, the preceptor leaves the meeting to medicate Mrs. Davis. Professor Long uses this opportunity to reinforce the importance of good communication among health care providers, particularly with the clinical preceptor and nurse educator. He assists Leslie in identifying an honest, alternative approach such as admit to her mistake, apologize to the patient, and work as quickly as possible with her nurse preceptor to administer pain medication to the patient. In situations in which the student is overwhelmed, Professor Long reinforces that students were instructed to contact him immediately. He emphasizes the danger to patient safety that incidents such as this can impose. The *content* here is both investigational and educational for the student, necessitating clinical judgment, problem solving, and critical thinking.

Professor Long further explains that falsifying the medical record and/or verbal report is a form of SAD and professional dishonesty that jeopardizes patient care and safety. He reminds Leslie that school policy stipulates a meeting at the college to discuss further actions. Documentation of the incident and current meeting will be placed in her student file, in keeping with college protocol.

SUMMARY

Implications of ignoring student academic dishonesty can be enormous. Desirable educational and professional outcomes can only be achieved through a faculty commitment to academic integrity during all phases of the nursing educational process. Academic integrity must be seen as an organizational priority and accepted as part of the mission, vision, and values of the school. A clear and consistent school policy that is well publicized and accepted by faculty can be used to guide PROACTIVE communication and effective interventions.

The SAD model, introduced earlier in this chapter, can be used to guide nursing school (and institutional) policies and procedures; discussion among students, faculty, and administrators; and decision making when SAD occurs. With some modifications, the SAD model is flexible enough to be adapted to both RN-BSN education as well as graduate nursing education.

Nurse educators are well positioned to promote academic integrity and discourage academic dishonesty through open and honest communication and through definitive action when cheating or other dishonest behavior is discovered. How effective they will be depends on the level of commitment and support that they receive from the college administration as well as their own personal commitment to their students and to their profession.

REFERENCES

American Nurses Association. (2001). *Code of ethics for nurses with interpretive statements*. Washington, DC: American Nurses Publishing.

Bailey, P. A. (1990). Cheating among nursing students. *Nurse Educator, 15*(3), 32–35.

Bailey, P. A. (2001). Academic misconduct: Responses from deans and nurse educators. *Journal of Nursing Education, 40,* 124–130.

Berger, J. B. (2001). Understanding the organizational nature of student persistence: Empirically based recommendations for practice. *Journal of College Student Retention Research Theory and Practice, 3*(1), 3–21.

Bradshaw, M. J., & Lowenstein, A. J. (1990). Perspectives on academic dishonesty. *Nurse Educator, 15*(5), 10–15.

Brown, D. L. (2002). Cheating must be okay—Everybody does it! *Nurse Educator, 27*(1), 6–8.

Daniel, L. G., Adams, B. N., & Smith, N. M. (1994). Academic misconduct among nursing students: A multivariate investigation. *Journal of Professional Nursing, 10,* 278–288.

Gaberson, K. B. (1997). Academic dishonesty among nursing students. *Nursing Forum, 32*(3), 14–20.

Graham, M. A., Monday, J., O'Brien, K., & Steffen, S. (1994). Cheating at small colleges: An evaluation of student and faculty attitudes and behaviors. *Journal of College Student Development, 35,* 255–260.

Harris, R. A. (2001). *The plagiarism handbook: Strategies for preventing, detecting, and dealing with plagiarism.* Los Angeles, CA: Pyrczak Publishing.

Hilbert, G. A. (1985). Involvement of nursing students in unethical classroom and clinical behaviors. *Journal of Professional Nursing, 1,* 230–234.

Hilbert, G. A. (1987). Academic fraud: Prevalence, practices and reasons. *Journal of Professional Nursing, 3,* 39–45.

Hilbert, G. A. (1988). Moral development and unethical behavior among nursing students. *Journal of Professional Nursing, 4,* 163–167.

Hoyer, P. J., Booth, D., Spelman, M. R., & Richardson, C. E. (1991). Clinical cheating and moral development. *Nursing Outlook, 39,* 170–173.

Jeffreys, M. R., & Stier, L. (1991). Student academic dishonesty: Issues for nurse educators. *Dean's Notes, 12*(5), 1–3.

Jeffreys, M. R., & Stier, L. (1995). SPEAKING against student academic dishonesty: A communication model for nurse educators. *Journal of Nursing Education, 34,* 297–304.

Jeffreys, M. R., & Stier, L. (1998). Student academic dishonesty. *Imprint, 45*(3), 48–49.

Kibler, W. L., Nuss, E. M., Patterson, B. G., & Pavela, G. (1988). *Academic integrity and student development: Legal issues and policy perspectives.* Asheville, NC: College Administration Publications.

McCabe, D. L., Trevino, L. K., & Butterfield, K. D. (2002). Honor codes and other contextual influences on academic integrity: A replication and extension to modified honor code settings. *Research in Higher Education, 43,* 357–378.

Merriam-Webster, Inc. (2003). *Merriam-Webster's Collegiate Dictionary, Unabridged Online.* Retrieved February 17, 2003, from http://www.m-w.com/home.htm

May, K. M., & Loyd, B. H. (1993). Academic dishonesty: The honor system and student attitudes. *Journal of College Student Development, 34*(2), 125–129.

National Student Nurses' Association, Inc. (1999). *Code of Professional Conduct.* Retrieved October 20, 2003, from http://www.nsna.org/pubs/pdf/Codeof ProfessionalConduct.pdf

National Student Nurses' Association, Inc. (2001). *Code of Academic and Clinical Professional Conduct.* Retrieved October 20, 2003, from http://www.nsna.org/ pubs/pdf/code-of-ac.pdf

National Student Nurses' Association, Inc. (1991). *Bill of Rights and Responsibilities for Students of Nursing.* Retrieved October 16, 2002, from http://www.nsna.org/ pubs/billofrights/asp

Osinski, K. (2003). Due process rights of nursing students in cases of misconduct. *Journal of Nursing Education, 42,* 55–58.

Prescott, P. A. (1989). Academic misconduct: Considerations for educational administrators. *Journal of Professional Nursing, 5,* 283–287.

Roberts, E. F. (1999). Nursing faculty's handling of academic dishonesty. *Nursing Connections, 12*(2), 13–22.

Scanlon, P. M., & Neumann, D. R. (2002). Internet plagiarism among college students. *Journal of College Student Development, 43,* 374–385.

Young, J. R. (2001, July 6). The cat-and-mouse game of plagiarism detection. *Chronicle of Higher Education,* pp. A26–27.

Chapter 16

Transition to Professional Nursing Practice: Emerging Issues and Initiatives

Judy Boychuk Duchscher

Across North America, health care systems have documented a shortage of qualified and committed registered nurses (RNs) (Canadian Nursing Advisory Committee [CNAC], 2002; Health and Human Resources and Services Administration [HHRSA], 2001). Despite countless and costly initiatives aimed at recruiting and retaining energetic, well educated, critically thinking, motivated, and caring RNs, the workforce continues to age. Alongside mounting evidence that the perception of nursing as a challenging, satisfying, and fulfilling vocation by society's youth is waning, North America is being left with a highly limited pool of RNs available to fill nursing vacancies that crosses cultural, geographical, and economic boundaries (Aiken et al., 2001).

Amid this crisis, health care communities continue to be challenged in their attempts to understand exactly what constitutes a quality work environment and how to provide a working context for nurses that fosters quality health care consistent with the values of the nursing profession (Aiken, Clarke, Sloane, & Sochalski, 2001; Buerhaus & Staiger, 1999). A recent report of nursing workforce trends in five countries (Canada, the United States, England, Scotland, and Germany) demonstrated strikingly consistent symptoms of distress suggestive of: (a) fundamental problems in the design of nursing work, (b) inadequate staffing quotas available to cope with elevated acuity and census figures, (c) increases in worker absenteeism and subsequent escalating costs of nursing care provision, (d) qualitative evidence of health care administrations that are out of touch with the voices of struggling nurses, and (e) reports of an increased tendency for younger nurses to show greater willingness to leave their hospital jobs (Aiken, Clarke, & Sloane, 2002). This disturbing picture of a decaying health care delivery system is expected to continue, if not escalate, as the long-predicted attrition rates of seasoned nurses are realized (HHRSA, 2001; CNAC, 2002). With almost half of the nursing workforce in North America over 45 years of age, and that number increasing exponentially (HHRSA, 2001; Canadian Institute for Health Information, 2001), it has been predicted that by 2011 Canada will experience a shortage of RNs upwards of 113,000 (Ryten, 1997), with the United States requiring a staggering infusion into their nursing work force of one million (Hecker, 2001).

Alarming statistics further inform us that 35–61% of new graduates (NGs) can be expected to change their place of employment or exit the nursing profession altogether within the first year of professional practice (Aiken, Clarke, Sloane, & Sochalski, 2001; Dearmun, 2000; Godinez, Schweiger, Gruver, & Ryan, 1999). In the U.S. alone, this attrition of nurses translates into costs averaging $50,000 per replaced nurse (Buerhaus & Staiger, 1999; Godinez, Schweiger, Gruver, & Ryan, 1999; Winter-Collins & McDaniel, 2000), and an even greater cost of increased patient mortality rates resulting from nurse burnout and job dissatisfaction (Aiken, Clarke, Sloane, Sochalski, & Silber, 2002).

Highly educated and intolerant of the "sink or swim" management style of many recruiting institutions, NGs are coming into the workplace with a greater loyalty to the nursing profession than the agency, a significantly higher self-esteem than graduates of other generations, and an unwillingness to tolerate a patriarchal and medically dominated health care management system that seeks to invalidate and devalue the nursing care they have committed their lives to delivering. The high turnover of new nursing staff in acute care is likely to continue unless steps are taken to recognize and provide support to resolve the issues inherent in what has been purported to be a traumatic and stressful transition of nursing students to professional nursing practice (Dearmun, 2000; Duchscher, 2001a; Gerrish, 1990; Godinez, Schweiger, Gruver, & Ryan, 1999; Kramer, 1974; Lathlean, 1987; Oermann & Garvin, 2002).

This chapter guides the reader in understanding the impact of an increasingly demanding work environment on the transition experience of the NG and the implications of shifting workloads and progressively more intense practice environments on the NG's professional self-concept, stress, and work satisfaction levels. The reader will gain insight into the impact of these workplace elements on the quality of patient care as well as an understanding of the critical relationship between senior nursing staff and novice nurses during the process of transition. Finally, this chapter suggests initiatives for both educational and service institutions to optimize their response to this growing issue in workforce recruitment and retention.

TRANSITION TO PROFESSIONAL PRACTICE FOR NURSING GRADUATES

The experience of transition to professional practice in NGs has been variably studied and reported in the literature, most notably in the work of Marlene Kramer (1966, 1968, 1974). Remarkably, almost four decades after the theoretical construct of "reality shock" in nursing was first published, many aspects of Kramer's original research have been substantiated as applying to the current transition of NGs to professional practice (Dearmun, 2000; Duchscher, 2001a; Godinez, Schweiger, Gruver, & Ryan, 1999; Horsburgh, 1989; Jasper, 1996; Kelly, 1998; Whitehead, 2001). Though the meaning of these alarming similarities remains speculative, they should pique our curiosity about the reasons for a consistently chaotic, unsupported, and painful transition experience to professional practice that leaves these recruits feeling overwhelmed, undervalued, and generally dissatisfied with their jobs (Blegen, 1993; Cowin & Jacobsson, 2002). Difficult elements of the transition process for NGs have survived purported advancements in the foundational education and practice of nursing, changes in health care delivery methods and enhancement of technologies, and an emphasis on quality care management throughout the acute care institutions of North America. This finding is undeniably puzzling and should be kept uppermost in the minds of readers as they navigate their way through the testimonies of professional socialization that follow.

Stages of Transition

Using Bridges' (1980) classic model of transitions as a framework, the NG transition experience can been seen as encompassing an *ending*, a *neutral phase*, and *reorientation*. The *ending* phase encompasses the first one to three months of professional practice and is characterized by a struggle to differentiate between educational orientation and practice reality, and is accompanied by letting go of familiar ways of being. Initially exhilarated by the arrival of a long-awaited goal, the new graduates' sense of euphoria is quickly replaced by *reality shock*, characterized by an impressive awareness of the contrasting differences between practicing nursing as a student and practicing nursing as a professional (Kramer, 1974). These disturbing discrepancies lead to profound feelings of vulnerability and moral distress (Kelly, 1998) as well as a necessarily linear and prescriptive approach of the novice to their unpredictable, inconsistent, and unfamiliar new practice world (Duchscher, 2001a).

An exceptionally traumatic time for the NG, crushing fear associated with the potential for practice incompetence and not being accepted by senior nurses overwhelms them (Duchscher, 2001a; Jasper, 1996; Kramer, 1974). Clearly lacking confidence in their clinical judgment and task performance, these NGs feel "marginalized" (Van Gennep, 1960, p. 11); they are neither nursing students nor professional practitioners. The excessive demands of this transition phase exhaust the NG emotionally, intellectually, and physically, leaving them with no more than a simple desire to get through the day "without killing anyone" (Duchscher, 2001a, p. 430).

Within 4–6 months, the NG commonly enters the *neutral* phase of their transition process, set apart by a sense of confusion, disequilibrium, and detachment brought on by the distortions of an idealized practice understanding. Confused and off-balance as a result of the traumatic disconnection between their educational and practical experiences, the NGs feel the need to disengage from their previous level of involvement in the practice environment. This sense of detachment allows the new nurse to fully experience the loss of *what was* while entertaining a dawning awareness of *what is*.

This may well be a pivotal time as the recruits crystallize their decisions around what "real" nursing is, what power they have and do not have as professionals, and the role they play in constructing the reality of their practice environments. They are more relaxed and multidimensional in their perspective and recognize the value of producing new responses to their issues. Successful progression through this stage is represented by a revised professional identity that assimilates select quality nursing care values held by the NG, with a respect for the structural and functional goals of the institution.

Bridges (1980) claimed that the *reorientation* stage of transition is expressed through a sense of renewed connectedness that comes from an "internal realignment" (p. 138). Feelings of connectedness are re-established within 6 months to a year through acceptance of a new reality and a stabilizing of emotions and intellect. Having tired of the confusion and uncertainty inherent in the previous stage, the NGs learn to accept their new responsibilities, gain a level of comfort with their own fallibility, mature in their professional relationships with clinical colleagues, and acquire a functional sense of their own professionalism relative to that of their colleagues (Duchscher, 2001a; Godinez, Schweiger, Gruver, & Ryan, 1999; Jasper, 1996; Kelly, 1998; Walker, 1998). Successful reorientation results in the return of the graduate to a new status or social position within the nursing unit culture, and a recognition that "the perfect job simply does not exist" (Kramer & Schmalenberg, 1977, p. 18).

EXPERIENCE OF TRANSITION IN NURSING GRADUATE

Wide variations of experience occur among individuals undergoing transition (Schumacher & Meleis, 1994). Several of Chick and Meleis's (1986) transition conditions are used here to provide substance and specificity for the understanding of the NG transition experience: expectations, meanings and sense of well being, level of knowledge and skill, and environment.

Expectations

The expectations of a transition experience can significantly impact one's perceptions of that process (Kane, 1992). In the nursing literature, Kelly (1996) postulated that the first year of professional nursing practice is like an obstacle course, with graduates experiencing their work as traumatic primarily because of unrealistic expectations that the NG will "hit the ground running." These expectations result from a seeming incongruency between the progressive clinical expectations provided through the course of their nursing education and those of senior nursing colleagues and nursing unit managers (NUM) in the new graduate's professional practice environment (Brown, 1999; Charnley, 1999). As has been noted frequently in interdisciplinary literature, "there is in every profession a gap between the culture of the profession transmitted in the teaching institution and the actualities of practice in sectors of the field" (Olesen & Whittaker, 1968, p. 297). This "silent dialogue" in the profession of nursing symbolizes those truths that are either lacking or hidden in both education and industry, but that serve to maintain a functional and even necessary tension between the polarized ideals of an altruistic service of care and the necessity of a capitalistic health care industry (Kramer, 1968; Olesen & Whittaker, 1968).

Evidence suggests that newly graduated nurses in acute care are confronted with what they perceive to be moral dilemmas in their practice (Duchscher, 2001a). Not uncommonly, recruits feel compelled to choose between:

- caring effectively *or* caring efficiently
- providing comfort, attending to needs of families, and advocating for patients self-determination *or* maintaining a powerfully fixed organizational structure and ordered routine
- being perceived as independent, capable practitioners by their colleagues *or* reaching out for needed assistance, exposing their naivete and ignorance, and risking the acceptance they so desire
- practicing the ideals that have been taught to them in their undergraduate education *or* assimilating the institutionally modified practice standards of the *real* world
- focusing on their own needs *or* attending to the ever-demanding, but unpredictable and unfamiliar needs of their patients
- fusing their understanding that while experience is key to their professionalization, they have little control over the nature, intensity, or quality of that experience.

A significant source of stress for the newly graduated nurse is the perception that senior nursing staff, clinical educators, and nursing unit managers have unrealistic expectations of the recruit's skill and knowledge (Brown, 1999). The nature of these unrealistic expectations may emanate from covert, albeit not entirely unexpected, value conflicts and role ambiguities inherent in a move from an educationally based, learner-focused care paradigm to the more functionally focused care paradigm of industry. A lack of formal acknowledgement of these conflicts may contribute to unrealistic clinical expectations by senior staff whose have long since adjusted to the altered workload and responsibility of professional practice, assimilated existing service values into their own personal care-value system, and possibly become desensitized to the impropriety of some of their collapsed values (Kelly, 1998). Concurrently, it may be that these senior staff have simply forgotten the intensity of this transition experience for the new practitioner. Finally, it is possible that the most recent changes in health care delivery being reflected in increases in acuity levels and reductions in staffing capabilities are profoundly impacting the quality of the nursing work environment, yet going unactualized by hospital administrators, managers, and clinical educators who have not made necessary adjustments to the orientation and ongoing clinical support programs for NGs in practice.

Meanings and Sense of Well-Being

Of particular consequence to theories of transition is the importance of understanding the meaning of that experience from the perspective of those experiencing it (Schumacher & Meleis, 1994). *Meanings* give voice to the wide range of emotions and the altered *sense of well-being* experienced during transition, and this voice articulates more clearly the effect of those transitions on one's life (Chick & Meleis, 1986).

Transitions have been noted as sources of stress and emotional distress (Schumacher & Meleis, 1994). This is undeniably the most strikingly consistent finding in the research on NGs making the transition to professional practice. The extraordinary, overwhelming, and phenomenally exhausting stress experienced by these neophyte nurses originates from a lack of confidence (Duchscher, 2001a), a sudden increase in responsibility and accountability (Horsburgh, 1989; Walker, 1998), a lack of clinical knowledge and skills (Tradewell, 1996; Walker & Bailey, 1999; Whitehead, 2001), unrealistic expectations by clinical colleagues (Oechsle & Landry, 1987), role conflict and role ambiguity (Jasper, 1996; Prebble & McDonald, 1997), value conflicts (McCloskey & McCain, 1987), and a lack of support (Hamel, 1990; Hartshorn, 1992).

Hamel (1990) and Horsburgh (1989) studied the transition period of NGs using ethnographic fieldwork research, concluding that the majority of stressors during the transition period were related to "fitting into the bureaucracy" and were typified by an overwhelming fear of failure, of total responsibility, and of making mistakes (Horsburgh, 1989, p. 614). New graduates described the tremendous pressure to conform to ward routines that were often viewed as ritualistic, and which interfered with the ability of the nurses to interact with and meet their patients' needs (Kelly, 1996). Concurrently, senior nursing preceptors in Brown's (1999) study admitted that "getting the work done by the end of the shift" was the most important criteria for NGs to successfully meet preceptor expectations during their orientation period. As Horsburgh articulated, "adjustment [to the nursing profession] meant the acceptance of nursing as [the] management of tasks" (p. 612). Associated with this acceptance for the NG was a tremendous sense of guilt and disappointment with this reality, manifested in a prevalence of moral distress or the perceived inability to live up to their moral convictions (Jasper, 1996; Kelly, 1996; Kramer, 1974).

Research-based evidence has suggested that formal complaints from NGs on the traumatic experience of this transition period is unlikely to occur (Duchscher, 2001a; Gerrish, 2000; Kelly, 1996). These NGs seem to believe that this is what life as a nurse is all about and they may fear retribution or reduced credibility if they voice concerns about, or provide resistance to, this initiation into professional practice. What is becoming clearer, however, is that workplace complacency regarding suboptimal practice standards and the moral residue that results from chronic moral distress will not likely be tolerated by this new generation of professionals (Aiken, Clarke, Sloane, & Sochalski, 2001; Charnley, 1999). In response to unresolved stressors and incongruencies in the workplace, it is highly possible that these NGs will simply leave hospital nursing or the profession altogether in search of a context that better matches their vocational aspirations (Cowin, 2002).

Level of Knowledge and Skill

The level of knowledge and skill relevant to the transition being experienced may be insufficient to meet the demands of the new situation (Chick & Meleis, 1986; Schumacher & Meleis, 1994). Anders, Douglas, and Harrigan's (1995) study of both baccalaureate and associate degree graduates supported this with an alarming 48% of health care agencies surveyed reporting that NGs did not meet their competency expectations. Of those, 84% could not adequately supervise ancillary staff, 39% could not collaborate with other members of the health care team, 53% could not organize their daily routine, 40% could not administer intravenous fluids safely and effectively, and 28% could not chart meaningful observations of their clients.

An interesting and prevalent, but perhaps not surprising, finding in research on NGs in practice is the significant discrepancy between the assessment of competence by employers of NGs and the graduates themselves. Graduates consistently asserted their practice competence at a higher level than that assessed by faculty and administrators (Failla, Maher, & Duffy, 1999). Ramritu and Barnard (2001) provided insight into the NGs conception of competence as "practising safely to prevent injury or harm" (p. 49). Participants in their study characterized safe practice as: following the standards outlined in policy and procedure manuals, performing fundamental nursing skills with a basic knowledge of practice principles, being aware of their limitations and asking for assistance, and using strategies to prevent harm to patients. This is interesting in light of alarming research by Khoza and Ehlers (1998) in which an average of 82% of senior professional nurses across a broad spectrum of practice areas claimed that the NGs they were working with did not render safe care to their patients. In related research, numerous authors have addressed the discomfort of NGs with basic technical or practical nursing skills (Benner, 1984; Dearmun, 2000; Jasper, 1996), managing a ward or supervising other levels of nursing staff (Horsburgh, 1989; Walker, 1998), dealing with dying patients or distraught family members (Kapborg & Fischbein, 1998; Maben & Macleod-Clark, 1998), and administering medications (Walker, 1998).

Numerous authors have identified the NGs' overall difficulty with prioritization of care, critical and analytical thinking, and clinical decision-making and judgment (Duchscher, 2003; Gerrish, 2000; Jasper, 1996; Lathlean, 1987; Walker, 1998). As previously outlined, several studies have reported the perception of reduced clinical skills among baccalaureate graduates compared with graduates of diploma and associate degree programs, while others have demonstrated comparatively advanced clinical decision-making capacity among graduates of university-affiliated nursing programs (Girot, 2000).

In a related study, Gerrish (2000) compared two time cohorts of British nursing graduates whose educational programs would be equivalent to the associate and baccalaureate nursing degree programs in North America. Congruent with Benner's (1984) depiction of the novice nurse, participants in both groups reported clinical situations where they knew *in theory* what action to take, but when faced with the *actual situation* were unable to act confidently. Although there may be a decided emphasis on classroom theory in baccalaureate nursing programs, these findings suggest that differences in the application of learned theoretical concepts to practice situations for NGs of varied programs may be unfounded. Assuming that all nursing education programs maintain a conceptual intent for the development of nursing praxis, the key to understanding the capacity of the NG to successfully apply theory to practice may lie in appreciating the mutual importance of both their foundational education and the environment within which they are hired to practice.

Environment

The importance of providing sufficient environmental resources to support a transition experience is a prominent theme in the literature. Imle (1990) conceptualized *organizational environment* as being the external resources outside of the person that supported them through the process of transition, while Braskamp and Maehr (1985) defined *organizational culture* as the underlying values and beliefs of an organization as perceived by its employees. For the NG, the experience of role socialization into professional nursing practice "marks the beginning of an acculturation process into the health care system" (Crowe, 1994, p. 105). Kramer (1974) added that the values and beliefs associated with what it means to be a nurse are either further developed or abandoned after the commencement of employment.

Informing this conceptual dyad is knowledge that within the acute care hospital environment, new nurses are immersed into a firmly entrenched, distinctively symbolic, and moral culture that exposes them to dominant normative behaviors working inherently to maintain existing power structures and support the practices of the health care organization (Crowe, 1994; Kramer, 1966). Duchscher's (2001a) participants described a prescriptive, intellectually oppressive, or at the least cognitively restrictive, working environment for nurses in acute care centres. Mohr (1995) concurred, claiming that the hospital environment tends to move NGs away from their ideal of professional nursing practice by emphasizing productivity, efficiency, and the achievement of institutionally imposed goals. The perceived inability to fulfill their professional and ethical responsibilities to their patients, and the moral distress and job dissatisfaction that ensues, have been cited as primary reasons for the attrition of nurses out of the nursing profession (Penticuff & Walden, 2000).

Kramer (1974) further contended that graduates who are not assisted in the successful socialization to their new working role may resolve the perceived incongruity by: diminishing or discarding ethical and practice standards for institutional routines and bureaucratic compliance; limiting their work commitment and turning their conflict inward, leading to work environment fatigue and burnout; expressing their discontent by "making waves" and contributing to a reduction in morale and an increase in unit dissention and discontent; or "going native" by aligning themselves with the institution, developing a pervasive disdain for a profession that led them to believe in an ethics and value-based practice ethos that they now recognize as *unrealistic* and *unachievable*. This failure to successfully adjust to the new organizational climate is one of the major factors leading to rapid NG turnover (Blegen, 1993).

FACILITATING A HEALTHY TRANSITION

Being "the new kid on the block" is never easy. Strategies to successfully integrate the new nursing graduate into professional practice must:

- acknowledge and bridge the inherent value discrepancies between academia and industry
- provide ongoing support for and nurturing of the high professional practice standards brought to the acute care environment by the NG
- provide consistent, structured, constructive, and goal-oriented feedback and supervised guidance of NGs
- cultivate a sense of belonging for these new professionals through formal mentoring and preceptored clinical orientation.

The following section incorporates these fundamental elements of a successful professional socialization process into NG transition initiatives for nursing education and practice environments.

Education Initiatives

The undergraduate nursing education experience of the NG is appropriately and necessarily idealistic, however, a bridge between the ideals taught in the classroom and the realities experienced in the workplace is required. Facilitating the development of praxis in undergraduate nursing students, moving senior students toward a more interdependent, critically thinking and reflective practice, and both anticipating and working to resolve NG socialization issues are good first steps in bridging the gap between education and industry.

Praxis

As Howkins and Ewens (1999) described, people make sense of their world by developing their own personal constructs, which they then use to test out explanations of their world. If their constructs do not provide meaning for their world, then they revise and reframe them so that they become meaningful. This synthesis of theory with practice, or *praxis*, is a desirable outcome of nursing education programs. Faculty with joint appointments as clinicians in a variety of work settings can assist senior nursing students in the synthesis of nursing theory into practice areas. Concurrent practice expertise allows faculty to model how students, as NGs, might go about modifying idealistic theoretical constructs for use in dynamic, unpredictable, and often resource-limited and time-constrained clinical practice contexts.

Peer Mentoring

The potential for fostering the move from dependent student to interdependent NG may lie in the concept of peer-partnered learning during senior undergraduate nursing education experiences (McAllister & Osborne, 1997). In a project involving student-student teaching and learning in undergraduate clinical nursing education, senior nursing students were helped to build on existing reflective abilities, to develop a sense of professional responsibility and accountability, and to advance personal leadership and facilitation skills (Duchscher, 2001b). In an approach coined *peer mentoring* by the author, students assumed the role of mentor to their peers in the context of their undergraduate, senior clinical practicum experiences. The purpose of peer mentoring was for students to exchange organizational, technical, structural, and clinical knowledge and feedback with each other, mimicking the interdependent collaborative environment of professional nursing practice and reducing the students' dependence on faculty supervised clinical practice and externally generated evaluative feedback.

Participants claimed that this experience was mutually supportive, cooperative, and collaborative, and acknowledged their knowledge and experience. As a result of mentoring their peers, participants described their practice as having grown in both diligence and precision, an increased confidence in making clinical practice decisions, and an enhanced sense of accountability for those decisions (Duchscher, 2001b).

Anticipatory Socialization

In early and seminal studies of behavioral and attitudinal changes in soldiers during WWII, Stouffer (1949) noted that those who successfully assumed a new status did so by acquiring the necessary behavioral characteristics, attitudes, and role orientations of that new position prior to formally making the change. Merton (1968) coined this premature adoption of an aspired identity as anticipatory socialization (AS). Kramer (1974) proposed this idea as the possible missing link in resolving existing professional-bureaucratic conflict for the new nursing graduate.

A subsequent program of AS for senior nursing students was born out of the recognition that improvements in the quality of patient care would only be brought about by nurses who worked within the care system to transform suboptimal health care delivery conditions through the integration of practice ideals into the realities of the work environment. As Kramer (1974) poignantly articulated, "the status quo will be maintained and fostered, not by indolent, uncaring nurses but rather by good nurses who do nothing" (p. 67).

In a visionary approach to bridging the theory-practice gap, Kramer set out to sociologically inoculate two classes of nursing students with the attitudes and role specific behaviors that would be required to successfully operationalize their professional values in the work setting. Two specific goals guided the AS program: (1) untried professional beliefs of the students were challenged, while they were provided concurrently with possible responsive statements or practices that could be used to protect their professional values and ethics, and (2) all possible dimensions of professional-bureaucratic role conflict and reality shock were presented to senior students, along with supplemental strategies used by a reference group of practicing nurses to successfully resolve any conflict.

A coordinated and collaborative effort is needed between education and industry to integrate transition-specific content into existing undergraduate curricula, develop and implement transition-specific courses or programs for senior nursing students, and address reality shock and socialization challenges in the job orientations of NGs. The prevailing stance in addressing issues inherent in the socialization process of the NG to professional practice should be that conflict and professional-bureaucratic issues are to be expected. Strategies aimed at heightening the awareness and establishing potential resolutions for these issues are presented in Table 16.1.

Practice Environment Initiatives

In a review of the issues underlying the current nursing shortage, Cowin (2002) asked how an educational system could be expected to prepare a nursing recruit for a workplace that is "fundamentally at odds with nursing care philosophy" (p. 6). Cowin further claimed that the salient point is that nursing knowledge is not the cause of poor nursing retention. Rather, it is the inadequacy of the work environment to nurture and develop the new employee that is at the heart of many losses of NGs. Strategies to optimize the socialization process of the NG are presented in Tables 16.2 to 16.4.

SUMMARY

The transition to professional practice for the NG is indisputably traumatic. This chapter provided a comprehensive and detailed description of the transition experience with the intent to foster a greater understanding of the breadth, depth, and scope of the experience of moving from student to professionally practicing nurse. It is hoped that the strategies presented will be used by nursing unit managers and educators alike, such that these energetic and idealistic new nurses can be assisted in navigating the unfamiliar health care contexts that we know to be veritable mine-fields of clinical intensity and organizational change. The goal of this facilitated transition to professional practice for the new graduate is the retention of a vital and optimistic professional nursing workforce that can ensure high-quality patient care and secure a more certain future for nursing professionalism that rests firmly in the values to which we aspire.

TABLE 16.1   Transition Strategies for New Graduates

- Transition programs that review the signs and symptoms of reality shock and cognitive overload expected in NG practice, providing strategies to cope with the stress and distress that ensues
- Inclusion of both education and service staff in the development and implementation of all anticipatory socialization content for transition programs
- Senior term courses or workshops to target professional practice issues such as:
    - Optimizing physician-nurse communication and minimizing interpersonal conflict in the workplace
    - Task organization and workload management in the clinical area
    - Facilitating interdisciplinary collaboration in patient care
    - Understanding and dealing with issues associated with different levels of nursing education preparation
    - Supervising ancillary and support staff
    - Negotiating professional-bureaucratic value differences and conflicts

- Reality-based, problem-focused learning approaches that balance academically initiated practice ideals with institutional context-based practice realities
- Discussion of characteristics and issues related to bureaucratic organizations and how to work within formalized institutional structures to actualize change and resolve conflict
- Development of working knowledge about professional identify formulation
- Encouragement of NGs to identify and select a mentor in the practice environment who has successfully integrated both professional and bureaucratic value systems
- Emphasis on understanding and developing individual change agent styles, acting as an advocate for patients within a competing practice value environment, and responding to expectations of others in the workplace

---

TABLE 16.2   Optimizing New Graduates' Workplace Culture

- Provide clear and realistic job interviews that include specific information related to job duties, tangible work benefits, leadership styles and nursing work routines, social climate of unit, evaluative expectations, and opportunities for career advancement
- Reduce perceived discrepancies between NG expectations and workplace opportunities
- Initiate regular focused meetings once or twice a month to provide structured feedback on NG's clinical progress
- Remain in touch with realities of the clinical practice environment and issues of nursing profession by getting involved in local professional nursing organizations and maintaining a high visibility on nursing units
- Maintain open door policy with all nursing staff, regularly meeting with individual nurses and as a group with all staff for career building, collaborative goal setting, and soliciting feedback on functional and relational aspects of workplace
- Have routinely scheduled "check-ups" with senior nursing staff responsible for mentoring and preceptoring new staff, providing guidance in leadership and clinical teaching strategies
- Pay attention to emerging professional needs of the NG, supporting and funding continuing education and clinical specialty advancement programs (i.e., telemetry experience, Advanced Cardiac Life Support training)
- Be direct, consistent, and honest in your approach
- Provide evidence of highly moral and ethical administrative practice, making visible the decisions required by management to secure an optimal nursing care delivery system
- Empower nursing staff by involving them in decision making that affects the nursing unit—find creative ways to allow staff to communicate their concerns and potential resolutions (e.g., suggestion boxes)
- Ensure easy access to Web-based clinical information and interactive computer programs for continuing education on all nursing units
- Build in time for practice reflection and continuing education of all nursing staff (e.g., regularly schedule a nurse who is responsible for assisting with morning care and spending the remaining shift time to deliver in-service education for staff on clinical issues)
- Encourage a relaxed workplace culture complete with more casual professional attire and exercise reasonable and unit-specific leniency related to body piercing and symbolic jewelry
- Provide for a more seamless connection between work and play—encourage interaction of staff through social gatherings, unit coffee parties, communication systems, and social networking (e.g., have a humor board in the coffee room, display photographs of staff with their families, celebrate birthdays and special occasions, recognize staff for professional and personal accomplishments)

TABLE 16.3   New Graduate Nursing Unit Orientation

- Provide for extended supernumerary staffing (outside of regular staffing quota) of NG to accommodate essential socialization needs of new employees for a minimum orientation period of 4 months
- Gradually and progressively introduce content related to unit-specific tasks, unit routines, and policies and procedures over the course of the orientation period
- Balance sequencing of theory and practice so that NGs are able to immediately apply content they are learning to practice situations
- Assist with development of concepts such as time management, workload organization, prioritization, decision making, and clinical judgment
- Plan for structured and frequent performance appraisals (e.g., begin daily and progress to weekly, biweekly, monthly, bimonthly, and then annually over the course of the first year)

TABLE 16.4   Assisted Transition Programs

- Assist in accurate appraisal and transmission of nursing unit's cultural norms and expectations by providing preceptoring (skill assistance) and mentoring (social and professional culture assimilation) of all NGs for the first year of professional practice
- Select mentors/preceptors intentionally based on the advanced nature of their clinical expertise, their competence in skill performance, capacity for patience, empathy and understanding, realistic perspective of expectations for NG practice, questioning attitude and openness to challenge, and willingness and ability to teach effectively
- Formally structure mentor/preceptor preparation programs to include basic communication strategies, supervision and evaluation techniques, adult learning principles, conflict resolution approaches, and anticipated transition issues of NGs in professional practice
- Schedule mentors/preceptors and NGs in corresponding shift schedules for the duration of the assisted transition to ensure one consistent mentor for each new graduate
- Encourage senior nursing staff to actively foster a sense of belonging by maintaining a welcoming and safe presence and providing frequent goal setting and feedback sessions on strengths and weaknesses in NG performance (minimum of weekly NG/mentor formal meetings)
- Compensate mentors/preceptors through individually and mutually identified reward and incentive programs (e.g., time in lieu, monetary honorariums, reimbursement for continuing education programs, advanced nurse titling)
- Visibly support critically based cognitive processing in clinical judgment and decision making of all nursing staff in the practice setting
- Encourage senior staff in their modeling of constructive change and independent decision making related to clinical practice issues

REFERENCES

Aiken, L., Clarke, S., Sloane, D., Sochalski, J., Busse, R., Clarke, H., et al. (2001). Nurses' report on hospital care in five countries. *Health Affairs, 20*(3), 42–53.

Aiken, L. H., Clarke, S. P., & Sloane, D. M. (2002). Hospital staffing, organizational support, and quality of care: Cross-national findings. *International Journal of Quality Health Care, 14*, 5–13.

Aiken, L. H., Clarke, S. P., Sloane, D. M., & Sochalski, J. A. (2001). An international perspective on hospital nurses' work environments: The case for reform. *Policy, Politics, & Nursing Practice, 2*, 253–261.

Aiken, L. H., Clarke, S. P., Sloane, D. M., Sochalski, J., & Silber, J. H. (2002). Hospital nurse staffing and patient mortality, nurse burnout, and job dissatisfaction. *Journal of the American Medical Association, 288*, 1987–1993.

Anders, R., Douglas, D., & Harrigan, R. (1995). Competencies of new RNs: A survey of deans and health care agencies in the state of Hawaii. *Nursing Connections, 8*(3), 5–16.

Benner, P. (1984). *From novice to expert: Excellence and power in clinical nursing practice.* Menlo Park, CA: Addison-Wesley Publishing.

Blegen, M. A. (1993). Nurses' job satisfaction: A meta-analysis of related variables. *Nursing Research, 42*(1), 36–41.

Braskamp, L. A., & Maehr, M. L. (1985). *Spectrum: An organizational development tool.* Champaign, IL: Metritech, Inc.

Bridges, W. (1980). *Transitions: Making sense of life's changes.* Reading, MA: Addison-Wesley.

Brown, P. L. (1999). Graduate nurses: What do they expect? *Kansas Nurse, 74*(5), 4–5.

Buerhaus, P. I., & Staiger, D. (1999). Trouble in the nurse labor market? Recent trends and future outlook. *Health Affairs, 18*, 214–222.

Canadian Institute for Health Information. (2001). Supply and distribution of registered nurses in Canada 2000. Available at: //222.cihi.ca/medrls/23may2001.shtml

Canadian Nursing Advisory Committee. (2002). *Our health, our future: Creating quality workplaces for Canadian nurses.* Ottawa, Ontario: Advisory Committee on Health Human Resources, Health Canada.

Charnley, E. (1999). Occupational stress in the newly qualified staff nurse. *Nursing Standard, 13*(29), 33–36.

Chick, N., & Meleis, A. I. (1986). Transitions: A nursing concern. In P. L. Chinn (Ed.), *Nursing research methodology: Issues and implementation* (pp. 237–257). Rockville, MD: Aspen.

Cowin, L. (2002). The effects of nurses' job satisfaction on retention: An Australian perspective. *Journal of Nursing Administration, 32*, 283–291.

Cowin, L. S., & Jacobsson, D. K. (2002). A growing health care crisis: The causes of the nursing shortage. *Collegian.* (In review)

Crowe, M. (1994). Problem-based learning: A mode for graduate transition in nursing. *Contemporary Nurse, 3*, 105–109.

Dearmun, A. K. (2000). Supporting newly qualified staff nurses: The lecturer practitioner contribution. *Journal of Nursing Management, 8*, 159–165.

Duchscher, J. E. B. (2001a). Out in the real world: Newly graduated nurses in acute care speak out. *Journal of Nursing Administration, 31*(9), 426–439.

Duchscher, J. E. B. (2001b). Peer learning: A clinical teaching strategy to promote active learning. *Nurse Educator, 26*(2), 59–60.

Duchscher, J. E. B. (2003). Critical thinking: Perceptions of newly graduated female baccalaureate nurses. *Journal of Nursing Education, 42*(1), 1–12.

Failla, S., Maher, M. A., & Duffy, C. A. (1999). Evaluation of graduates of an associate degree program. *Journal of Nursing Education, 38*, 62–68.

Gerrish, K. (1990). Fumbling along. *Nursing Times, 86*(30), 35–37.

Gerrish, K. (2000). Still fumbling along? A comparative study of the newly qualified nurse's perception of the transition from student to qualified nurse. *Journal of Advanced Nursing, 32*, 473–480.

Girot, E. A. (2000). Graduate nurses: Critical thinkers or better decision makers. *Journal of Advanced Nursing, 31*, 288–297.

Godinez, G., Schweiger, J., Gruver, J., & Ryan, P. (1999). Role transition from graduate to staff nurse: A qualitative analysis. *Journal for Nurses in Staff Development, 15*, 97–110.

Greenwood, J. (2000). Critique of the graduate nurse: An international perspective. *Nurse Education Today, 20*, 17–23.

Hamel, E. (1990). An interpretative study of the professional socialization of neophyte nurses in the nursing subculture. Doctoral thesis, College of Education, University of San Diego, San Diego, CA.

Hartshorn, J. (1992). Evaluation of a critical care nursing internship program. *Journal of Continuing Education, 23*(1), 42–48.

Health and Human Resources and Services Administration (HHRSA). (2001). *The RN population: National sample survey of RNs.* Washington, DC: U.S. Department of Health and Human Resources.

Hecker, D. J. (2001). Occupational employment projections to 2010. *Monthly Labour Review, 124*(11), 57–84.

Horsburgh, M. (1989). Graduate nurses' adjustment to initial employment: Natural field work. *Journal of Advanced Nursing, 14*, 610–617.

Howkins, E. J., & Ewens, A. (1999). How students experience professional socialization. *International Journal of Nursing Studies, 36*, 41–49.

Imle, M. A. (1990). Third trimester concerns of expectant parents in transition to parenthood. *Holistic Nursing Practice, 4*(3), 25–36.

Jasper, M. (1996). The first year as a staff nurse: The experiences of a first cohort of Project 2000 nurses in a demonstration district. *Journal of Advanced Nursing, 24*, 779–790.

Kane, J. J. (1992). Allowing the novice to succeed: Transitional support in critical care. *Critical Care Nursing Quarterly, 15*(3), 17–22.

Kapborg, I. D., & Fischbein, S. (1998). Nurse education and professional work: Transition problems? *Nurse Education Today, 18*, 165–171.

Kelly, G. (1996). Hospital nursing: 'It's a battle'! A follow-up study of English graduate nurses. *Journal of Advanced Nursing, 24,* 1063–1069.

Kelly, B. (1998). Preserving moral integrity: A follow-up study with NGs. *Journal of Advanced Nursing, 28*(5), 1134–1145.

Khoza, L. B., & Ehlers, V. J. (1998). The competencies of newly qualified nurses as viewed by senior professional nurses. *Curatonis, 21*(3), 67–76.

Kramer, M. (1966). The NG speaks. *American Journal of Nursing, 66,* 2420–2424.

Kramer, M. (1968). Role models, role conception, and role deprivation. *Nursing Research, 17*(2), 115–120.

Kramer, M. (1974). *Reality shock: Why nurses leave nursing.* St. Louis: CV Mosby Co.

Kramer, M., & Schmalenberg, C. (1977). *Path to biculturalism.* Wakefield, MA: Contemporary Publishing, Inc.

Lathlean, J. (1987). Are you prepared to be a staff nurse? *Nursing Times, 83,* 25–27.

Maben, J., & Macleod-Clark, J. (1998). Project 2000 diplomates' perceptions of their experiences of transition from student to staff nurse. *Journal of Clinical Nursing, 7,* 145–153.

McAllister, M., & Osborne, Y. (1997). Peer review: A strategy to enhance cooperative student learning. *Nurse Educator, 22*(1), 40–44.

McCloskey, J., & McCain, B. (1987). Satisfaction, commitment and professionalism among newly employed nurses. *Journal of Nursing Scholarship, 19,* 20–24.

Merton, R. K. (1968). *Social theory and social structure.* New York: Free Press.

Mohr, W. K. (1995). Values, ideologies, and dilemmas: Professional and occupational contradictions. *Journal of Psychosocial Nursing, 33*(1), 29–34.

Oermann, M. H., & Garvin, M. F. (2002). Stresses and challenges for new graduates in nursing. *Nurse Education Today, 22,* 225–230.

Oeschsle, L., & Landry, R. (1987). Congruity between role expectations and actual work experience: A study of recently employed RNs. *Western Journal of Nursing Research, 9,* 555–571.

Olesen, V. L., & Whittaker, E. W. (1968). *The silent dialogue: A study in the social psychology of professional socialization.* San Francisco: Jossey-Bass.

Penticuff, J. H., & Walden, M. (2000). Influence of practice environment and nurse characteristics on perinatal nurses' responses to ethical dilemmas. *Nursing Research, 49,* 64–72.

Prebble, K., & McDonald, B. (1997). Adaptation to the mental health setting: The lived experience of comprehensive graduates. *Australian and New Zealand Journal of Mental Health Nursing, 6*(1), 30–36.

Ramritu, P. L., & Barnard, A. (2001). New nursing graduates' understanding of competence. *International Nursing Review, 48,* 47–57.

Ryten, E. (1997). *A statistical picture of the past, present, and future of registered nurses in Canada.* Ottawa, Ontario: Canadian Nurses Association.

Schumacher, K. L., & Meleis, A. I. (1994). Transitions: A central concept in nursing. *IMAGE: Journal of Nursing Scholarship, 26,* 119–127.

Stouffer, S. (1949). *Studies in the social psychology of World War II.* Princeton, NJ: Princeton University Press.

Tradewell, G. (1996). Rites of passage: Adaptation of nursing graduates to a hospital setting. *Journal of Nursing Staff Development, 12,* 183–189.

Van Gennep, A. (1960). *The rites of passage.* London: Routledge & Kegan Paul.

Walker, J. (1998). The transition to registered nurse: The experience of a group of New Zealand degree graduates. *Nursing Praxis in New Zealand, 13*(2), 36–43.

Walker, J., & Bailey, S. (1999). The clinical performance of new degree graduates. *Nursing Praxis in New Zealand, 14*(2), 31–42.

Whitehead, J. (2001). Newly qualified staff nurses' perceptions of the role transition. *British Journal of Nursing, 10,* 330–339.

Winter-Collins, A., & McDaniel, A. (2000). Sense of belonging and NG satisfaction. *Journal for Nurses in Staff Development, 16,* 103–111.

Chapter 17

The Nurse Educator Role in Staff Competency

Magdalena A. Mateo and Eileen McMyler

Nurse educators in clinical settings assume vital roles in the development of staff to provide safe and efficient care to patients and their families through orientation, ongoing competency development, and staff development programs. Several strategies are used to address these components. First, collaboration is needed with personnel in the human resources department who are involved in recruitment and orientation of staff, with nurse managers who are knowledgeable in the skills necessary to perform the job, and with staff who are in a unique position to participate in planning and implementing orientation, competency, and staff development programs. Second, is the delineation of staff responsibilities and the feasibility of methods for programs to determine staff clinical competencies. Once clinical competence is assured, resources can be used to develop the next level of clinical practice including staff leadership skills.

A sufficient number of competent staff is paramount to patient safety. The Institute of Medicine (IOM) stressed safety problems in the hospital in relation to inadequate staffing, problems of communicating vital information between care providers, and the need to serve an increasingly complex and diverse patient population (Anthony & Preuss, 2002; IOM, 2000). The problem of not having sufficient staff means that current staff should be more efficient, effective, and competent (Buerhaus, Needleman, Mattke, & Stewart, 2002). To ensure the ability of staff to provide safe care to patients, institutions continuously search for ways to enhance their orientation, competency, and staff development processes.

In addition to reviewing the literature, a valuable venue is networking with educators in other settings. This is an excellent and timely way to learn current trends in orientation, competency, and staff development programs. Knowledge of methods used by colleagues can then be assessed for feasibility in relation to one's setting. The purpose of this chapter is to present strategies used in evaluating staff competency and development in orientation and throughout employment. A graduate assistant of the first author contacted several hospitals to inquire about their practices in relation to these programs. Ideas from nurse educators who responded to questions about practices in their organization are included throughout the chapter. Exhibits are used to present examples of program components and forms that can be adapted by other educators.

ESTABLISHING AND MAINTAINING STAFF COMPETENCY

Emphasis on quality of care, cost effectiveness, and use of technology require that programs be conducted efficiently using the least amount of resources. Considerations should be given to determining topics that should be covered during and after orientation; identifying strategies for dealing with a new staff when orientation is not going according to plan; documenting, assessing, and measuring the progress of staff toward competence; and developing staff. Galt (2000) identified the importance of using feedback from staff about what was helpful in orientation and what should be changed to get the most out of "orientation dollars." Direct observation of practice using procedural guidelines or policies as the standard is the preferred way of determining if staff is competently performing a skill. However, it can be time consuming because of the logistics of having someone available to observe the staff person performing the skill and then to document that observation.

The success of orientation and competency programs, an ongoing process, depends on successful collaboration among nurse educators who provide education programs, staff in leadership positions who ensure maintenance of staff competency, the preceptor, and the staff member (Miller, Flynn, & Umada, 1998). Job descriptions and performance appraisals that include maintenance of competencies and further professional development are essential. A good working relationship with management to support time for these activities is vital. Communication between hospitals and schools of nursing to keep abreast of curriculum and clinical experiences that prepare nurses to fulfill job requirements should be maintained to promote successful transition from the student to the registered nurse (RN) role.

ORIENTATION PROGRAMS

Teaching techniques used in orientation and people involved in the process vary because of differences in organizational structures and resources. Depending on the size of the organization, there may be a new employee orientation program sponsored by the Human Resources (HR) department, a nursing department orientation, and a unit orientation. Assuming HR covers new employee information, it is likely to be on benefit information, introduction to core values of the institution, safety information, employee policies about dress code, payroll, and any diversity or mutual respect policies of the organization. The nursing department orientation would cover more department-specific topics that are relevant to all nursing staff. Unit orientation would focus on the clinical environment, the team, competencies for meeting job requirements, and day-to-day job specific information. Table 17.1 illustrates topics covered in employee orientation.

A new staff's successful completion of orientation depends partially on assessing learning needs for the skills that will be required in the specialty practice while acknowledging the breadth of work experience the RN may bring to the new setting (Figure 17.1). It is important to use the preceptor's knowledge and expertise in identifying important skills required in the specialty area of nursing practice (Biancuzzo, 1994). This builds collaboration and ensures that pertinent topics are covered.

During the planning phase, identifying the unit goals for orientation and then linking them to the orientee's goals is the first challenge. The second challenge is to schedule times for evaluation of performance in fulfilling job responsibilities and of critical thinking, technical, and interpersonal skills. These challenges can be addressed through careful planning and collaboration among the preceptor, new RN, nurse manager, and nurse educator. It also is prudent to consider the cultural background of the new employee when selecting staff to work as a preceptor.

TABLE 17.1 Examples of Topics for New Employee Orientation by Human Resources Department, by Department of Nursing, and on Clinical Unit

Human resources department	Department of nursing	Clinical unit
Introduction to mission, values and core principles	Time cards or payroll information	Meet preceptor, manager, educator, staff
Dress code	Overview of department	Orient to area
Benefits	Staff roles in department	Review orientation schedule
Safety	Medication administration	• Shifts and weekends
Infection control	Emergency response	• Class days
Security	Resources:	
Diversity		Progression of direct patient care activities
Mutual respect	• Transcultural resources	
Parking	• Patient education resources	• Number of patients
	• Physical therapy	• Acuity level of patients
	• Diabetes resources	
	• Discharge planning	Review orientation objectives
		Evaluate ability to meet job requirements
	Regulatory information	Identify competencies required in job description
	• Vulnerable adult	
	• Advance directives	Assess ability to do competencies required
	Risk management strategies	Individualize action plan to meet staff's identified needs
	Expectations	Assess progress in meeting orientation objectives
	• Patient classification	
	• Floating	
	• Accountability and delegation	• Develop action plan if performance does not meet expectation
	Hospital-wide protocols	
	• Chemical dependence	Wrap-up orientation
	Computer applications	

Name: _____ Date: _____

On the following pages, nursing activities have been listed that reflect the role and responsibilities of a Registered Nurse specific to work area. The tool includes an assessment of what the orientee needs and how the competency is demonstrated. The educator will discuss your responsibilities as an orientee and those of staff on the unit to ensure that the tool is completed correctly.

NEEDS ASSESSMENT

The needs assessment will assist you and your preceptor to identify your learning needs and plan your orientation on your work area. As you review each of the nursing activities listed, check if you would like additional content/instruction beyond the orientation classes, additional practice opportunities, or neither of these.

COMPETENCY DEMONSTRATED

You will need to demonstrate your competency with each of the activities listed. Competency is achieved when:

- You are able to carry out the activity independently.
- The activity is based on appropriate nursing standards, guidelines, policies, and procedures that reflect sound nursing practice.
- Both you and your preceptor mutually agree that you have demonstrated competency.

As you demonstrate your ability to carry out each of the activities, you and your preceptor will sign your initials and date. If an activity does not occur during the orientation period, indicate *opportunity not available (ONA)* and incorporate into goals set at end of orientation.

FIGURE 17.1   RN needs assessment and competency tool.

(continued)

FIGURE 17.1 *(continued)*

NEEDS ASSESSMENT				COMPETENCY DEMONSTRATED	
Do you need additional:					
	INSTRUCTION	PRACTICE	NEITHER	Date demonstrated and initials of preceptor/double assigned nurse Competency Validation codes D = Demonstration E = Explanation & Discussion	
				Initials	Date
I. Specific Work area					
A. Demonstrate complete patient assessment. Identify necessary components: heart sounds, breath sounds, cultural component, etc. Include necessary age appropriate assessment considerations.					
1. Demonstrate use of equipment used during assessment. List out equipment that will be used, e.g., special scales, thermometers, pumps.					
2. Demonstrate understanding of medications used in specialty, e.g., indication, administration. List out medications.					
3. Demonstrate understanding of psychosocial issues involved with specialty patient population. List out items, i.e, family visiting issues, etc.					
B. Demonstrate understanding of resources available to assist with assessments. List out specific resources staff should be accessing, e.g., diabetic nurses, pharmacy, clinical specialist.					

FIGURE 17.1 *(continued)*

NEEDS ASSESSMENT				COMPETENCY DEMONSTRATED
Do you need additional:				
	INSTRUCTION	PRACTICE	NEITHER	Date demonstrated and initials of preceptor/double assigned nurse Competency Validation codes D = Demonstration E = Explanation & Discussion Initials Date
C. Demonstrate safe handling precautions when working with patients receiving cytotoxic agents.				
D. Verbalize understanding of standard precautions				
1. Demonstrate the second tier of the infection control precautions for a. VRE				
b. TB				
E. Demonstrate giving a complete and accurate report to the nurse who will be receiving your patient assignment. List out components of necessary communication.				
F. Demonstrate procedures done on the unit. List out procedures, e.g, NG insertion, chest tube management, drain management, etc.				
G. Demonstrate accurate and timely documentation. List out components of documentation.				
H. Verbalize understanding/demonstrate processes needed for specific patient population, i.e, care of the diabetic patient, post op patient, post procedure patient.				
II. Specific work area--often staff work in different areas				
A. Demonstrate needed skills to function in the work area, list out specific skills required.				

FIGURE 17.1 *(continued)*

NEEDS ASSESSMENT				COMPETENCY DEMONSTRATED
Do you need additional:				
	INSTRUCTION	PRACTICE	NEITHER	Date demonstrated and initials of preceptor/double assigned nurse Competency Validation codes D = Demonstration E = Explanation & Discussion Initials Date
B. Demonstrate preparing the patient for dismissal. Identify components required.				
C. Verbalize understanding/demonstrate scheduling responsibilities. List out specific responsibilities.				
D. Demonstrate closing the work area.				
1. Count narcotics according to guidelines				
2. Restock supplies				
3. Clean up unit				
4. Lock unit				
5. Drop off responsibilities for charts, patient materials.				
III. Other work areas or specific equipment				
A. Demonstrate responsibilities that are specific to additional work areas where the staff person will work. List the responsibilities.				
VII. My goals for nursing orientation are: (Have the orientee write goals for orientation so you can assess how you should prioritize your approach.)				

_____ has completed the unit orientation program and has successfully demonstrated the ability to perform the basic skills required of a Registered Nurse in the work area

_____Orientee   Date _____
_____Preceptor   Date _____
_____Educator   Date _____
_____Nurse Manager   Date _____

Documentation of staff competency assessment beginning with orientation is required. The 2002 Joint Commission on Accreditation of Healthcare Organizations (JCAHO) Hospital Accreditation Standards address the competence of employees and the responsibility of leadership to ensure that competence. This principle is illustrated in the following excerpts from JCAHO (2002):

> HR 3   The leaders ensure that the competence of all staff members is assessed, maintained, demonstrated, and improved continually.
>
> HR 3.1   The hospital encourages and supports self-development and learning for all staff.
>
> HR 4.3   The hospital regularly collects aggregate data on competence patterns and trends to identify and respond to the staff's learning needs.
>
> HR 5   The hospital assesses each staff member's ability to meet the performance expectations stated in his or her job description. (pp. 235–237)

The documentation process for the employee file is shown in Table 17.2. Aspects to consider when providing constructive feedback during orientation are in Table 17.3.

When an orientee does not meet expectations, it is necessary that the performance be discussed immediately with the RN. The RN, preceptor, nurse manager, and educator should review areas in which the performance is not up to expectations and discuss what needs to be revised in the orientation plan. Discussions should be documented to ensure that everyone is clear on the major points identified at the meeting (Fahje, McMyler, & Mateo, 2001).

Teaching Strategies Used in Orientation

In addition to classroom instruction, the following strategies are used in orientation as reported by nurse educators from various settings:

1. Individualized pathways with exit competencies
2. Skills stations
3. Videotapes either developed by the hospital or commercially available such as those by Dorothy Del Bueno. With this strategy, vignettes are presented to which the orientees respond; the preceptor or nurse educator then reviews the responses.

TABLE 17.2   Documentation of Orientation for Employee File

Orientation plan	Orientation objectives Employee's orientation schedule Identified classes needed to meet orientation objectives Identified competencies required to do the job—competency tool completed and on file Successful completion of orientation Identified goals for employee after orientation until first performance review Areas of interest in specialty Areas of interest in leadership development
Feedback during orientation (at scheduled intervals) [If concerns arise more frequent meetings will occur—either orientee or preceptor can initiate additional meetings.]	Review of objectives of orientation • Are objectives being met? • Do the preceptor and orientee agree that objectives are being met? • **If not**, what are the discrepancies? • What needs to be put into place? • Can the two come to agreement on plan to resolve the discrepancy? Assessment of competent performance of identified skills using criteria, e.g., procedural guidelines, policies, and equipment manuals
Review of orientation progression	Is acuity of patients for whom orientee is caring increasing? Is number of patients for whom orientee is caring increasing? Are aspects of care needed for patient, e.g., assessments, treatments, and medications, getting done? Is documentation accurate and complete? Is orientee able to manage unplanned events? Is orientation paperwork getting done?
Assessment of orientation progression	Do orientee and preceptor agree on how orientee is progressing? • **If not**, discussion needs to occur (Provide specific examples where care does not meet expectations) • **If yes**, discuss continued progression

TABLE 17.2 *(continued)*

Forms used for feedback sessions	May be general or specific. (If unit preceptors are not comfortable giving constructive feedback, more specific forms are helpful)
Orientation modification	Identify action and follow-up plans for areas of concern
Wrap-up	At end of orientation time frame, i.e., when all objectives for orientation have been met, it is important to acknowledge that orientee has successfully completed orientation Inform orientee of suggestions preceptor has to function more independently Ask about goals for first 6 months to 1 year in area • Discuss plan for meeting goals. • Confirm plan to place orientee on the unit schedule

4. Satellite TV programs such as the GE TiP-TV Programming (GE Medical Systems, 2003), which also can be used for ongoing competencies
5. Computer-assisted instruction and Web-based training and education such as that offered by HealthStream (2003)
6. Clinical time with an assigned nurse, ideally a preceptor, to facilitate progression toward increasing complexity of patient assignments in terms of acuity and numbers of patients.

Selecting, Preparing, and Compensating Preceptors

Preceptors are used widely in implementing orientation programs although the criteria for designating a staff member as a preceptor vary (Abruzzese & Quinn-O'Neil, 1996; Fahje, McMyler, & Mateo, 2001). Criteria for selecting a RN as a preceptor include:

1. Experience in the clinical setting, with the number of years depending on the unit staff available
2. Educational preparation at the bachelor's level depending on the mix of RN staff

TABLE 17.3   Example of Form for Providing Constructive Feedback During Orientation

Aspects of orientation	Areas of strength	Areas for growth	Action plan
Objectives			
Progression of patient acuity assignment			
Increase in number of patients assigned			
Demonstration of competencies identified in job description or orientation tools			
Documentation in patient's medical record			
Management of patient assignment: • Medications given • Treatments done • Accurate report to oncoming nurse • Documentation reflective of patient assessment/care			

3. Successful completion of preceptor classes, training, or workshop
4. Recommendation from the nurse manager
5. Support of other staff
6. Successful performance appraisals
7. Effective communication and interpersonal skills
8. Ability to teach
9. Interest in being a preceptor

Preparation for preceptors vary as well; however, if a formal preceptor program exists, class topics would likely include:

1. Teaching and learning styles
2. Communication styles
3. Adult learning principles
4. Orientation tools used in the institution
5. Techniques for giving and receiving feedback
6. Problem-solving skills in the clinical setting
7. Strategies if orientation goals are not being met (Abruzzese & Quinn-O'Neil, 1996; Fahje, McMyler, & Mateo, 2001).

The second author's institution has one class that staff attend before assuming the preceptor role. After the first year of precepting, staff are encouraged to attend another class that builds on the content from the first one and focuses on some of the challenges faced in the preceptor role including the difficulties of giving constructive feedback when orientees are not meeting expectations.

Compensation for being a preceptor varies across different institutions. This is driven in part by philosophy—that developing colleagues is part of everyone's job and that all nurses, even those who are not preceptors, should support orientation in some way such as by taking additional patients or modifying their schedules. Resources to design and implement a formal preceptor program also are a factor (Czerwinski, Blastic, & Rice, 1999). Compensation for preceptors may be a differential when working with an orientee or when paid for time to participate in education programs designed to increase skills as a preceptor. Whatever the environment, having experienced staff available to orient new employees and evaluate their progress is crucial.

Changes in Orientation Programs

The changing healthcare environment requires new knowledge and skills among employees to enhance the delivery of patient care. In our survey of nurse educators, the following major changes to orientation programs were reported:

- Inclusion of a work style assessment by the orientees and preceptors to improve understanding of differences in personality and how nurses approach their work
- Expansion of orientation to meet the needs of new graduates who are increasingly going into more specialized areas of practice

such as critical care. More hands-on clinical experiences are provided as part of the orientation

- Movement toward a paperless record system and an increase in the use of computer technology for documenting nurses' competencies and gaining access to medical records and resources
- Addition of programs, for example a two-day workshop, for nursing assistants to review concepts for care of patients and practice skills
- Fewer lectures in classes and increased use of interactive teaching methods

COMPETENCY PROGRAMS

Organizations are responsible for ensuring that staff are competent because patients deserve the best possible care (Boylan & Westra, 1998; Del Bueno & Buyer, 2001). Several issues are important when establishing a competency program: accountability, implementation, skills required for the job, skill level of staff, and evaluation and documentation.

Accountability

Nurse managers, nurse educators, and staff share accountability. Nurse managers and educators are responsible for ensuring that topics required for delivery of safe patient care are included in competency programs. Scheduling and unit staffing must be considered when assessing staff if validation methods other than direct observation of skills are used. The nurse manager plays a part in approving the staffing numbers or empowering charge nurses to hire staff. The nurse manager is ultimately responsible for holding staff accountable for developing and maintaining competencies and would initiate corrective action if the staff refused to submit necessary confirmation that competencies were completed. When the nurse manager sets clear expectations and follows through when deadlines are not met, noncompliance is usually not an issue.

Nurse educators are in charge of coordinating competency programs. Staff who serve as preceptors and those who are informal leaders on the unit are often asked to participate in peer evaluation of competency and documentation of the evaluation. Nurses have an important responsibility in gaining competence, by attending educational programs and completing other types of learning activities, by completing competency assessments and demonstrations, and by assisting with tracking required paper work.

Implementation

The implementation of a competency program requires that the educator identify relevant topics (De Onna, 2002), decide on methods of validating competency, and then develop the performance criteria for the methods chosen (Tracy & Summers, 2001). This includes assuring that patient care needs are met during scheduled competency programs so that staff can attend.

Nurse educators and nurse managers need to collaborate to determine the best time to plan and implement programs while meeting frequency requirements of the JCAHO and other regulatory agencies. The frequency of offering competency programs varies. Competency programs are implemented at different time intervals depending on the nature of the work area. Some medical-surgical skills may be demonstrated on a yearly basis while critical care areas may require competency assessment and demonstration more frequently. The decision on frequency depends on hospital policies, quality data that are being collected that highlight a problem area, and outside regulatory agencies. New equipment and changes in policies and procedures often dictate the initiation of a competency assessment and demonstration on skills.

Each staff member is expected to attend competency programs. Scheduling staff to attend programs, however, can be challenging. Competency programs should be repeated, programs with skills lab should be provided around the clock throughout a week or more, and make-up sessions should be offered. When there is limited staff, nurses can attend programs on their day off, but should be paid for their time. Staff must complete identified competencies to receive merit raises, a reason why the nurse educator communicates with the nurse manager on the status of staff completing the designated competencies. If necessary, staff can be denied opportunity to work until the competency is completed, although this rarely occurs.

Competencies

There are several ways to determine the skills required for competency. First, the educator should consider what skills are necessary for providing safe patient care in a clinical area, particularly when there is a change in the patient population or new technology. Second, the educator should identify high-risk and low-frequency procedures or techniques such as medical procedures in an area devoted to care of patients with psychiatric problems. Procedures that are done infrequently require that competency evaluation be held more often. Third, practice guidelines from professional organizations and requirements of accrediting bodies such as the JCAHO suggest skills to be evaluated for competency. Lastly, the educator should ask for staff input, review changes in policies and procedures within the organization, and identify problem areas on a unit and in a setting as other strategies for identifying skills for competency programs.

Skill Level of Staff

Competency is defined by JCAHO (2002) as an evaluation of a person's ability to perform. This implies that the scope of services offered by a facility, in a specific area of practice, and the job title of staff should be included when planning programs. The clinical experience of a person may or may not be adequate for practice in the setting. For example, when a new graduate nurse is hired as a staff member in an emergency department, an extended orientation plan is needed, as compared with a nurse with considerable clinical experiences in other areas of nursing practice including the emergency room.

Evaluation and Documentation

Having yearly performance appraisals that relate to the competency-based job description is a critical component of a competency program. For annual competencies and those required more often, it is helpful to use standard forms for evaluation and documentation. Table 17.4 provides an example of a competency evaluation form.

Methods for validating and documenting staff competency include:

- Posttest following a class, after viewing a videotape, or after an educational program
- Demonstration of skills, for example, at skills stations or on the unit

TABLE 17.4   Example of a Competency Evaluation—IV Pump

IV Pump

RN

Name: _____

Objectives

List the desired objectives of the check-off.

The participant will be able to:

- Load and unload the tubing set into the IV infusion pump.
- Program a medication infusion (250 cc bag at 10cc/hr)

Use information contained in the operator's manual and quick reference guides.

Demonstration Criteria—all criteria must be met

Pump Selection

- Verbalizes criteria used for selecting type of pump to use
- Heparin/Insulin continuous infusion = Single Channel Pump

Tubing Sets

- Identifies tubing sets for type of infusion being started

Battery Operation

- Verbalizes when pump should be plugged in
- Plugged in at all times except during transport
- Locates indicator on panel that verifies that pump is plugged in.
- Locates Battery Charge indicator on panel display.

Modes of Functioning

- Identifies different modes of the pump
- Demonstrates changing mode setting

    - At start up
    - After pump has been in use (turning pump off/on)

TABLE 17.4 *(continued)*

Loading the Tubing Set

- Demonstrate correctly loading the primary tubing set into pump

Programming an Infusion

- Demonstrate entering an infusion for which there is an order
- Start the infusion and verify that it is infusing as programmed
- Demonstrate how to change the rate and volume to be infused for infusion

Alarms and Alerts

- Locate and identify status indicator lights
- Identify, silence, and correct alarms
- Demonstrate how to adjust volume of alarms

Miscellaneous Pump Features

- Identify and demonstrate special features

Unloading Tubing Sets

- Demonstrate removing the tubing set from pump
- Verbalize failure situations when tubing would have to be removed to instill fluids

All components as designated above have been met to demonstrate competency.

(RN Evaluator Signature)

Date

- Peer review of the competency using identified criteria
- Direct observation of practice using procedural guideline
- Case study/discussion group—after reading a vignette, staff can be asked to discuss problems, possible approaches, and what they would do
- Exemplars—after being informed of a competency, for example, providing a safe environment for a patient after surgery, staff can

be asked to identify and discuss interventions they would implement.

- Presentations by staff highlighting the nurse's competency
- Quality monitor review, using standardized tools, to confirm the absence or frequency of a problem (Tracy & Summers, 2001).

STAFF DEVELOPMENT

Programs that are directed at further developing the staff's competencies strengthen an organization's ability to recruit and retain staff. Recruitment efforts are enhanced when potential employees notice the creative efforts undertaken by staff working in the organization. Staff who continue to grow professionally will be inspired to seek job advancement opportunities within and outside the organization and have high job satisfaction, which is a major contributor to retention.

Similar to orientation and competency programs, staff development programs are resource intense. However, if nurses provide quality patient care and continue to build their skills, this helps retention, thereby allowing resources to be diverted from orientation to staff development. Through staff development programs, nurses can move into leadership roles, also contributing to retention. The culture and resources of the organization influence unit staffing, which is the foundation on which all programs, orientation, competency, and staff development, are built. Whether nurses are given access to resources and are able to participate in programs to enhance their skills depends on the culture of the organization.

Staffs are encouraged to pursue professional development by attending continuing education (CEU) programs, participating in online learning, and completing other activities to improve knowledge and skills. Attending CEU programs provides the staff with a chance to network with RNs from other institutions. By networking, nurses can learn about trends in the delivery of patient care in settings other than their own. Organizations vary in their method of providing staff the opportunity to attend conferences outside of their institutions. For example, an organization may offer financial support through scholarships.

Opportunities also can be provided for nurses to develop their management and leadership skills such as serving as a charge nurse, becoming a preceptor for new staff or nursing students, and chairing committees. The nurse educator can serve as a cochair on a unit committee with a staff. By doing this, staff can learn the processes for conducting effective meetings, developing and accomplishing agendas during meetings, and communicating with committee members. Membership in a department committee permits the staff to gain a perspective of the organization beyond one's unit.

Aside from leadership skills, opportunities for staff to develop skills as an educator can be offered, for example, by teaching a program with guidance from an experienced educator. By participating in planning, implementing, and evaluating an educational program, the staff learn the intricacies of teaching others and gain knowledge and skills that can be applied to patient and staff education in the future. As part of their development in the area of education, staff are encouraged to pursue continuing education, specialty certification, and higher education.

SUMMARY

The nurse educator has a vital role in preparing staff to provide safe and up-to-date patient care. This role is most visible in activities related to orientation, competency, and staff development programs. These programs are not provided in isolation but are best accomplished through collaboration with colleagues within and outside the organization. Along with changes in health care systems is the need to continually search for different and more effective ways to *accomplish vital programs.*

ACKNOWLEDGMENT

The authors thank Rebecca Sanford, RN, MS, for contacting several hospitals to survey their practices on orientation, competency, and staff development programs.

REFERENCES

Abruzzese, R. S., & Quinn-O'Neil, B. (1996). Orientation for general and specialty areas. In R.S. Abruzzese (Ed.), *Nursing staff development: Strategies for success* (2nd ed.) (pp. 259–280). St. Louis: Mosby.

Anthony, M. K., & Preuss, G. (2002). Models of care: The influence of nurse communication on patient safety. *Nursing Economics, 20*, 209–214, 248.

Biancuzzo, M. (1994). Staff nurse preceptors: A program they "own." *Clinical Nurse Specialist, 8*, 97–102.

Boylan, C. R., & Westra, R. (1998). Meeting joint commission requirements for staff nurse competency. *Journal of Nursing Care Quality, 12*(4), 44–48.

Buerhaus, P. I., Needleman, J., Mattke, S., & Stewart, M. (2002). Strengthening hospital nursing. *Health Affairs, 21*, 123–132.

Czerwinski, S., Blastic, L., & Rice, B. (1999). The synergy model: Building a clinical advancement program. *Critical Care Nurse, 19*(4), 72–77.

Del Bueno, D., & Buyer, D. J. (2001). Beware: The cost of competence. *Nursing Economics, 19*, 247–257.

De Onna, J. (2002). DACUM: A versatile competency-based framework for staff development. *Journal for Nurses in Staff Development, 18*, 5–11.

Fahje, C. J., McMyler, E., & Mateo, M. A. (2001). When new employee orientation doesn't go as planned: "It is time for plan B . . . but, what is plan B?" *Journal for Nurses in Staff Development, 17*, 137–143.

Galt, R. G. (2000). The value of training and orientation programs in large medical organizations. *Journal for Nurses in Staff Development, 16*, 151–156.

GE Medical Systems (2003). *TiP-TV Programming and Sponsorship Opportunities: How you can Benefit from Partnering with GE TiP-TV.* Retrieved February 24, 2003, from http://www.gemedicalsystems.com/education/tv/benefit.html

HealthStream (2003). HealthStream Home Page. Retrieved February 24, 2003, from http://healthstream.com/hco/acute/index.html

Institute of Medicine (2000). *To Err is Human. Building a Safer Health System.* National Academy Press. Retrieved February 24, 2003, from http://www.nap.edu/catalog/9728.html

Joint Commission on Accreditation of Healthcare Organizations (JCAHO) (2002). *Hospital accreditation standards: Accreditation policies standards intent statement* (pp. 235–237). Oakbrook Terrace, IL: JCAHO.

Miller, E., Flynn, J. M., & Umada, J. (1998). Assessing, developing, and maintaining staff's competency in times of restructuring. *Journal of Nursing Care Quality, 12*(6), 9–17.

Tracy, J. S., & Summers, B. G. (2001). *Competency assessment: A practical guide to the JCAHO standards.* Marblehead, MA: Opus Communications.

Chapter 18

Preparing New Faculty for Teaching: Caring Coach with a Vision

Janet Hoey Robinson

As Americans face a severe nursing shortage, new faculty are needed in schools of nursing. Popular media have pointed to nurse educators to increase the workforce supply as one solution to this multifaceted problem. Nursing educational institutions need visionary, pragmatic leaders to transform the work culture for faculty to prepare the number of nurses needed to meet society's demand.

The ability of nursing programs to increase the numbers of graduates is compounded by a critical nurse faculty shortage. Faculty shortages affect enrollments in nursing programs. The American Association of Colleges of Nursing (AACN) Annual Report (2001) indicated that 5,823 qualified applicants were turned away from nursing programs in the United Stated in the 2000–2001 academic year due to insufficient numbers of faculty, clinical sites, classroom space, and clinical preceptors, and because of budget constraints. Thirty-eight percent of responding schools cited the faculty shortage as a reason for not accepting qualified applicants in baccalaureate programs. Of these, 44.7% reported that their inability to recruit qualified applicants was due to competition with clinical agencies (AACN, 2001). Higher compensation in clinical settings and as researchers and consultants attracts nurse educators from academic settings. Another reason given for faculty shortages was budget constraints that limited the hiring of new faculty (83%). Strategies to attract nurse educators must include economic incentives or the shortage will worsen.

The nurse faculty shortage will increase as more educators retire in the next ten years. The median age of nursing faculty is 51 years (AACN, 2001). Only about 50% of nurse faculty have doctorates; of those with doctorates, the average age of professors is 55.9, associate professors 53.2, and assistant professors 50. The National League for Nursing (2002) reported in a study of 491 institutions in sixteen southern states and the District of Columbia that there were 425 unfilled faculty positions. Kimball and O'Neil (2002) reviewed 16 selected national reports, white papers, and issue briefs written in 2000 and 2001, to analyze the nurse shortage for the Robert Wood Johnson Foundation and found the current nursing shortage has a different nature than previous ones and requires different solutions. One of the strategic efforts they recommended was "reinventing nursing education and work environments to address the needs and values of—and to appeal to—a new generation of nurses" (White, 2002, p. 311). Nursing schools need aggressive recruitment plans, multifaceted orientation programs and caring leaders to direct, mentor, and develop nurse educators of the future.

The purpose of this chapter is to describe the role of the academic leader in preparing new faculty for teaching. The term "academic leader" refers to department chairs, program directors, deans, assistant or associate deans, and other nurse administrators responsible for faculty orientation and development. The definition of faculty used in this chapter includes teachers in all levels of nursing programs.

This chapter focuses on how academic leaders can create solutions to problems reported in the literature. Most academic leader position descriptions include responsibilities for recruiting, orienting, guiding and evaluating new faculty. Michaelangelo looked at pieces of marble and saw masterpieces in them. Academic leaders must look at new faculty in the same way.

ACADEMIC LEADERS ARE KEY TO SUCCESS

The academic leader is the key to successful faculty development; he/she needs to be *a caring coach with a vision*. Coaches are defined as "trainers" and "tutors" that prepare individuals and groups ready for events (American Heritage Dictionary, 1997).

The needs of new faculty can be met by an effective coaching leader. The academic leader's power emerges from an ability to shape the culture in which the academic leader and faculty work (Hecht, Higgerson, Gmelch, & Tucker, 1999). Academic leaders are key to changing work culture. The work culture needs to espouse values conducive to student learning and teaching competence. Academic leaders need to care passionately about how students learn and how faculty can learn to teach effectively. Developing new faculty individually and facilitating their integration into the group as a whole is key in building healthy productive work environments.

Brandt (1994) combined insights from care theory and leadership theory in describing individuals who could transform the work environment in practice. The same caring leadership philosophy can be applied to nursing education. Caring leaders can educate, motivate, encourage and work with faculty to promote a quality education for students and job satisfaction for faculty. Valuing and empowering nurse educators fosters their autonomy and creativity. Caring leaders recognize the difference between excellence and perfection, and understand the importance of personal integrity. Academic leaders can expect the best effort of new faculty but also should be prepared for novice mistakes. Coach Krzyzewski, a legendary Duke University basketball coach, said, "Hunger not for success, but for excellence. And don't let anyone else define excellence for you" (Krzyzewski, 2000, p. 220). Caring leaders as coaches are needed to introduce new faculty to academe.

Academic leaders can change work environments to improve feelings of connectedness. Boice (2000) spent 25 years studying qualitatively the experiences of new faculty in academia and found that being new was associated with pervasive feeling of loneliness. Misunderstanding effective ways to work and socialize was associated with failure and misery. New faculty did not feel supported when they were new.

NEEDS OF NEW FACULTY

New faculty need advice and instruction on their new role. They need to be prepared for the academic milieu and coached on the rules of play in the institution. Novice faculty often do not understand the expectations of academia and need help in setting priorities and creating a path for success. Along the same line, experienced faculty who transfer to new institutions need assistance in understanding and succeeding in their new environments.

The needs of new faculty depend on their background and current teaching assignment. Many new faculty arrive at nursing schools and staff development positions without any previous teaching experience and without any formal educational preparation for a teaching role. They are most often advanced practice nurses, expert clinicians who seek a career change. These new faculty are often unprepared for the expectations of students, colleagues, administration, and clinical agencies.

Siler and Kleiner (2001) completed a phenomenological study on the experience of novice and experienced faculty in the first year in a new faculty position and found four themes in novice faculty's experience: expectations, learning the game, being mentored, and fitting in. Novice faculty did not feel prepared for their role and were not socialized for the requirements of academia. They found the work culture unfamiliar and incongruent with what they expected from their former student perspective. Workload was heavier than novices imagined and assuming primary course responsibility was most challenging. After receiving initial help with the syllabus and test preparation (the tasks of teaching), novice faculty had trouble finding answers to their questions. In this new role, novice faculty were concerned about how effective they were as teachers and were less focused on the scholarship and service parts of their job. "Previous experience in nursing did not, and could not, prepare them for their first year as faculty" (Siler & Kleiner, 2001, p. 401).

ACADEMIC LEADERS ARE UNIQUE COACHES

Conceptualizing academic leaders as coaches is a strategy to foster better role transition for new faculty. Academic leaders who make teaching assignments, and orient and evaluate new faculty are in a unique position to foster role development. The author has been an academic leader for the last 9 years as an associate director of curriculum and instruction, a department chair, and an associate dean of a graduate program. She, like the participants in Boice's (2000) and Siler and Kleiner's (2001) studies, experienced loneliness and frustration and longed for effective mentoring as a new faculty at several institutions.

The author developed and uses a "caring coach with a vision" philosophy and leadership style to foster the development of new faculty in their teaching role. She believes academic leaders play a significant coaching role in helping new faculty in several areas:

- welcoming the team
- socialization/becoming a team player
- focusing on the drills and skills
- offensive play
- defensive play
- integrity of the teaching sport

WELCOMING THE TEAM

Great coaches demand hard work from their players; they expect them to be contributing members of the team. Shula, the Miami Dolphins legendary football coach said coaching is a matter of motivating people to work hard and to prepare to play as a team (Shula & Blanchard, 1995). Becoming a member of the team starts with recruitment and orientation and being welcomed on the team.

Recruitment

Recruiting and hiring the right mix of faculty is critical to leadership. The academic leader needs to know and understand current faculty to know what kind of person is needed in the department. Initiating trust with new faculty starts with recruitment and hiring. An example of early trust happened between a department chair and prospective candidate who had multiple contacts with each another. The faculty group suggested that the candidate be invited to campus before a funded position was available. While the academic leader extended an invitation on behalf of the group, she let the prospective candidate know that it might not be in the person's best interest, in terms of her time, to come before a position was budgeted. The academic leader promised to contact the candidate as soon as the position was officially available. This candidate was contacted the day the position was announced and eventually was hired. Part of the reason the candidate said she accepted the position was the honesty she felt in communicating with the department chair at the time of the first contact.

Orientation

The faculty group must plan and activate collective responsibility for various kinds of orientation a new faculty member needs. It really does "take a village to raise a child." The academic leader must oversee the process but find ways for all faculty and staff to participate; everyone needs to be vested in the new faculty's success. One department chair enlisted five people to help with this process for a new faculty. An experienced faculty was assigned as the orientation mentor, the course leader assisted with the didactic orientation, two faculty were in charge of clinical site orientations, and one was assigned to help with documenting teaching effectiveness and developing a teaching portfolio.

The academic leader has a responsibility to create an environment where new faculty can feel part of a team. One index of the health of a group is its ability to take in a new member. Academic leaders must have aggregate assessment skills and communicate their findings with the group and, especially, with new faculty. Faculty as a group must be part of recruiting candidates into the institution and must be part of the decision making process to hire new educators. When faculty have a vested interest in bringing people on the team, they are more ready to welcome new members and create an environment for success.

SOCIALIZATION/BECOMING A TEAM PLAYER

Being valued as a team player is as integral to a nurse educator's success as it is to a professional or college athlete. Academic leaders need to monitor how new faculty become members of the team or are socialized. Siler and Kleiner (2001) found novice faculty were not socialized for the requirements of academia. Novices need to be socialized, taken out to lunch and accompanied to social functions where presence is important.

Socialization is key to success on many levels. New faculty need an opportunity to interact with experienced faculty. Interactions can be as simple as reacting to a campus event or planned discussions such as grading a particular test. The author routinely meets with new faculty for lunch two times each semester during their first year. This leader also makes sure other groups are meeting routinely with the novice faculty. Attempts to make new faculty comfortable at campus-wide events include accompanying them and indicating if any specific dress is needed at an event. One new faculty described her personal horror at arriving at a holiday party in professional work attire only to be greeted by her colleagues in cocktail attire. These embarrassing moments should not occur. New faculty need to learn team values and the importance of forming alliances and the unwritten rules of play.

Team Values

Institutions subscribe to unique value sets, but all educational cultures value "hard work," "presence," and "team spirit." Discussions of these values, including the mission of the institution, should take place in recruiting conversations, job interviews, and orientation sessions. A faux pas often made by new faculty is to comment that the academic atmosphere is relaxed compared to clinical practice. If experienced faculty perceive that the new faculty's teaching assignment is not as challenging as clinical practice, they might try to show that person how "tough" teaching can be. Preparation for teaching in the classroom and clinical setting is an all-encompassing responsibility that involves a lot of hard work. Being socialized into academia also involves hard work.

Teams value the balance of varied talent and experience. Coaches know one of their critical skills is balancing the right numbers of people playing. Academic leaders can help new players assess where the institution is going and where they fit in the group. Sometimes this means a new player has to "sit on the bench" and watch someone else move the ball. The role of the coach in helping new faculty become part of the team is to point out the team plan and where various members fit into the overall plan. New players may be as good as seasoned ones, but may have to wait until their turn to play comes up. An academic leader needs to point out the importance of new members handing over the ball over to the "lead scorers" in the beginning.

Forming Alliances

The importance of understanding the system is often underestimated. Forming alliances with colleagues is important. It also is wise to befriend administrative and secretarial staff whose collective wisdom about the operational level of systems facilitates pragmatic practice. They can make suggestions for consultation, and they often know who will be helpful and who will put up barriers. The academic leader can point out who are the significant people in the institution for new faculty to get to know. The academic leader can suggest a list of people and groups who are important to know for a new faculty member and identify them with a priority plan.

Forming alliances also will help the new person understand the unwritten rules of play. The academic leader, faculty, and staff must attempt to identify and communicate unwritten rules for new faculty. For example, attending fall convocation might be advertised as an invitation to new faculty in an institution in which attendance is actually mandatory. All cultures have unwritten rules; identifying and articulating them is an important part of preparing new faculty for their role.

FOCUS ON DRILLS AND SKILLS

Coaches spend a great deal of time running their players through the basic moves needed for team play. Coaches expect players to be at every practice, follow the rules, and go through the drills. Coaches assume responsibility for assessing what each player knows and for teaching individuals what they need to know for success. Novice nurse educators, like new players, need help with the basics, for example, how to write a learning objective, develop a syllabus, prepare and deliver a lecture, prepare media for presentation, write test questions, evaluate students' clinical performance, and develop Web-enhanced courses.

Developing Competencies

In addition to assisting new faculty in developing skills for teaching, the academic leader's goal is to identify their strengths and limitations, and support the novice in developing competencies for teaching. The "new kid on the block" is often too vulnerable to ask for help. Academic leaders know who has taught courses before and planned similar educational experiences for students and can help negotiate assistance for the new faculty without causing a loss in self-confidence.

The academic leader can create ease in describing what is not known. For example, one can say, "None of us likes starting from scratch; these lecture notes may not be what you'll want to use, but at least they give you an idea of what someone else did." The academic leader models trust and helps create a partnership where honest communication is evident. The academic leader uses coaching skills in getting the more experienced team members to mentor novice teachers.

Academic leaders can motivate faculty to teach effectively by helping them accept that pedagogy is an area in which all faculty can help one another (Lucas, 1994). For example, a department chair facilitated a planned discussion with faculty on creative approaches to classroom teaching with the Internet. Three faculty volunteered to share their experiences, and the department chair quietly invited a fourth member who was the newest in the group to be part of the panel. The supportive interactions that occurred during this panel discussion heightened feelings of camaraderie by all and helped the novice faculty feel part of the team.

Importance of Feedback

Coaches also need to validate skill level and give new faculty feedback on their development as teachers. This process may include clinical and classroom visitation. Validating teaching skills is different from summative evaluation. Academic leaders should observe new faculty at their best, at a time and place selected by the faculty. Asking for an invitation to a class with content that a person enjoys teaching and has effectively developed for presentation is a better choice than showing up at a time more convenient to the academic leader's schedule. The goals of any visit are observation, skill validation, and the opportunity to give positive feedback in teaching effectiveness so the faculty feels competent in the role and knows how to improve performance.

OFFENSIVE PLAY

Coaches are best in directing offensive play. While many say that it does not matter if you win or lose, it is how you play the game, all sports enthusiasts know winning is more fun. Offensive play is about winning. Success in any game is about scoring points and establishing a winning record. Scoring points in academia relates to facilitating student

:arning. Teaching a class on a new topic, writing appropriate test questions, and having students score well on the examination are examples of measurable student learning. Academic leaders need to oversee this process to ensure the integrity of the curriculum in the institution.

New faculty want to be perceived as effective teachers by students, colleagues, and administrators. Teaching assignments need to be based on faculty skill sets as well as institutional needs. Where possible, new faculty can work with experienced faculty to facilitate role transition and learn the effective ways of fostering student learning and performance.

Positive Student Evaluations

Faculty who get high student evaluations on their teaching effectiveness "score points" and experience success. Students measure the worth of faculty by their knowledge of content, presentation skills, clinical practice abilities, their availability, and how they grade students. New faculty need to be knowledgeable about the content they are teaching and skilled in presenting it to students. Students want faculty who are organized and present content clearly, not teachers who present confusing information and are unsure of the content. In clinical practice, teachers who exhibit competence are rated higher than those who appear more tentative and lacking in clinical skills. Faculty who are available and foster student interaction are often evaluated higher than those who are difficult to contact and not available in the clinical setting. Students who perceive grading is fair also rate faculty higher on evaluations. Nursing students have many needs in their own learning process and look for faculty mentors to lean on. Academic leaders can encourage new faculty to develop the competencies that students use to measure the worth of their teachers and assume the role of a caring educator who provides the support needed by students.

One of the areas in which new faculty need assistance is how to encourage student learning and performance in a way that will result in positive student evaluations. From the author's perspective, new faculty are often evaluated negatively by students if they seem too tentative, are either too tough or too lenient, and rigid or disorganized. The academic leader can advise new faculty about the importance of timing in evaluation, for example, not asking students for feedback on the last day of class (they are too tired) or the day of an exam (they are too stressed). Courses in which feedback is sought throughout the semester provide valuable information for teachers to improve their performance and identify where students are learning and not learning. Listening and responding to concerns of students throughout a course prevents negative evaluations at the end. An academic leader can teach new faculty the art of requesting useful, evaluative feedback from students.

Positive Peer Evaluations

Colleagues evaluate peers as contributing team players by their ability to master the teaching drills and skills. Most institutions have formal peer evaluation processes in place. Colleges and universities with tenure and promotion policies have a peer review process that is often threatening for a novice educator. The academic leader needs to carefully explain this process to novices.

In institutions with peer visitations, it is helpful if the academic leader can be present when peer feedback is sought. Peer evaluators may need reminding that giving positive feedback is more effective than negative, and the goal is to promote faculty development. New faculty may need help interpreting constructive criticism; letting novices know that certain faculty are "harder to please" may help them better understand the process. The author saved an early negative peer evaluation of herself to share with new faculty to let them know being initiated into a new group and a new role is often problematic. Though the focus of this chapter is on the teaching role, peer evaluation may include assessment of service, clinical practice, and scholarship components of the faculty role, which are often less understood by the new educator.

Positive Evaluations by Academic Leader

Summative evaluations of new faculty are completed by the academic leader at periodic intervals. Written evaluations are part of an individual's permanent file and may be the basis for tenure and promotion decisions, contract renewal, and merit raises. It is important for new faculty to articulate and write attainable goals early in the first year of employment. The academic leader is expected to provide tips in writing goals with reasonable outcomes. The leader needs to foster new faculty success while protecting the integrity of the institution's goals.

Depending on the academic setting, criteria based on rank must be met in teaching, service, scholarship, and in some settings clinical practice. Often, novice faculty set the highest priority on teaching effectiveness and put less effort into service and scholarship goals. Depending on the institution, this may be acceptable. If new faculty also are evaluated on service and scholarship, they need to find ways to meet minimal expectations in those areas. Like a coach making sure a new player "gets the ball" some of the time in the game, new faculty need to be given opportunity to meet service goals with appropriate committee assignments. Academic leaders can make sure individuals are on a committee that will introduce them to some of the workings of the institution while not exploiting their naive position. Leaders also can suggest areas for novice involvement in scholarly activity within the institution or community.

Developing a Professional Portfolio

Getting the ball, scoring points, and establishing a winning record are necessary offensive plays that new faculty must learn to be successful in their educator role. One of the most important skills the academic leader can teach a novice faculty person is how to establish and document his or her own winning record. Developing professional portfolios is an art and not one usually developed in clinical practice. Providing examples of good models is an effective strategy as are frequent focused meetings throughout the year to monitor progress. Faculty also demonstrate success in offensive play with positive student, peer, and administrative evaluations and with evidence of aggregate learning taking place in the courses they teach.

DEFENSIVE PLAY

Coaches know defensive play is as critical to success as offensive play. In academia, defensive play protects the individual from attack and puts the team (faculty) in a position to score offensively. Three defensive skills that all faculty need to understand are how to protect their reputation, the importance of squelching rumors early, and picking one's battles.

Protecting One's Reputation

Academic leaders are in an optimal position to help new faculty protect their initial reputations at institutions. Reputation is an important commodity for new faculty; when it is attacked, self-esteem and feelings of competency are challenged. Leaders are in a position of knowing the personality of groups and can warn a new person of possible conflicts. For example, if students are used to getting handouts with every lecture and a novice faculty lecturing for the first time did not prepare handouts, he or she can be "attacked" by the students in a matter of minutes. It is the coach's responsibility to make the "unwritten institutional practices" known to new faculty.

Nursing applauds assertive behaviors in students until they are directed at faculty as facilitators of learning. Students are consumers of learning. They expect a lot of faculty and compare novices with experienced teachers, quick to point out their deficiencies. Academic leaders need to help new faculty develop assessment skills in "reading the crowd" so they are prepared for defensive play. Classroom groups are poised and ready for attack on a myriad of items. New faculty need to learn to balance what students want with what they believe students need. Academic leaders need to keep lines of communication open with new faculty and encourage dialogue about new faculty's perceptions of their reputation from students.

Squelching Rumors

Squelching rumors early is another defensive play. An example of the importance of this play occurred when a new faculty member told a student group that there would be a grade penalty, a loss of 2 points a day for a maximum of 20 points, for assignments turned in late. By the time the news was shared across student groups, the students reported they would lose 20 points a day for any late assignments and decided to petition the administration for too strict a penalty. The academic leader met with the new faculty member and encouraged a broadcast e-mail to the class to clarify the course policy. It also was an opportune time to discuss the importance of written communication when grading was concerned and to discuss the need to specify all grading policies in the course syllabus to avoided this type of response in the future.

Picking One's Battles

Picking one's battles is another critical skill for novice faculty. Entering a new environment is threatening for a professional who is used to being competent in a former role or in a similar role at another institution. The academic leader can help new faculty with acculturation. It is easy for new faculty to compare cultures with a former place where one experienced competence and success; often the comparison is not complementary to the new place. Voicing less than optimal judgments, however, breeds opposition. Academic leaders can help new faculty chose carefully what they are going to object to by giving suggestions about whether an issue is worth confrontation. Confrontation and strong opposition need to be done in context and with a clear perspective of the work culture. Academic leaders have an obligation to not let a new person set him or herself up in a known volatile area.

INTEGRITY OF THE TEACHING SPORT

Coaches have an ethical responsibility to make sure the game play is fair. Fairness is important in grading issues and in dealing with critical judgement of others. New faculty need guidance about how to grade and then how to defend their actions. Coaches need to teach players to define what is acceptable and unacceptable play and how to deal with referee calls. The integrity of the sport depends on the critical judgment of others who are not part of the team. In academic settings, these other judges or referees include high level administrative leaders and accrediting agencies.

Grading

Grading student work is one of the most challenging parts of the teaching role. Societal expectations for high grades has put pressure on students and faculty. Students challenge faculty routinely on the validity of test items and their grades. Novice faculty are particularly vulnerable to student challenges about grades. Academic leaders need to orient new faculty to developing appropriate test items, item analysis software programs, and how to use the results of tests. Ideally, experienced faculty can model the art of dealing with students after examination grades have been posted.

A good example of role modeling occurred when a senior faculty member and new teacher were questioned by several students about items on a test. The senior member suggested that the novice teacher tell the students that she would keep their written notes about the items and if the question they contested made an overall difference in their course grade at the end of the semester, she would give them the benefit of the point. This quieted the students and helped the novice faculty's reputation as a listening and fair teacher. Academic leaders can work with new faculty to discuss specific issues associated with grading such as reliability of testing, how to determine course grades, how to deal with late assignments, and what to do with tests when students are absent because of illnesses and similar events.

Deciding that a student did not meet the course or clinical objectives, and must repeat the course or leave the nursing program, is one of the most serious decisions a faculty can make. The threat of violence is real as was evidenced by the loss of three faculty lives at the University of Arizona in the Fall of 2002 (Boychuk-Spears, 2002). Yet, the public depends on educators as gatekeepers for safe nursing practice. Novice faculty may have a difficult time judging clinical competence and rating performance because they have not seen as many learners in the same situation. In a litigious society, it takes courage to issue a failing grade. New faculty need a coach in this situation and colleagues with whom to share their decision-making process. Clinical papers can be read and graded by colleagues for inter-rater reliability. Documentation is key to clinical grading, and academic leaders are in a great position to teach new faculty and mentor them on how to document and judge clinical performance.

Outside Judges

Coaches get individuals to play the game, but referees make the decisions about who scored and what points counted. All teams are accountable for judgments by others; some calls are tough to live with, but acceptance is part of the game. In nursing education, integrity is an essential element in all parts of the teaching-learning process. Referees assess penalties and watch for illegal play. The institution's high-level administrative leaders and outside accrediting agencies are academic referees.

High-level demonstrative leaders make decisions on contracts, workload, merit increases, and course and office assignments. Some decisions make sense and others are difficult to understand. Some decisions involve a peer process with input into the decision making while others do not. New faculty often do not understand why things happen. Academic leaders are hired by high-level administration to carry out the mission of the institution; in effect, they are university or college cheerleaders.

The academic leader may experience conflict between institutional goals and individual new faculty goals. For example, when there is a freeze on hiring for new positions, the academic leader may have to ask a new faculty to take on added responsibility. The decision to freeze hiring is out of the coach's power to control; this situation is akin to the conflict between coaches and referees in the sports arena. The coach can argue, scream, and yell but risks having a technical foul called on his or her team. If the coach does not protest the decision, faculty may assume the coach agrees with the call. The team ultimately has to follow the referee's call. Helping new players deal with perceived unfair calls is an art that can be fostered by caring coaches.

Nurse educators are expected to implement programs that meet accreditation standards and produce safe graduates who will provide competent, ethical nursing care to society. Getting ready for an accreditation and being able to speak to standards is an anxiety-producing experience for new faculty who are still learning about the institution and their faculty role. Academic leaders need to spend time orienting new faculty to this process and help them feel comfortable in their role. New faculty need to be coached and prepared for others questioning their judgment; they need to pay attention to the outside referees and be willing to live with their decisions.

CONCLUSIONS

Administrators are hired to provide creative leadership and vision. Conceptualizing one's role as a coach who prepares players for a winning

season is a unique way to operationalize one's vision for nursing education. Academic coaches can mentor faculty by recruiting, orienting, and
socializing new members on the team. Academic coaches can facilitate
new faculty becoming team players and can help them focus on the
drills and skills of teaching. They can help new faculty keep the fans
happy by directing their offensive and defensive play while protecting
the integrity of the teaching sport. Fostering success in new faculty will
increase retention, draw other qualified experts into nursing education,
and increase the number of new practitioners for society.

REFERENCES

American Association of Colleges of Nursing. (2001). *AACN Annual Report: Annual
State of the Schools.* Washington, DC: Author.
American Heritage Dictionary (3rd ed.) (1997). Boston: Houghton Mifflin Company.
Boice, R. (2000). *Advice for new faculty members.* Boston: Nihil Minimus Allyn
and Bacon.
Boychuk-Spears, T. (2002). Threats on campus: Need for faculty response. *Journal
of Psychosocial Nursing, 40*(12), 20–22.
Brandt, M. A. (1994). Caring leadership: Secret and path to success. *Nursing Manage-
ment, 25*(8), 68–72.
Hecht, I., Higgerson, M. L., Gmelch, W. H., & Tucker, A. (1999). *The department
chair as academic leader.* Phoenix: Oryx Press.
Kimball, B., & O'Neil, E. (2002). *Health care's human crisis: The American nursing
shortage.* Robert Wood Johnson Foundation, San Francisco: Health Workforce
Solutions. Retrieved November 6, 2002, from http:/www.rwjf.org
Krzyzewski, M. (2002). *Leading with the heart: Coach K's successful strategies for
basketball, business and life.* New York: Warner Books.
Lucas, A. (1994). *Strengthening departmental leadership: A team-building guide for
chairs in colleges and universities.* San Francisco: Jossey-Bass.
National League for Nursing. (2002). *The nursing faculty shortage: National League
for Nursing Perspective.* Presentation to the National Advisory Council on Nurse
Education and Practice. April 11, 2002. Retrieved December 16, 2002, from
http:www.nln.org/slides/speech/htm
Shula, D., & Blanchard, K. (1995). *Everyone's a coach: You can inspire anyone to be
a winner.* New York: Harper Business.
Siler, B., & Kleiner, C. (2001). Novice faculty: Encountering expectations in acade-
mia. *Journal of Nursing Education, 4,* 397–403.
White, K. M. (2002). Health care's human crisis: The American nursing shortage.
Policy, Politics & Nursing Practice, 3, 309–312.

Chapter 19

Using the Holistic Paradigm in Teaching

Bonnie W. Duldt-Battey

The primary role of teachers is to coach winners. In this chapter winners are defined as well-informed individuals who know where they are going, who are capable of critical thinking to determine how to get there, and who are persuasive in convincing followers of the worthiness of the goal. To coach winners, teachers need to view students as *holistic beings*, who are aware of their own *life mission*, and who *communicate persuasively*. No matter what content is being taught, these three factors are the core of teaching to influence the professional nursing culture (Meehan-Hurwitz, 2002) and to effectively prepare our nursing students for their practice in the 21st century.

Consider how nursing was practiced at the beginning of the 20th century in comparison with practice at mid-century and today. Who among nurse educators in 1900 could have anticipated the knowledge and skills nurses would need? Nurses had to rise to the challenges of the polio, influenza, and tuberculosis epidemics, and the health care advances associated with World War I and II. The development of new areas of practice such as hospice and intensive care nursing also provided challenges. These and many more historical events played a crucial role in changing how nursing was practiced.

Educators today need to be aware of the potential advances in health care practices of the future and prepare our students for meeting the challenges of the 21st century. In doing so, we need to "let go" of the content and focus on the students as holistic beings.

The purpose of this chapter is to describe one approach to applying the holistic paradigm to teaching. Not intended as a final answer, this is offered as an initial guideline for nurse educators. This chapter describes holism as it applies to humanizing communication in the teacher-student relationship, to forming a "spiritual connection" with students, and to encouraging students to think critically and communicate persuasively. Students' evaluative comments are included to document the effectiveness of applying the holistic paradigm to teaching.

STUDENT AS HOLISTIC BEING

With the many practical and pressing details of teaching to which educators must attend, it is sometimes difficult to stay aware of one's own and students' holistic nature. My thesis for this chapter is this: *If* the holistic paradigm can be incorporated into the educator's perspective of students, *then* students will tend to perceive others, including their clients, in a holistic manner. Consequently, there may be a higher probability of providing holistic care to clients. To view students as holistic beings requires an understanding of holism and holistic discord:

> One can appear to be physically "healthy" yet not be "whole." To be "whole" implies completeness, to be undivided, uncut, unbroken, perfect, all in one piece . . . as a harmonious melody, tones in "accord" with one another. In contrast, poor health is like a clash of tones or musical "discord." (Duldt & Pokorny, 1999, pp. 27–28)

Students in touch with their harmonious and whole selves are healthy, energetic, alert, and self-motivated. They anticipate successful completion of the academic work and expect to make significant contributions to society in the future. Educators' interactions with such students are primarily those of mentor or facilitator.

Conversely, students experiencing holistic discord may exhibit anger, resentfulness, guilt, hopelessness, despair, self-doubt, and depression. Such students may be disconnected from their spiritual path, significant relationships, goals and purposes for life, and awareness of bodily signals of distress. Holistic discord is reflected in academic settings by behaviors that include crying, complaining, grieving over losses, just "sticking it out," or withdrawal demonstrated by not participating in class, absences, or tardiness. These students may appear disinterested, bored, lacking in self-confidence, and/or overly distressed.

The educator's role with these students may include that of motivator, comforter, limit setter, and leader. It is challenging to teach a student who is suffering holistic discord. My proposal is this: *If* educators view the student as "spiritually depleted" rather than psychologically resistant, *then* they may intervene creatively at the spiritual level by applying the holistic paradigm to the student's unique situation.

Spiritual Dimension of Holism

The spiritual dimension of holism is common to all humans. The four elements of the spiritual dimension are one's values, meanings, relationships, and goals or life mission (Duldt & Pokorny, 1999, pp. 27–28). Some students may express their spirituality in the practice of an organized religion and faith community. Although religion is an expression of spiritual life, it is not the only way to be spiritual. Students should be encouraged to reflect upon and to define the dimensions of their own spirituality in relation to these four elements.

First, values are the principles the student considers to be the most important in life. Values can emerge out of a faith tradition or a spiritual path, or from living what one considers a principled life. Values include how the student regards the self, the body, and life, as well as how one cares for others, including family, friends, and community. Students formulate professional values related to their potential contribution to nursing.

Second, meanings are the holistic implications of what is happening. How will additional education affect the student's body, mind, and spirit? What will be different in the student's life when she/he has a degree in nursing? What will completing this course or this degree mean in the way the student cares for patients or clients? How will the student's life change?

Third, relationships can begin, be maintained, or end. What is the ultimate relationship in the student's life? Does the student believe in a creator, god, or god(s)? What are the student's relationships with other people? Which relationships are most important? How do relationships change as this educational process proceeds? Who will be supportive, understanding, and helpful, and who will not? Which relationships will change? Which will end? Who cares whether or not the student completes the course or program and obtains a degree in nursing?

Finally, what is the student's goal or mission in life? What is the student called to do? Will this mission in life be achieved? In the given situation, course, or program, what skills and abilities will the student need to achieve potential? What can the student achieve in terms of personal and professional goals? What will the student be doing a year from now, in five years, or in ten years? What does the student need to change to achieve these goals?

As the student progresses through the educational program in nursing, change is not only occurring in the areas of knowledge and skills (body and mind) but also in the student's spiritual dimension. It is helpful for faculty to recognize and honor the transformative changes occurring in students as they move through the educational process. For faculty to support the student's consideration of these ideas, the teacher–student relationship needs to be carefully defined.

TEACHER–STUDENT RELATIONSHIP

Health care professions in general, and nursing as a discipline and profession in particular, are basically humanitarian—that is, concerned with and caring about the well-being of other people. Nursing students gain their first experiences by interacting with teachers, working with clients, and interacting with other health professionals in clinical contexts. Unfortunately, given the increasing stress of clinical practice in this context, students see and sometimes experience dehumanizing communication and interactions. During my years of experience in nursing education, I have known of frustrating, even unpleasant, student-faculty encounters that leave both participants puzzled, offended, and annoyed.

Applying the Humanizing Nursing Communication Theory to the educational context involves interaction patterns that include communing, asserting, confronting, conflicting, and separating (Duldt, 2001a, 2001b). The continuum of attitudes in humanizing and dehumanizing interactions follows:

Humanizing	Dehumanizing
Dialogue	Monologue
Individual	Categories
Holistic	Parts
Choice	Directives
Equality	Degradation
Positive Regard	Disregard
Acceptance	Judgment
Empathy	Tolerance

Authenticity	Role-playing
Caring	"Care-less"
Irreplaceable	Expendable
Intimacy	Isolation
Coping	Helpless
Powerful	Powerless

I have found that communing with one student at a time in each personal interaction increases the incidence of humanizing interaction patterns in my encounters with students (Duldt, 2001a). *Communing* refers to the intimate, two-way or dialogical communication that occurs "between" people who are aware of each other's presence. It is a subjective event that occurs between people, that is, "being there" and "being with." Communing is the element that makes nursing a humanistic interaction. Conversely, if unidirectional or nondialogical communication is used, then it becomes dehumanizing.

Communing consists of a subset of four elements that are the heart of humanistic communication: *trust, self-disclosure, listening,* and *feedback. Trust* is an attitude involving perceptions, feelings, and behavior. It is defined as one person relying on another. This person risks potential loss in attempting to achieve a goal when the outcome is uncertain. In this case, the potential for loss is greater than the potential for gain if trust is violated (Patton & Giffin, 1977, p. 431). Elements of trust include reliability (the student can depend on the educator to do something helpful), expertness (the educator has special skill and/or knowledge relevant to the issue), and dynamism (the educator is open and frank in judgments).

The educator trusts that the student is willing to learn. The student is reliable in completing assignments, has considerable expertise in scholarly study, and is open and frank in consideration of new knowledge.

When students *self-disclose,* they are risking rejection in telling how they feel and think regarding here and now events relevant to the course of studies. Trust is present when students trust the educator enough to disclose something about themselves and their concerns related to learning. This is valuable information for the instructor, and the disclosed facts and/or feelings can become the database necessary for the educator to design individualized teaching strategies and approaches specific to each student.

Listening requires the instructor to give full attention to the student's messages and deliberately try to understand what is being conveyed.

The educator, in a humanizing communication mode, needs to actively listen and provide the student relevant feedback, both facts and feelings. For authentic dialogue to ensue, the student needs to reciprocate in kind.

Feedback involves the educator (a) describing the student's communication patterns (or behaviors) and humanizing or dehumanizing attitudes, and (b) giving one's evaluation or feelings about the topic or issue. The manner in which feedback is given to students is critical to the teacher-student relationship. The student's self-perception is "I see me," and students see themselves as mirrored in the faculty's response: "I see you seeing me." These self-perceptions are the ground out of which a validating communication process can grow. Faculty need to label students as worthy of being heard, thereby validating their self-image. The greater the similarity between the student's self-perception and the educator's perception of the student, the greater the tendency for students to see educators as attractive role models. The more attractive the faculty, the greater the student's desire to become a member of the professional group. This process is a critical for successful recruitment and retention of members for any group or profession.

In summary, trust, self-disclosure, listening, and feedback characterize communing, which is the heart of a humanizing teacher-student relationship. These elements are necessary to the development of a relationship in which students and faculty are validated, respected, understood, and satisfied. When each person holds the other in high regard, humanizing communication behavior occurs to a significant degree. Trust, self-disclosure, and feedback are the tripod on which humanizing communication stands. Listening is in the center because it is the core of communicating; one listens before responding (Duldt, 2001a, 2001b; Hersey & Duldt, 1989).

The teacher–student relationship needs to be in a humanizing mode to explore the spiritual dimension of life. The teacher needs to ask the student to consider how the spiritual dimension is expressed in their lives. The spiritual dimension includes four major elements, that is, the values, meanings, relationships, and goals or mission in life.

LIFE'S MISSION—THE SPIRITUAL CONNECTION

I teach a three-credit graduate course entitled "Ethics in Health Care." This course provides an example of how to connect with the student's spiritual dimension and acknowledge the student's holistic dimension, particularly in regard to their life mission. My role as a faculty member is to present theories and principles of ethics and persuasion in the first few class sessions. Students choose topics from a list of ethical issues for seminar discussions and papers.

The theoretical basis for identifying the student's life mission is Victor Frankl's (1984) book, *Man's Search for Meaning*. Frankl, a psychiatrist, proposed that when a person has a reason for living and a mission to complete, he/she can survive incredible adversities. According to Frankl (1984), meaning is the primary motivational force in human beings (p. 121). Activating whatever has meaning for that student is tapping into the student's spiritual dimension. This is a key component of my role as educator in this course. There may be many ways to do this. The following describes one approach I use.

At the first class, many students do not know each other. Often the instructor will ask the students to introduce themselves. In developing relationships, it is important to focus on one person at a time, getting to know that person well. For this reason, I ask that students interview a person they do not know and present this person to the class. In the interview, individuals are asked to identify their most significant achievement, excluding children and family. After a noisy, ten-minute interlude of interviewing, the presenting begins. As each individual's significant accomplishments are shared with the large group, there are often applause and supportive remarks in recognition of that which has been achieved.

Second, I place the following verse of a *Lutheran Book of Worship* (International Commission of Worship, 1978) hymn on the overhead projector:

> O God, O Lord of Heaven and Earth.
> Your living finger never wrote that life should be an aimless mote,
> A deathward drift from a futile birth.
> Your word meant life triumphant hurled in splendor through Your
>   broken world.
> Since light awoke and life began,
> You made for us a holy plan. (M. Franzmann, 1907–1976)

Acknowledging the multiplicity of religious beliefs, I suggest the variety of terms that can be used for God, such as Jehovah, Allah, Creator, and so on. It has been my observation that most religions propose some reason for human life; even those who do not believe in some version of a Creator seem to have direction to their life. Some of the students have never thought about this, or they have struggled with what they were doing with their life. Others are confident in stating what they expected to accomplish.

Third, I ask the students to assemble themselves in groups of two or more and identify (self-disclosing) their "mission" in life. What does each of them expect to accomplish in life? Another noisy, ten-minute interlude occurs, and the discussions are often more intense. This time, however, I do *not* ask for individuals to reveal their mission. To publicly discuss one's mission is too much pressure for some students, particularly those with little idea of where they are headed. Instead, I use the following questions for discussion:

1. What is the relationship between what you are learning, your practice, and your life's mission?
2. What scholarly skills have you learned?
3. What are the most important principles you have learned?
4. What has changed you the most?
5. What do you still need to know?

Finally, students choose one seminar topic to present either as an individual or in a small group. I suggest they "follow their heart" and choose the topic that is most relevant to their life's mission. Before the end of the class, the students seem to be unusually focused on the assignments. As the instructor, I try to stay out of their way and let them grow.

COMMUNICATE PERSUASIVELY

Winners are people who become or are leaders. As educators, we prepare our students for potential leadership roles in society. Leadership is "the *process of influencing* the activities of an individual or a group in efforts toward goal achievement in a given situation" (Hersey & Duldt, 1989, p. 9). To influence or persuade is to communicate through argument, reasoning, or appeal so that the individual or group is convinced and changed in opinion and/or feelings. This is done in an ethical manner. Leadership is a holistic and humanistic behavior involving critical thinking skills, knowledge, and creativity. Persuasive leadership is democratic in assuming that, when exposed to all sides of an issue, people *can* make responsible decisions.

In communicating, students can practice the persuasive leadership skill of painting a picture of potential future realities for nursing. In classroom presentations with supportive audiences, students have opportunities to develop professional commitment to positions and develop credibility by publicly articulating a stand on an issue. Presentations involving argumentation and persuasive communication need to include holism, giving consideration to the spiritual aspects of the issues they study: values, meanings, relationships, and goals or life's mission.

Students appreciate any personal attention and specific feedback faculty can provide to help them develop skills in applying critical thinking and holistic perspectives to persuasive communication, whether written or oral presentations. Although some students may not need this, for those who have not stood before a group to speak, who have not written an argumentative term paper, or who have not studied debate and argumentation, faculty feedback increases the probability of the student's academic success. For students returning for advanced degrees, the challenge of writing a formal argumentative paper needs to be a positive experience that instills confidence and self-reliance.

Telling stories of successful persuasive situations in clinical practice helps students relate course content to real life events. For example, one major issue nurses face is the assignment of responsibility for patient care—for how many patients can one nurse safely provide care? One ICU nurse used this argument with her manager when asked to assume responsibility for three more patients: "*If* I take over the care of these three new patients, *then* which three of my current patients do you want me to turn over to someone else? I already have a full load assignment for safe care." In a similar approach, another ICU nurse told her manager: "*If* you are sending more patients to my area, *then* send licensed persons to take care of them because we already have full assignments for all of our nursing staff." Both nurses stated they had been successful in avoiding excessive patient care assignments without being accused of abandonment or insubordination.

Finally, students learn better when humor is included in the classroom discussion. The topics of discussion in this ethics course are so distressing and laden with human misery that a comical paradox can lighten the atmosphere for a few moments. For example, one day the discussion turned to an obstetrical ethical problem requiring the attention of an ethics committee. The pregnant patient's uterus was infected, and the questions concerned abortion, hysterectomy, or both. After a lively discussion, I, a semiretired, gray-haired instructor, indignantly stated, "Well, I won't have my babies at that hospital!" Laughter dissolved the morbid discussion momentarily so that we could all take a moment to reconsider our responses.

THE EVALUATION

Final student evaluations suggest that exploring their personal mission during the course affirms that they have a mission, and this awareness enables them to connect with the content of the course. The nonthreatening classroom atmosphere fosters dialogue and the open exploration of ethical issues and the many different opinions on those issues.

One student stated she had not realized she could take a position on an issue and support it to influence others. Argumentation and persuasive communication skills are considered important by students. Students also noted that no one had ever related their spirituality (values, meanings, relationships, and goals or life mission) to the content. One student, a psychiatric nurse, noted that the manner in which the teacher interacted with students set the tone for the way relationships developed in the class.

SUMMARY

In the end, educators begin to appreciate that they are not coaching students to *become* winners but are coaching students who are *already* winners. When educators focus on students' holistic essence, particularly their values, meaning, relationships, and goals or life mission, students' spirits are released. Applying a holistic paradigm to nursing education holds the potential of graduating students who are energetic, motivated, and optimistic, and who treat others with the same respect with which they were treated.

REFERENCES

Duldt, B. W. (2001a). *Anatomy of a theory, A computer assisted instruction program about nursing and health care theories* (Lesson 12). Springfield, VA: Duldt & Associates.

Duldt, B. W. (2001b). *Humanizing nursing communication theory and theory of nursing communication ethics.* Retrieved February 18, 2003, from http://www.gmu.edu/ departments/nursing/graduate/duldt

Duldt, B. W., & Pokorny, M. (1999). Teaching communication about human sexuality to health care providers. *Nurse Educator, 24*(5), 27–32.

Frankl, V. E. (1984). *Man's search for meaning.* New York: Washington Square Press.

Hersey, P., & Duldt, B. W. (1989). *Situational leadership in nursing.* East Norwalk, CT: Appleton-Lange.

International Commission of Worship: Lutheran Church in America, American Lutheran Church, The Evangelical Lutheran Church of Canada, and The Lutheran Church Missouri Synod. (1978). *Lutheran book of worship, Hymn #319.* Minneapolis: Augsburg Publishing House, and Philadelphia: Board of Publications, Lutheran Church of America.

Meehan-Hurwitz, J. (2002, April 4). *Press release: Nursing profession unveils strategic plan to ensure safe, quality patient care and address root causes of growing shortage.* Retrieved April 10, 2002, from http://www.nursingworld.org/ rerealnews/

Patton, B. R., & Giffin, K. (1977). *Interpersonal communication in action* (2nd ed.). New York: Harper & Row.

SUGGESTED READINGS

Duldt, B. W. (1998). Coaching winners: How to teach critical thinking. In *SmartPrim, A computer assisted instructional program about critical thinking, term papers and speeches: Instructor's manual* (pp. 38–50). Springfield, VA: Duldt & Associates.

The Center for Leadership Studies. (2003). Home page. Retrieved March 1, 2003, from http://www.situational.com/

Gelb, M. J. (2002). *Discover your genius: How to think like history's ten most revolutionary minds.* New York: HarperCollins.

Myss, C. (2001). *Sacred contracts: Awakening your divine potential.* New York: Harmony Books.

Index

Contents of Volume 1

ORDER FORM

Save 10% on Volume 3 with this coupon.

____ Check here to order the *Annual Review of Nursing Education,* Volume 3, 2005 at a 10% discount. You will receive an invoice requesting prepayment.

Save 10% on all future volumes with a continuation order.

____ Check here to place your continuation order for the *Annual Review of Nursing Education.* You will receive a prepayment invoice with a 10% discount upon publication of each new volume, beginning with Volume 3, 2005. You may pay for prompt shipment or cancel with no obligation.

Name _____

Institution _____

Address _____

City/State/Zip _____

Examination copies for possible adoption are available to instructors "on approval" only. Write on institutional letterhead, noting course, level, present text, and expected enrollment (include $4.00 for postage and handling). Prices slightly higher overseas. Prices subject to change.

Mail this coupon to:
SPRINGER PUBLISHING COMPANY
536 Broadway
New York, NY 10012